Issues in Children's and Families' Lives

Series Editor:

Thomas P. Gullotta, *Child and Family Agency of Southeastern Connecticut, New London, CT*, USA
Herbert J. Walberg, *University of Illinois at Chicago, Chicago, IL*, USA
Roger P. Weissberg, *University of Illinois at Chicago, Chicago, IL*, USA

More information about this series at http://www.springer.com/series/6110

Carl G. Leukefeld • Thomas P. Gullotta
Editors

Adolescent Substance Abuse

Evidence-Based Approaches to Prevention and Treatment

Second Edition

Research Assistance by Jessica M. Ramos

A Sponsored Publication of the Child & Family Agency of Southeastern Connecticut.

Springer

Child & Family Agency of Southeastern Connecticut, Inc.
It's About Children

Editors
Carl G. Leukefeld
University of Kentucky
Lexington, KY, USA

Thomas P. Gullotta
Child and Family Agency of Southeastern Connecticut
New London, CT, USA

ISSN 1572-1981
Issues in Children's and Families' Lives
ISBN 978-3-030-08054-9 ISBN 978-3-319-90611-9 (eBook)
https://doi.org/10.1007/978-3-319-90611-9

This Springer imprint is published by the registered company Springer Nature Switzerland AG
The registered company address is: Gewerbestrasse 11, 6330 Cham, Switzerland

Bernie Gullotta, Beloved Son
October 29, 1983–February 25, 2018
Bernie, Yes all cats do go to heaven.

Acknowledgments

Tom and Carl would like to thank Jessica Ramos for her dedicated and insightful contributions that made this book possible. Thank you Jessica!

Contents

Editors and Contributors

About the Editors

Carl G. Leukefeld is a professor and chair of the Department of Behavioral Science and founding director of the Center on Drug and Alcohol Research at the University of Kentucky. He is also the Bell Alcohol and Addictions Endowed Chair. He came to the University of Kentucky in 1990 to establish the Center on Drug and Alcohol Research from the National Institute on Drug Abuse (NIDA), where he filled administrative and research positions. He was also the chief health services officer of the United States Public Health Service. Dr. Leukefeld has published articles, chapters, books, and monographs. He has taught undergraduate, graduate, and medical students.

Thomas P. Gullotta (Tom) retired as the Chief Executive Officer of Child and Family Agency of Southeastern Connecticut in 2015 and as a member of the Psychology and Education Departments at Eastern Connecticut State University in 2014. His scholarship encompasses the co-authorship of two college textbooks, the founding editorship of *The Journal of Primary Prevention* (Kluwer/Academic 1980–2000), co-editor, Advances in Adolescent Development: An Annual Book Series (Sage 1985–2000), editor, Prevention in Practice Library: A Monograph Series (Plenum, 1996–2001), and senior editor, Issues in Children's and Families' Lives: A Book Series (Springer 1990–present). In addition to authoring nearly 100 chapters, papers, or reviews, he has co-edited or authored over 30 volumes devoted to illness prevention/promotion of health for the treatment of children, adolescents, and families. Tom was the senior editor for the first edition of the *Encyclopedia of Primary Prevention and Health Promotion* (Kluwer/Academic, 2003) and returned to that same role for the four-volume second edition of that reference work published in late 2014. Currently, he is the senior advisor to Serve Here CT and the Chairman of the Town Council in his hometown of Glastonbury, CT.

About the Contributors

Joie Acosta, Ph.D. is a senior behavioral scientist at the RAND Corporation with a degree in Community and Cultural Psychology from the University of Hawaii, Manoa. She specializes in participatory research and evaluation of health promotion, prevention and intervention, and community development projects. She has 11 years of experience developing and conducting community-based research and strategic planning at the local, state, and national level and has worked with hundreds of community health organizations to improve their ability to use information to improve their efforts. Dr. Acosta is currently the PI on an NIH R01 assessing the effectiveness of Restorative Practices, a whole school positive youth development intervention. She is also co-PI on two NIH R01's funded to evaluate Getting To Outcomes, an implementation support intervention to improve the implementation of evidence-based programs.

Tanvi Ajmera is a public health advisor in the Child, Adolescent and Family Branch of the Center for Mental Health Services at the Substance Abuse and Mental Health Services Administration (SAMHSA). In this role she provides program oversight, guidance, and leadership to recipients of grants, contracts, and cooperative agreements who utilize a system of care approach to better serve children and adolescents nationwide. Prior to joining SAMHSA, Tanvi worked as a clinician in India.

Andrea L. Alexander is a licensed clinician in Maryland with 30+ years of experience in the child and adolescent service delivery system. At present she is a public health advisor in the Child, Adolescent and Family Branch at the Substance Abuse and Mental Health Services Administration (SAMHSA). In this role she provides program oversight, guidance, and leadership to recipients of funds who utilize a system of care approach to address behavioral health issues for youth, young adults, and families. Prior to joining SAMHSA, Ms. Alexander held leadership positions in state and local government and nonprofit agencies. She has utilized her knowledge of implementation science and the nuances of each child serving agency to coach recipients through the delivery and evaluation of services within a system of care framework. She received her Master of Science in Marriage and Family Therapy at the University of Maryland and maintains a small clinical practice.

Kadie Ausherbauer, M.S. is a doctoral student in the Department of Family Social Science (Couple and Family Therapy specialization) at the University of Minnesota. Her research interests focus on mechanisms of self-regulation development in children in early care-giving systems, specifically co-regulation and parent–child synchrony. She is interested in multiple levels of parent–child synchrony, including psychophysiological as well as behavioral markers of synchrony. She has a translational science lens for this work, particularly from the perspective of development and evaluation of preventive interventions for families under stress with a family systems perspective on resilience.

Pamela C. Baumer, M.A. is a research associate at Chestnut Health Systems for the past 7 years, has helped prepare the annual SAMHSA/CSAT Summary Analytic GAIN data sets, and has assisted in analytic requests and requests to use pooled GAIN data for secondary analysis. She also co-authored the GAIN Evaluation Manual, a guide for evaluators using GAIN data, as well as research presented at the Joint Meeting on Adolescent Treatment Effectiveness, NADCP, and published in the *Journal of Substance Abuse Treatment*. Her research interests include employee motivation, satisfaction, and turnover and their impact on organizational performance.

Gary M. Blau, Ph.D. is a licensed clinical psychologist and chief of the Child, Adolescent and Family Branch at the federal Substance Abuse and Mental Health Services Administration. In this role he provides national leadership for children's mental health and for creating "systems of care" across the United States. Dr. Blau has over 70 publications and is the editor of eight books. He has received numerous awards for his work, including the Rock Star Award, presented by Youth M.O.V.E., for "being a true champion for the youth movement and advocate for youth voice." This award has now been named the "Dr. Gary Blau Award." He also received the HHS Secretary's Award for Meritorious Service for his national leadership in children's mental health. He is happily married to his best friend, Gwenn, and they are incredibly proud of their children, Jennifer and her husband, Riley (and their sons, Logan and Evan), and Andrew and his wife, Kristina.

Martin Bloom retired from the University of Connecticut to a life devoted to art, primary prevention, and research. He co-edited (with Tom Gullotta) the *Encyclopedia of Primary Prevention and Health Promotion*, 2nd edition (2014); *Client-Centered Evaluation: New Models for Helping Professionals* (with Preston Britner, 2012); and various other professional activities including art. When will he ever learn?

Andria M. Botzet, M.A. has worked at the University of Minnesota, Department of Psychiatry, in the Center for Adolescent Substance Abuse Research as a Project Coordinator for a variety of topics related to addiction. She has worked on multiple projects that address adolescent substance use, including a longitudinal assessment of the progression of substance use, studies on the efficacy of a Brief Intervention, and gambling assessment studies. She was a primary contributor in the development of Mpower, a new Screening, Brief Intervention, and Referral for Treatment (SBIRT) program designed to address mild-to-moderate adolescent substance use. She also serves as the lead therapist on that intervention. Ms. Botzet additionally works as a psychotherapist in the Marriage and Family Therapy field. She and her husband have three children, who continually challenge her to grow and continue learning.

Shaun I. Calix is an assistant professor in the Department of Psychology at Cameron University in Lawton, OK, and the coordinator for the Family and Child Studies degree program. He received his Ph.D. from the University of Missouri in 2013 and his M.S. in Marriage and Family Therapy in 2005. His research interests lie in adolescent and emerging adult development, substance abuse, sexual scripts and attitudes, and fatherhood. He has published and presented in the areas of emerging adulthood, divorce education, and substance abuse.

Kristen Chalmers has a Bachelor of Science degree in Psychology from the University of Minnesota. She has assisted in research at several psychology labs at the University and did her senior project on Climate Change Denial Determinants.

Matthew Chinman, Ph.D. is a senior behavioral scientist at the RAND Corporation and a research scientist at the VA Pittsburgh Healthcare System. Dr. Chinman has a degree in clinical/community psychology from the University of South Carolina. Dr. Chinman leads a program of research focusing on the implementation of evidence-based practices, which centers around the Getting To Outcomes® (GTO) model and implementation support intervention. This work has been supported with CDC, SAMHSA, VA, and NIH funding. GTO has been adopted by SAMHSA, CDC, VA's National Center for Homelessness among Veterans, and several states agencies to support their own work in the areas of drug prevention, underage drinking prevention, homelessness, and teenage pregnancy prevention. Dr. Chinman has published and presented extensively on Getting To Outcomes research and implementation science more broadly. More information about GTO at: http://www.rand.org/health/projects/getting-to-outcomes.html.

Michael L. Dennis, Ph.D. senior research psychologist and director of the GAIN Coordinating Center at Chestnut Health Systems in Normal, Illinois, and adjunct professor in the Department of Psychiatry and Behavioral Science at the Northwestern University Feinberg School of Medicine in Chicago, has conducted substance use treatment- and justice-related research since 1985. His focus has been on methodology, measurement, adolescent treatment, recovery management, and life course issues through old age. He was the principal investigator (PI) of the Cannabis Youth Treatment experiment coordinating center; has served as the director, PI, or co-PI of over two dozen clinical trials and coordinating centers; and has published more than 250 articles, chapters, and manuals.

Barbara Estrada, M.S. is the Software Manager and Senior Evaluator at Chestnut Health Systems, Lighthouse Institute. Ms. Estrada manages the software development, support, and data management teams responsible for the development and maintenance of cloud-based software applications that allow over 4700 providers to conduct screening and assessment, to use clinical decision support systems reports, and to manage aggregate data. As a senior evaluator she was instrumental in the development of the GAIN clinical decision support applications and training which helps clinicians to interpret GAIN data in order to guide clinical decision making, and facilitate clinical treatment planning and level of care placement at the individual level. Ms. Estrada is also the lead developer of a comprehensive training that teaches program managers and evaluators to use data for program planning, implementation, management, and sustainability.

Andrew J. Finch, Ph.D. is associate professor of the Practice of Human and Organizational Development at Vanderbilt University. Dr. Finch co-founded the Association of Recovery Schools in 2002. Among his numerous published works on recovery and education are *Starting a Recovery School* (2005) and *Approaches to Substance Abuse and Addiction in Educational Communities: A Guide to Practices that Support Recovery in Adolescents and Young Adults* (2010), for which he was a co-editor. For 9 years, he worked for Community High School in Nashville, one of the early schools for teens recovering from alcohol and other drug addictions and a school he helped design and open in 1997. He also helped found Vanderbilt University's collegiate recovery program in 2007 and currently serves on its advisory committee. His most recent projects include a recovery school outcomes study, funded by NIDA, and a recovery high school history, to be published by Oxford University Press.

Mark A. Fine is professor and chair in the Department of Human Development and Family Studies at the University of North Carolina at Greensboro and was previously at the University of Missouri Columbia from 1994 to 2011, serving as Department Chair from 1994 to 2002. He was editor of *Family Relations* from 1993 to 1996 and was editor of the *Journal of Social and Personal Relationships* from 1999 to 2004. His research interests lie in the areas of family transitions, such as divorce and remarriage, early intervention program evaluation, social cognition, and relationship stability. He has published almost 200 peer-reviewed journal articles, book chapters, and books. He serves on the editorial boards of seven peer-reviewed journals in family studies, personal relationships, and human development. In 2000, he was selected as a Fellow of the National Council on Family Relations.

Kevin C. Garrett, Ph.D. is assistant professor and the clinical director of the M.S. Marriage and Family Therapy program at the Oregon Institute of Technology. He is an AAMFT Approved Supervisor. The majority of the time he contributed to this book chapter, he served as assistant professor in the Department of Psychology at Cameron University. He was and is a Licensed Marital and Family Therapist (LMFT) in Oklahoma and an Oklahoma State Approved LMFT Supervisor. Prior to this, he worked at a community mental health center in Wyoming for 5 years. In Wyoming, he worked with individuals, couples, and families presenting with many issues, including life-threatening crises and those affected by adolescent substance abuse, who were often involved in the juvenile justice system. His research interests include self-care; medical issues and their influence on patients' families; the interplay of poverty, depression, and suicidal ideation; and trauma's effects on individuals and couples.

Rachel Gonzales-Castaneda, Ph.D. is an associate professor of psychology at Azusa Pacific University. She also serves as an associate research psychologist at UCLA Integrated Substance Abuse Programs. She has extensive training in designing and evaluating prevention and treatment programs that address substance use disorders. She currently serves as the project director for the SBIRT Student Training grant funded by SAMHSA. In addition, she serves as the PI on a large, multi-program evaluation of the youth system of care in LA County funded by the Department of Public Health.

Thomas P. Gullotta (Tom) retired as the Chief Executive Officer of Child and Family Agency of Southeastern Connecticut in 2015 and as a member of the Psychology and Education Departments at Eastern Connecticut State University in 2014. His scholarship encompasses the co-authorship of two college textbooks, the founding editorship of *The Journal of Primary Prevention* (Kluwer/Academic 1980–2000), co-editor, Advances in Adolescent Development: An Annual Book Series (Sage 1985–2000), editor, Prevention in Practice Library: A Monograph Series (Plenum, 1996–2001), and senior editor, Issues in Children's and Families' Lives: A Book Series (Springer 1990–present). In addition to authoring nearly 100 chapters, papers, or reviews, he has co-edited or authored over 30 volumes devoted to illness prevention/promotion of health for the treatment of children, adolescents, and families. Tom was the senior editor for the first edition of the *Encyclopedia of Primary Prevention and Health Promotion* (Kluwer/Academic, 2003) and returned to that same role for the four-volume second edition of that reference work published in late 2014. Currently, he is the senior advisor to Serve Here CT and the Chairman of the Town Council in his hometown of Glastonbury, CT.

Arit Harvanko, M.S. is a Ph.D. candidate in the University of Kentucky's Departments of Psychology and Behavioral Science. He specializes in behavioral pharmacology research and his graduate work has focused on abuse liability of electronic cigarettes and other drugs of abuse. Mr. Harvanko's work has also examined associations between personality and drug abuse vulnerability and treatment.

Anna Hemze is an undergraduate student at the University of Minnesota. She will graduate in spring of 2018 with a Bachelor of Arts degree in Psychology, and minors in Neuroscience and Family Violence Prevention. Her primary academic interests include stress and trauma related to abuse and has volunteered at organizations that provide assistance to survivors of trauma.

Sarah Hunter, Ph.D., (Psychology, UCSB) is a senior behavioral scientist at the RAND Corporation. She has led formative, process, and summative evaluations at regional, state, and national levels in the areas of substance use and related community public health issues for nearly 20 years. She has also assisted in the development and testing of an implementation support tool, called "Getting to Outcomes®," that has been demonstrated to assist substance use prevention staff better plan, implement, evaluate, improve, and sustain programming. Dr. Hunter is considered an expert in the emerging field of implementation science. As such, she has served as core faculty for the Implementation Research Institute at Washington University and as a standing study section member for the National Institute of Health's Dissemination and Implementation Research in Health review committee. Dr. Hunter also serves as faculty for the Pardee RAND Graduate School where she teaches Program Evaluation.

Pamela S. Imm, Ph.D. is a community psychologist affiliated with the University of South Carolina and the Lexington/Richland Alcohol and Drug Abuse Council in Columbia, South Carolina. Dr. Imm has worked as an evaluator with various local, state, and national agencies including the Center for Substance Abuse Prevention, the Center for Substance Abuse Treatment, and the Community Anti-Drug Coalitions of America. She is a frequent presenter at national conferences and co-author of the award-winning empowerment evaluation manual: *Getting to Outcomes (GTO): Methods and Tools for Planning, Self-Assessment, and Accountability*. Updated versions of the Getting to Outcome series, including Preventing Underage Drinking, are published by the RAND Corporation. In 2015, she was awarded the Distinguished Contribution to Community Practice Award by the Society for Community Research in Action, a division of the American Psychological Association. She received her doctorate in clinical-community psychology from the University of South Carolina.

Thomas H. Kelly, Ph.D. is the Robert Straus Professor and Vice Chair of the Department of Behavioral Science in the College of Medicine; Professor of Psychiatry, Psychology and Nursing; and a faculty affiliate of the Center for Drug Abuse Research. He serves as Associate Dean for Research in the College of Nursing and Director of Research Education, Training and Career Development for the Center for Clinical and Translational Science. Dr. Kelly is a clinical behavioral pharmacologist examining drug–behavior interactions and assessing biobehavioral factors associated with individual differences in drug abuse vulnerability. His current research combines clinical pharmacological and neuroimaging methodologies to examine neurobiologically based personality dimensions on vulnerability to drug abuse.

Magdalena Kulesza is an associate behavioral scientist at the RAND Corporation. She received her Ph.D. in clinical psychology from Louisiana State University and trained at Brown University Medical School. Prior to joining RAND, she completed her postdoctoral fellowship at the University of Washington. Her work has focused on three specific areas: (1) conducting randomized controlled trials to evaluate the efficacy of brief interventions in reducing harm and high risk behaviors among college students who use alcohol and/or other drugs; (2) assessing the impact of stigma on help-seeking and well-being of individuals coping with substance use-related problems; and (3) understanding the relationship between public opinion, stigma, and access to services among individuals coping with substance use-related problems.

Carl G. Leukefeld is a professor and chair of the Department of Behavioral Science and founding director of the Center on Drug and Alcohol Research at the University of Kentucky. He is also the Bell Alcohol and Addictions Endowed Chair. He came to the University of Kentucky in 1990 to establish the Center on Drug and Alcohol Research from the National Institute on Drug Abuse (NIDA), where he filled administrative and research positions. He was also the chief health services officer of the United States Public Health Service. Dr. Leukefeld has published articles, chapters, books, and monographs. He has taught undergraduate, graduate, and medical students.

Sarabeth Leukefeld Biermann, Ph.D., M.S.W. is a lecturer at the University of Kentucky College of Social Work where she teaches Social Welfare Policy, Ethics, Theory, and Practicum Seminar courses. Dr. Biermann's practice experience includes in-home therapy with children and families, providing case management services for young mothers receiving TANF, program coordination for college students receiving TANF, and managing program evaluations of women's residential substance abuse treatment. She has also been involved in federally funded research projects and program evaluations.

Emily K. Lichvar, Ph.D. is an applied developmental psychologist and is currently a public health advisor in the Child, Adolescent and Family Branch of the Center for Mental Health Services at the Substance Abuse and Mental Health Services Administration (SAMHSA). In this role she provides program oversight, guidance, and leadership to recipients of grants, contracts, and cooperative agreements who utilize a system of care approach to better serve children and adolescents nationwide. Prior to joining SAMHSA, Dr. Lichvar held academic appointments at Washington State University in the Inland Northwest and at Manhattan College in New York City. She worked for 6 years at the National Center on Addiction and Substance Abuse (CASA) at Columbia University. There she worked on research and programs pertaining to prevention and treatment for adolescents with behavioral health problems. She received her B.A. in psychology from the University of Delaware, M.A. in clinical psychology from Teachers College, Columbia University, and Ph.D. in applied developmental psychology from Fordham University.

Michelle R. Lofwall, M.D. is an associate professor of behavioral science and psychiatry at the University of Kentucky (UK). She is board-certified in psychiatry and addiction medicine and is the medical director of the Straus Clinic, an outpatient addiction treatment clinic in the UK Center on Drug and Alcohol Research. Her clinical work, teaching, and research are focused in the area of substance use disorders, with a focus on medications development for opioid use disorder, integration of addiction treatment into general medical care, and health provider training and education to prevent and treat substance use disorders.

Katherine R. Marks is a postdoctoral fellow in the Department of Behavioral Science at the University of Kentucky. Her research focus is on the recovering process from substance use disorders, with a particular interest in women and environmental factors that can support recovering outcomes. Dr. Marks has also conducted research on cognitive and pharmacological interventions for substance use disorders. Dr. Marks holds a Ph.D. from the University of Kentucky in experimental psychology.

Catherine A. Martin, M.D. is the Dr. Laurie L. Humphries Endowed Chair and the Division Director of Child and Adolescent Psychiatry. She currently and has been funded to investigate individual differences in drug effects of drugs of abuse. She has been funded to explore novel therapies for smoking cessation including pharmacotherapies and family and behavioral interventions. She is involved in the training of clinical researchers locally and nationally as part of the NIDA: AACAP K12 program and the K12 BIRCWH (Building Interdisciplinary Research Careers in Women's Health) program. She collaborates with other scientists in the College of Medicine and is currently implementing a statewide grant to train providers and treat adolescents with substance use. She sees patients and supervises residents and medical students in the psychiatry as well as lectures to these same groups.

Peter Panzarella is a private consultant to federal and state governments. He serves on the nonprofit board of Multidimensional Family Therapy (MDFT) International. Peter retired as the state director of Substance Abuse Services for the Connecticut Department of Children and Families in 2013. In 2007, he received special recognition awards for collaboration from the National Center on Substance Abuse and Child Welfare, and in the same year another Government award for Facilitation and implementing Evidenced-Based Practices by the Joint Meeting on Adolescent Treatment Effectiveness. He is licensed as Alcohol/Drug and a Professional Counselor in Connecticut. He has two master's degrees—a Master of Arts in Community Psychology from Lesley University and a Master of Science in Administration from State University of New York College at Buffalo—and a Bachelor of Science in Psychology from State University of New York College at Buffalo.

Timothy F. Piehler, Ph.D., L.P. is an assistant professor in the Department of Family Social Science at the University of Minnesota. He researches the etiology and prevention of substance use and conduct problems in children and adolescents. His work seeks to identify moderators and mechanisms of response to family and youth-focused preventive interventions with a goal of developing increasingly targeted and personalized intervention strategies. Dr. Piehler is a member of the Institute for Translational Research (ITR) in Children's Mental Health and the Center for Personalized Prevention Research (CPPR) at the University of Minnesota.

Mark E. Pierce was born in Albuquerque, NM. He attended undergraduate university at NYU where he majored in Neural Science with minors in Chemistry and Mandarin Chinese. He followed this with a Master's in Cognitive Neuroscience at the University of Sussex, England. He is currently a fourth-year medical student at the University of Kentucky College of Medicine, applying for Neurology and mixed Neurology-Psychiatry residencies, and is currently working with the American Academy of Neurology on a project to make neuroscience education available to elementary school students.

Robert W. Plant, Ph.D. is a licensed clinical psychologist who received his masters and Ph.D. degrees from the University of Rochester and completed psychology fellowships at Yale University Medical School. Dr. Plant is the Senior Vice President for Analytics and Innovation at Beacon Health Options and has held various positions overseeing behavioral health programs and statewide systems for the State of Connecticut and various private nonprofit organizations. Professional and research interests include self-determination theory, real-world implementation of evidence-based practice, measurement-based care, health equity, treatment of opioid use disorders, and research using "big" data. Recent publications include the *Handbook of Adolescent Behavior Problems* (Gullotta, Plant, & Evans, Springer, 2015) and national presentations at the American Academy of Child and Adolescent Psychiatry 2017 Annual Conference and the 31st Annual Research & Policy Conference on Child, Adolescent, and Young Adult Behavioral Health.

Jessica M. Ramos received her B.A. in Psychology from Eastern Connecticut State University. She is a Research Assistant at Child and Family Agency of Southeastern Connecticut and has been employed there for the past 21 years. Jessica has assisted in the editorial process of 22 books on the topics of primary prevention and health promotion. She is also responsible for reviewing clinical cases for quality assurance. Ms. Ramos enjoys working for the agency and has not used a sick day for 13 consecutive years, since 2005.

Abner O. Rayapati is an assistant professor of psychiatry at the University of Kentucky. He serves as Vice Chair of Clinical Operations and Director of Consult Services within the Department including Addiction, Emergency, ECT, and Transplant, along with having an inpatient service. He joined the faculty after completing his general psychiatry residency and fellowship in child and adolescent psychiatry at the University of Kentucky. Beyond his clinical responsibilities, he is active in grant-funded research through collaboration with the Center of Drug and Alcohol Research. His interests include ADHD, substance use disorders, and the impact of psychological trauma on neuro-development. He treats substance use disorders for inpatients and outpatients across the life span including the specialized care of opioid dependence in pregnancy.

Zili Sloboda, Sc.D. President, Applied Prevention Science International, was trained in mental health and epidemiology at the Johns Hopkins University Bloomberg School of Public Health. She is an expert on the prevention of substance use by adolescents and has broad experience in research related to at-risk youth. She has been a member of the faculty at Johns Hopkins University Bloomberg School of Public Health, the University of Illinois School of Public Health and Abraham

Lincoln School of Medicine, and the University of Akron. She served as the director of the Division of Epidemiology and Prevention Research at the National Institute on Drug Abuse and was a founder of the Society for Prevention Research. She is well published in the area of substance use epidemiology and prevention.

Sally Stilwell is a current graduate student at Florida State University's College of Social Work. Prior to this, Sally obtained her bachelor's degree in psychology from the University of South Florida. During her education, Sally has completed several internships in substance use and mental health for adults, youth, and children. These experiences have included working in direct service as well as in administration, research, policy, and funding at the county, state, and national level.

Randy Stinchfield is a clinical psychologist who worked for 24 years at the University of Minnesota Medical School and is a consulting psychologist to a number of treatment and research agencies. Dr. Stinchfield has conducted clinical studies and survey research in the area of addictions with both adult and youth samples. His research on classification accuracy of DSM-IV diagnostic criteria for Pathological Gambling is credited as the rationale for lowering the diagnostic threshold in DSM-5. Dr. Stinchfield serves on the editorial boards for the *Psychology of Addictive Behavior*, *Journal of Gambling Studies*, *International Gambling Studies*, and the *Journal of Gambling Issues* and is an ad hoc editorial reviewer for the *Journal of Consulting and Clinical Psychology*, *Addiction*, *American Journal on Addictions*, *Addictive Behaviors*, *American Journal of Psychiatry*, *Canadian Journal of Psychiatry*, *American Journal of Public Health*, *Canadian Journal of Public Health*, and the *Journal of Clinical Psychology* among others.

William W. Stoops, Ph.D. is an associate professor in the Department of Behavioral Science at the University of Kentucky. He holds joint appointments in Psychiatry and Psychology and directs the Regulatory Knowledge and Support Core at the University of Kentucky Center for Clinical and Translational Science. Dr. Stoops' research has focused on the behavioral pharmacology of stimulant drugs, including methamphetamine, as a way of modeling, developing, and improving treatments for stimulant use disorder. His work combines human laboratory and clinical trial methods to advance promising treatments along the intervention development continuum. He has also conducted research evaluating the behavioral pharmacology of prescription opioids and cigarettes and has recently built a portfolio of research that relies on mTurk technology to assess cognitive behavioral performance of drug users throughout the United States.

Justin C. Strickland is a doctoral student in the behavioral neuroscience and psychopharmacology program at the University of Kentucky. His work focuses on using human laboratory techniques to understand the behavioral and pharmacological mechanisms contributing to cocaine and other drug use disorders. His research emphasizes an interdisciplinary approach by combining techniques and theoretical perspectives used in the experimental analysis of behavior, neuroscience, and behavioral economics. He is particularly interested in the role that exteroceptive and interoceptive drug cues play in the development of drug use disorders and their resistance to treatment interventions.

Ken C. Winters, Ph.D. is a senior scientist at the Oregon Research Institute and also an adjunct faculty in the Department of Psychology (Clinical Science and Psychopathology Program), University of Minnesota. Dr. Winters was a professor in the Department of Psychiatry at the University of Minnesota for 25 years, and founded and directed during that period the Center for Adolescent Substance Abuse Research (CASAR). Dr. Winters received his B.A. from the University of Minnesota and a Ph.D. in psychology (Clinical) from the State University of New York at Stony Brook. His primary research interests are the assessment and treatment of adolescent drug abuse.

Amy M. Yule is board-certified in adult, child, and addiction psychiatry. She is the medical director of the Addiction Recovery Management Service at Massachusetts General Hospital and an instructor at Harvard Medical School. Her research interests include risk factors associated with the development of a substance use disorder in adolescents with psychiatric illness and risky behaviors in adolescent substance users. She was a recipient in 2016 of a career development award from the American Academy of Child and Adolescent Psychiatry funded by the National Institute of Drug Abuse (5K12DA000357-17) to evaluate medication treatment for youth with substance use disorders co-occurring with bipolar disorder.

Introduction

Thomas P. Gullotta and Carl G. Leukefeld

This second edition of Adolescent Substance Abuse updates the progress made in treatment and prevention interventions for the misuse of substances since the first edition. It adds specific new treatment and prevention chapters in addition to examining the social, behavioral, and biological factors contributing to misuse. The applauded standardized chapter format used in the first edition that identifies evidenced-based approaches that work, might work, and do not work is maintained when appropriate. This second edition of Adolescent Substance Abuse is a thoughtful thorough distillation of the research on substance abuse treatment and prevention that offers clear guidance to students, practitioners, researchers, and policy-makers in the treatment and prevention of substance abuse.

This book is about how some young people use substances to intensify or alter perceptions, feelings, and understandings. On one level, the purpose of this volume is straightforward: identify and share those practices that appear to be most efficacious. To this end, we asked the respected and talented teams of scholars that worked on this project to identify evidence-based treatment and prevention practices. These practices are provided clearly in the chapters that introduce the reader to the subject area before delving into the details of those treatment and prevention techniques. On another level, the editors of this volume want the reader to appreciate the need to be persistent in youth-focused substance misuse prevention and treatment activities as well as being mindful of changing adolescent needs.

To that end, this volume opens with two foundational chapters that ground the uninitiated reader in the complexity of associated issues. In the first chapter, Gullotta

T. P. Gullotta (✉)
Child and Family Agency of Southeastern Connecticut, New London, CT, USA
e-mail: tpgullotta@aol.com

C. G. Leukefeld
Department of Behavioral Science, Center on Drug and Alcohol Research, University of Kentucky, Lexington, KY, USA
e-mail: cleukef@uky.edu

C. G. Leukefeld, T. P. Gullotta (eds.), *Adolescent Substance Abuse*, Issues in Children's and Families' Lives, https://doi.org/10.1007/978-3-319-90611-9_1

makes it clear that the desire of humankind has always been to intensify or alter perceptions, feelings, and understandings to achieve some futile understanding of the unpredictable events surrounding them. With time these transporting means to other worlds lost their imagined foretelling, religious or medicinal powers and entered the realm of personal recreational use. Every substance discussed in this book has at one time been legally used and at another time been prohibited from use—including coffee!

For example, King Charles II of England banned coffee houses in 1675, as did several other European monarchies. Those who ignored the royal decrees were beaten (Emboden, 1979). The kick in coffee is provided by caffeine that is commonly added to over-the-counter drinks in some beverages in outrageous amounts. Some of these substances like tobacco, alcohol, and coffee have reentered society with differing degrees of regulation.

Presently, US drug policy is to deny legitimate access to tobacco and alcohol until youth reach the legal age when use is permitted. Other substances, some legal and others not, are more rigidly administered (prescription drugs) or prohibited (e.g., cocaine). The difficulty becomes, as Kandel and her associates established decades ago (1975), that tobacco and alcohol can be the entry-level substances to other illegal drugs. The availability of these entry-level substances in most households in the Americas and the marketing of these substances by those who profit from their sale is a guarantee that this book will not lose its usefulness anytime soon which is exemplified by the current increase of heroin and opioid prescription drug misuse, related overdoses and deaths, the so-called US "opioid crisis."

In Chap. 2, Kelly and his colleagues expand on this point by providing the reader with a biological explanation for the power of caffeine, nicotine including E-cigarettes, alcohol, and opioids on the individual. Their review clearly establishes the rewarding, calming, or numbing aspects these chemicals exert on the brain.

With this knowledge as a backdrop, the reader is introduced by Baumer and her associates in Chap. 3 to the characteristics and treatment needs of substance misusing adolescents and young adults. After reviewing the literature on prevalence, course, and correlates of substance misuse, Baumer et al. use two large treatment data sets to describe the demographics, substance use, and comorbidity characteristics of youth and how substance use treatment varies by substance problem, treatment systems, and levels of treatment. Findings for practice support other studies that multi-morbidity is the norm for youth presenting to treatment in addition to high rates of victimization. Consequently, it is important for treatment to be trauma informed. A key implication is the need for more comprehensive clinical assessments, which includes risk and treatment need.

In Chap. 4, Winters et al. examine the substance abuse treatment literature by identifying promising psychosocial and pharmacological interventions. Using their review and a meta-analysis of the literature on substance use disorder treatment among adolescents, the authors examine research studies that focus on adolescents as the primary target of an intervention or treatment, includes drug use as an outcome, and incorporates a structured evaluation. From this review, recommendations are made.

Continuing this effort, in Chap. 5, Calix, Garrett, and Fine follow this discussion with an examination of the differing degrees of success family-based treatment has in treating adolescent substance abuse and dependence. The authors provide detailed descriptions of family-based therapeutic interventions, guiding theoretical frameworks, components of the therapy, and research evidence in support of multisystemic therapy, multidimensional family therapy, and functional family therapy. The authors describe a promising family treatment approach that integrates cognitive-behavioral therapy with functional family therapy. An overview of brief strategic family therapy is provided with attention to the therapeutic process, components of treatment, and supporting research evidence. Family-based interventions that have not been supported by research literature are also described.

Lichvar et al. discuss adolescent residential evidence-based treatment approaches in Chap. 6. The authors point out that significant knowledge gaps exist in determining those interventions in residential treatment that matter. They highlight inconsistencies raised in the literature on the general effectiveness of residential treatment as a therapeutic milieu and limitations in the research on residential treatment outcomes which include low participation rates, low follow-up rates, and limited quality assurance. Despite these limitations, the emergence of some promising evidence-based approaches for adolescent residential treatment over the recent years including the Minnesota Model (12-steps), The Multidisciplinary Professional Model, The Seven Challenges, and the Therapeutic Community is discussed. In addition, evidence-based models that have demonstrated success in community and home settings such as cognitive-behavioral therapy, motivational enhancement therapy, and some family models are described for their potential application in residential settings.

Lofwall and Yule expand this discussion in Chap. 7 by focusing on adolescent opioid and prescription misuse and abuse treatment in the context of the current and ongoing US opioid epidemic. This misuse is associated with over prescriptions of opioids by health care providers and the increased availability of heroin. The authors emphasize the need for comprehensive individual assessments including collateral information and urine toxicology. Although there is limited research on the use of medication assisted treatment with adolescents as well as misconceptions about substituting one addiction for another, Lofwall and Yule recommend that medication assisted treatment should be considered for youth with an opioid use disorder. This treatment includes methadone, buprenorphine/naloxone, and extended release naltrexone.

In Chap. 8, Strickland and Stoops add to the discussion of treatment and prevention by focusing on cocaine, amphetamine, and methamphetamine use problems for the individual user and society. The authors examine the literature and history of stimulant use and misuse as well as clinical effects and the limited adolescent outcome research and conclude that stimulant misuse remains a significant public health concern particularly for adolescent developmental trajectories. Since stimulant research is limited the stimulant prevention and treatment literature is scant. The authors indicate that prevention and treatment approaches for adolescent alcohol, tobacco, and cannabis could be tailored for adolescent stimulant users to incorporate individual, peer, family, and community factors.

The promise of self-help and mutual help activities for adolescents is the focus of Chap. 9. Leukefeld Biermann and Leukefeld indicate that self-help/mutual help can be a promising approach for adolescent substance misusers and that self-help/mutual help can be an intervention for everyone who misuses substances. Adolescent self-help/mutual is described as a safe no cost group process, including 12 steps, spiritual or other grounding, in which peer youth involved in substance misuse along with sponsors and/or mentors mutually support recovering youth to deal with cravings, life stressors, and to promote change. US treatment utilization data are presented to highlight the limited adolescent self-help information currently available, which is in addition to the limited adolescent self-help/mutual help research, particularly controlled trials.

The next three chapters are concerned with prevention and health promotion approaches to substance use in childhood and adolescence. That is, how do we develop the capacity (promotion) of young people to resist the lure of drug misuse and how do we prevent that misuse. Bloom and Gullotta begin this discussion in Chap. 10 by providing the reader with an understanding of the concept and examples of how primary prevention and health promotion work. The authors describe five technologies as essential components of any effective prevention effort. These are education, promotion of self-competency, natural caregiving, impacting change at the community organization and systems level, and redesigning the social environment.

An area with ties to competency and prevention is recovering. Marks and Leukefeld present recovering as a process rather than an outcome—recovery. Chapter 11 by Marks and Leukefeld also includes an overview of selected factors related to adolescent recovering from substance use, examines a way of thinking about recovering and presents factors that can support recovering. Recovering is defined as a process of change through which an individual achieves improved heath, wellness, and quality of life. Using a bio/psycho/social/spiritual framework, the recovering process includes residential and/or outpatient treatment which can be involuntary, coordinated individualized services using community resources, emphasis on adolescent strengths and resiliencies within the adolescents social context (family, friends, and school), in addition to using environmental factors to support recovering.

In Chap. 12, Sloboda emphasizes the importance of school prevention intervention programs for adolescent substance abuse. She states the need for these efforts by noting that the possession of tobacco and alcohol by persons under the age of 18 is illegal, and that research indicates that the use of tobacco and alcohol increases the risk for later, more extensive drug use. Sloboda reviews the historical context for the development of school-based prevention programs, the developing body of research on their effectiveness, and the impact of these approaches on adolescent use of tobacco, alcohol, and illicit substances.

In Chap. 13, the prevention and health promotion approaches shift to a broader community focus. Namely, what larger community organization/system interventions might alter the availability of these to commonly available substances. Imm et al. provides the reader with valuable insights on ways to intervene in the system to achieve effective change.

This volume concludes with the lessons we learned as editors in this process and as practitioners and scholars in this field for several decades. This volume contains both good and sobering news. The good news is that progress has been made to improve the likelihood that young people can be treated successfully. This book documents that fact and can be used by practitioners and program developers at local, county, and state levels to implement those practices. The good news is also that substance misuse can be prevented, and this book clearly demonstrates that fact. The prevention and health promotion examples provided and similar efforts should be copied and implemented elsewhere.

The sobering news is that if we are correct and that humankind has forever sought the means to transport itself to altered states of consciousness then problems associated with substance misuse will remain. If we are correct in believing that tobacco and alcohol can be a stepping-stone or gateway drugs to more serious drug misuse for some, then our society must continually reseed itself with new generations of evidence-based treatment and prevention interventions. This means that we cannot ignore promising treatment, health promotion, or prevention activities as they are developing. Drug misuse at any age by any group is a problem that if ignored will grow worse. It calls for a reconceptualization of the tactics to manage drug misuse and associated problems. The first step is to heed the advice of the talented scholars in this volume. The second step is returning the phrases "harm risk reduction" and "distribution of consumption" to our lexicon and expanding on the evidence-based interventions discussed in this book.

References

Emboden, W. (1979). *Narcotic plants: Hallucinogens, stimulants, inebriants, and hypnotics, their origins and uses*. New York, NY: Macmillan.

Kandel, D. B., & Faust, R. (1975). Sequence and stages in patterns of adolescent drug use. *Archives of General Psychiatry, 32*, 923–932.

A Selected Social History of the Stepping-Stone Drugs and Opiates

Thomas P. Gullotta

In the mid-1970s, Denise Kandel and her colleagues (Kandel, 1981; Kandel & Faust, 1975; Kandel, Kessler, & Margulies, 1978; Kandel, Yamaguchi, & Chen, 1992) published a series of papers establishing a sequence in the pattern of use of substances by adolescents and debunking the prevalent belief that marijuana was the stepping-stone drug to heroin use. More recently, scientists examining the effects of alcohol on the brain have offered partial evidence in confirmation of Kandel's original thesis (National Institute on Alcohol Abuse and Alcoholism [NIAAA], 2008). Regrettably, this information has been ignored by generations of policymakers and their appointees to federal and state departments responsible for the prevention of substance abuse. In a volume dedicated to examining evidence-based approaches to the prevention and treatment of adolescent substance misuse, it is useful to trip down memory lane and revisit Kandel and her associates' findings and further to place three of these stepping-stone drugs into a broader social historical perspective. By so doing the reader of this volume hopefully will appreciate the challenges that confront society as it attempts to reduce the misuse of substances by its youth. Lastly, we examine heroin, the drug at the end of drug abusers journey and those man-made concocted opiates that rival heroin in their destructive abilities.

The Sequence of Adolescent Drug Use

American colonists whether English or Dutch loved their drink, preferably intoxicating. Struyvesant reported that "Almost one full fourth of the town of New Amsterdam [New York]" was occupied by "houses for the sale of brandy, tobacco,

T. P. Gullotta (✉)
Child and Family Agency of Southeastern Connecticut, New London, CT, USA
e-mail: tpgullotta@aol.com

C. G. Leukefeld, T. P. Gullotta (eds.), *Adolescent Substance Abuse*, Issues in Children's and Families' Lives, https://doi.org/10.1007/978-3-319-90611-9_2

and beer" (Struyvesant cited in Child, 1896, p. 17). Whether smoking a pipe and downing a pint in a tavern to the stories of headless horsemen or attending the ordination of the new minister in a New England village, alcohol quenched the thirst of those in attendance. Consider this invoice for the community gathering accompanying an ordination in 1785:

Thirty bowls of punch before the people went to meeting.
Ten bottles of wine before they went to meeting.
Forty-four bowls of punch while at dinner.
Eighteen bottles of wine.
Eight bowls of brandy.
Cherry rum and cider [quantity not mentioned] (Child, 1896 pp. 55–56).

Given this long infatuation with intoxicating beverages, it is not surprising that Americans in their condemnation of drug abuse overlook the connection between those substances and alcohol.

The work of Denise Kandel and her associates (e.g., Kandel & Faust, 1975) was the first to establish a well-defined pathway to illicit drug use. Using representative samples of New York State high school students, these researchers established that the overwhelming majority of youth who used marijuana (98%) began with beer and wine. "Drug use begins specifically with beer and wine … These are the 'entry drugs' into the continuum of drug use" (Kandel & Faust, 1975, p. 931).

The second step toward illicit drugs in their model was either the use of stronger alcoholic beverages followed by cigarette smoking or cigarette smoking followed by stronger alcoholic beverages. In either instance this could then lead to the third stage of marijuana use and then to the fourth stage of other illicit drug use.

The authors caution, "while the data show a very clear-cut sequence in the use of various drugs, they do not prove that the use of a particular drug infallibly leads to the use of other drugs higher up in the sequence" (Kandel & Faust, 1975, p. 931). At each stage individuals choose to stop and not use the next drug in the sequence.

While this last observation remains true, advances in neuroscience point to the heightened risk individuals experience along this pathway. Combine this increased biological risk with life events whether of a medical, social, or personal nature and the risk of addiction rises. Having identified the stepping-stones into illicit drug misuse as beer and wine, tobacco, and marijuana, what we know about these substances from a social historical context is discussed next.

Beer: The Staff of Life

> Lager Beer: A friendly drink,
> A healthy drink, A family drink, A national drink. (Late nineteenth-century poster, in Burnham, 1993)

At an eatery that brewed its own beers I sampled bread made from the grain left over from the beer-making process. That act of consumption completed a circle albeit in reverse that has gone on for thousands of years. Beer or "liquid bread" was likely discovered as the by-product of bread making by our ancient Neolithic ancestors (Tannahill, 1973 p. 63). Through a process of trial and error our distant relatives found that raw grain was made digestible by allowing it to sprout in water, then dried and ground into meal. Incidentally, this wet mixture was porridge. Left in an old earthen vessel filled with nooks and crannies harboring bacteria, this porridge would start to ferment after several days as the bacteria (yeast) consumed the sugars released by crushing the grain. The by-products released by the bacteria happened to be CO and alcohol, producing a porridge that was both filling and mildly intoxicating.

Draw off the liquid from this mixture and the resulting product is nutritious beer. Tannahill (1973) informs us that the ancient Sumerians allotted 40 oz. of this brew to a worker daily. That is a tad more than a half-gallon a day. Beer mattered as much for the Egyptians whose Goddess Hathor was the deity responsible for its presence on earth. Not only was it a food and a beverage, but it was also a medicine appearing as an ingredient in 118 of the 600 prescriptions found in the ancient Egyptian medical text, Papyrus Ebers (Brown, 2003).

Beer as nourishment continued to recent times. For example, before pasteurizing milk became popular its consumption by children and others could be deadly. This was especially true of the milk provided to large cities like New York and Chicago where the cows that provided milk to these cities were often confined in unsanitary disease-ridden warehouses where tubercular animals quickly spread the infection to all. Thus, statements like, "You can depend on the beer, but you can't tell about the milk you get down here," speak to reasons why parents gave beer to their children to drink (Burnham, 1993, p. 60).

Despite America's propensity for alcoholic beverages and the growth in popularity of beer with the influx of immigrant groups like the Germans who brought their taste for it from the Old World to the New, concern for its harm to individuals and families grew. This minority of voices gathered strength as Saloons multiplied and more potent distilled alcoholic beverages appeared. One need only compare Hogarth's etching of a society consuming beer with the plate of that same society downing gin to understand the growing worry.[1]

In the USA, this concern reached a crescendo in 1916 with enough antidrinking candidates elected to Congress to pass a national prohibition amendment. By 1919, the necessary majority of states had ratified the 18th amendment that it became law. Interestingly, Burnham (1993) contends that due to wartime restrictions in 1916 on grain for food rather than alcohol, prohibition was essentially in place by 1918. The notorious Saloons in which most drinking occurred had virtually disappeared and the country appeared ready to accept prohibition.

[1] During the thirteenth century, the process of distillation became known in Europe. Distilled beverages were treated as medicines called aqua vitae (water of life). By the 1500s, aqua vitae was associated with criminal activity in England. In the mid 1600s, gin was developed in Holland by distilling grain with juniper berries.

More interesting still is that prohibition did not totally prohibit alcohol consumption! The Volstead Act that defined the 18th amendment "explicitly permitted religious groups to use wine, physicians to prescribe alcohol, and private citizens to own and drink it even to make small quantities of wine and beer for home use" (Burnham, 1993, p. 27). Thus, those with wealth stocked their cellars with distilled spirits. The immigrants brewed their own beer or as my Italian grandmother did crushed her own grapes in a wine press I still own, deposited the sweet liquid into oak barrels for bacteria to feed upon and transform into wine. The losers in this were the cash-rich distillers and the poor who had frequented the now closed Saloons. As we know, this experiment was not to last long. Change occurred and prohibition was repealed not because of the rise in the criminal element and the "Speak Easy" but because of the loss of tax revenue and the effective lobbying of cash-rich disgruntled distillers (Burnham, 1993).

Sobered by their recent experience, the distillers and their distributors launched a media campaign to redefine the role of beer and other alcoholic beverages in American life. Using magazines, sporting events, and even toys, beer was taken out of the Saloon and the back room where men were grudgingly permitted to retire after supper for a smoke and a drink to the dining room table where it was consumed in front of the family. In time, mom was seen toasting her smiling husband with a foaming glass herself. Billboards spoke to the allegiance of a beer to a ball team, and I was known to stuff the ballot box in favor of my favorite Reingold Beer Beauty as a child of 9 as I played with my toy Budweiser Wagon piled high with kegs pulled by several handsome plastic white horses. The keg temporarily disappeared to be replaced by bottles and cans in a six-pack that has been replaced over time by the 12-, 18-, and now 24-can case.

With the end of prohibition, consumption of beer and other alcoholic beverages gradually grew and with it returned the problem of men, women, and, shortly, youth unable to manage their drinking. Prior to prohibition, this problem was identified with the substance and its dispensing location—the Saloon. The distillers and their distributors were not to make this same mistake again. Home, the family picnic, and other G-rated celebrations would be the venues for consumption. Alcoholism was gradually redefined not as a societal issue but as an individual problem. Rather than consider distribution of consumption approaches that would limit the availability of alcohol, the focus was now on genes and the psychological fallings of that man, woman, or youth (Burnham, 1993).

In place of setting a limit on the alcoholic beverages to be consumed, the public was told to designate a driver. Appealing to individual responsibility that rings so true in a society that worships rugged individualism shifted responsibility from the makers of conveniently packaged cases with carrying handles containing cans or bottles with pop top or twist off caps and newly formulated "fortified" alcoholic beverages to the flawed soul unable to exercise control over the command to "Pick a pair of six packs—Buy Bud." Any attempt to refocus the discussion toward limiting alcohol consumption was dealt with harshly by this cash-rich powerful beer and alcohol lobby. For example, in 1995, the long brewing resentment of the beer industry against the Center for Substance Abuse Prevention found expression in its successful efforts to significantly reduce the agency's drug prevention effort in a newly elected Republican Congress. As Kuntz (1995, p. A12) reported in the *Wall Street Journal*, "Soon after the House passed its last major spending bill this month, Coors Brewing Co. sent two cases of beer to the office of the subcommittee that wrote the measure. The alcohol beverage industry has good reason to be grateful. The bill would gut the Center for Substance Abuse Prevention, an agency the industry says promotes an antidrinking message threatening to its bottom line."

Presently, the message to the public is to drink in moderation but to purchase in bulk. The effects of this mixed message on youthful drinkers can be measured in one sense by data that indicate 23.1% of 8th graders, 42.2% of 10th graders, and 61.5% of 12th graders reported trying alcohol in 2017 (Johnston, O'Malley, Miech, Bachman, & Schulenberg, 2017, Table 1, Trends in Lifetime Prevalence). The source of this information is the *Monitoring the Future* survey that has been undertaken with graduating seniors since 1975 and extended to other students in the 1990s. Now, 61.5% of 12th graders tasting alcohol is nothing to be particularly proud of considering that the drinking age is 21 except that the grandparents of those youths who graduated in the class of 1979 reported that 93% of them had tried alcohol. Of course, those grandparents will likely fondly recall that the legal drinking age was 18 in most states in 1979. Thus, compared to their grandparents the graduating student in 2017 is less likely to have ever tried alcohol, but as the child who drank beer in place of milk would be quick to share—circumstances color the picture significantly.

Tobacco

"The most sovereign and precious weed that ever the earth tendered to the use of man" (Ben Johnson, 1598, cited in Shoemaker, 1898, p. xi).

While the Old World introduced small pox to the New World, "Montazuma's revenge" might better be considered syphilis and tobacco to the Europeans. The first is believed to have been returned to Europe by a less than virtuous Columbus and his crew, and the second is briefly mentioned in his log as "a few dried leaves which must be something of importance to these people" (Burns, 2006, p. 16). While syphilis spread quickly across Europe and reached epidemic proportions within a few years of its arrival, the use of those "few dried leaves" was considerably slower. Its introduction to England is credited to Sir John Hawkins, English sea captain and slave trader, who is said to have seized the crop in a raid along the Florida coast noting that:

> The Floridians when they travel have a kind of herb dried, who with a cane and an earthen cap in the end, with fire, and the dried herb put together, do suck through the cane the smoke thereof, which smoke satisfieth their hunger, and therewith they live four or five days without meat or drink. (Burns, 2006, p. 22).

It was not Hawkins, however, but Sir Walter Raleigh whose friendship with Queen Elizabeth I popularized the use of tobacco in England and earned him the distinction of a brand of cigarettes to be named after him centuries later.

Like nearly every newly discovered New World plant, tobacco was touted for its medicinal qualities. In the Old World, tobacco smoke, paste, or parts of the plant would be applied to every imaginable orifice or laid on to relieve pain, cure emotional distress, or treat sickness. Similarly, in England from 1573 to 1625 it was believed to be a helpful treatment for heart pains, snake bites, fever, exhaustion, and the Black Plague. None other than the great diarist Samuel Pepy recorded:

> This day … I see in Drury Lane houses marked with a red cross [denoting the presence of the Plague]…which was a sad sight to me … It put me into an ill conception of myself and of my smell, so I was forced to buy some roll tobacco to smell an chaw, which took away the apprehension. (Burns, 2006, p. 27)

As with every great discovery, it would not be the medicinal benefits (sic) but the entertainment aspects of tobacco that would endear this plant to society. In taverns and coffee houses across Old and New Worlds the active ingredient in tobacco would work its magic of calming its consumer and subduing his hunger.

That ingredient, nicotine or more properly nicotiana, was named after the Frenchman Jean Nicot who first described the medicinal properties of the substance in 1559 (Austin, 1979). The addictive characteristics of nicotine, being as it is commonly inhaled into the lungs thus enabling its rapid passage to the brain, led the then Surgeon General C. Everett Koop in 1988 to caution that "the pharmacologic and behavioral processes that determine tobacco addiction are similar to those that determine addiction to drugs such as heroin and cocaine" (Byrne, 1988, p. 1143).

But concern about this noxious weed was evident centuries earlier. It was prohibited in the Massachusetts Bay Colony in 1632 and several years later in Connecticut. In the mid 1600s, The Roman Catholic Church concerned with the growing use of tobacco by its clergy and parishioners and the calming effects resultant from its use sought to refocus its following on more salient issues like death, damnation, and the like. Thus, papal bills prohibiting the use of tobacco under penalty of expulsion from the church were enacted. This ban remained in effect for roughly 100 years (Goodman, 1994).

In Russia, tobacco was called "the devil's plant" in the 1600s. The Russian Czar, no slouch at having his word taken seriously, saw thousands put to death who ignored his decree prohibiting its use (Goodman, 1994).

Even the English monarch James I who followed Queen Elizabeth I to the throne saw no good in this plant and tried by means of taxation to eliminate its presence on English soil. In 1604, the year after his coronation, he had published anonymously *A Counter-Blaste to Tobacco*. In it, he concluded that tobacco was:

> a custom loathsome to the eye, hateful to the nose, harmful to the brain, dangerous to the lungs, and in the black stinking fume thereof, nearest resembling the horrible Stygian smoke of the pit that is bottomless. (James, 1604/1932, pp. 34–35)

Actually, what may have been driving James I mad was the reality that the tobacco England was consuming was coming from the Spanish settlements of the

New World. In the sense of balance of trade payments, tobacco was costing the England what imports from China is costing the USA today.

Enter into this scenario the American Colonies and, in particular, Virginia. In the 1500s, the Virginia colony was a small destitute community with a history of repeated financial failure behind it. There is evidence that James I was growing tired of the financial drain Virginia was having upon the Mother Country, but this disappointment and simultaneous concern over tobacco's noxious harm vanished with the development in Virginia of a tobacco similar in quality to that being imported from Spain. Soon the revenues from the sale of Virginia tobacco erased any concern of either quelling tobacco's use or possibly disposing of this previously nonproducing asset (Virginia).

Tobacco was consumed in the colonies and in the early years of the republic by crushing the dried leaves and igniting them in a pipe, rolling the leaves and igniting them (a cigar), compacting the leaves into a tight mass and biting off a small portion which was then chewed (a chew or chaw), or, as was popular in Europe, pulverizing the leaf into a very fine powder and inhaling it through the nostrils (snuff).

The development of the cigarette must be credited to Spain. The story of its invention was that discarded cigars were gathered by the poor and the waste tobacco deposited onto paper which was then rolled, crimped, and smoked. The advantage of the cigarette over the cigar or pipe was time. A good pipe or cigar was a leisurely affair spent in contemplation of writing the next verse, savoring the aroma of a fine brandy, or attending to the learned argument of a fellow coffee house philosopher. The popularity of the cigarette was made on the battlefield. First, in the ill-fated British experience in the Crimean War and later by its export from England to the USA in the Civil War (Goodman, 1994; Wagner, 1971).

Recall that the active ingredient in tobacco is nicotine, a substance which when inhaled into the lungs travels quickly to the brain and produces a sense of calm and relaxation by interacting with brain neurotransmitters like serotonin and dopamine. Imagine being Steven Crane's (1895/2001) young protagonist, Henry Fleming, in the *Red Badge of Courage* marching forward with friends and neighbors as the unit's leader rushes before them waving his sword above his head attracting to his motions soft masses of lead-like yellow jackets to a fall picnic. These stinging insects of death flatten on contact tearing into a face or punching a hole into flesh that cries out as it writhes on the dampened crimson ground. Still, the line of which you are a part advances slowly worming its way across the battlefield turned cemetery. The cigarette was the perfect fortifier for such a suicidal venture. Alcohol would impair motor control, cloud vision, and numb rather than stir the body to action. Better the quickly consumed cigarette to impart just enough calm before the butchery. With the close of conflict between the states, the cigarette found a home off the battlefield and in the rapidly industrializing USA. In a world where time is money, its advantages of quickly induced calm and quenched hunger favored its use over the pipe or cigar and it was cleaner than the chaw whose residue could be found nearly everywhere as this visiting Englishman observed:

> We discussed these important questions until my companions paired themselves off into their respective beds. I selected the cleanest corner of that had been least spat upon—and lay down on the floor with my carpet-bag for a pillow. (Anonymous, 1863, p. 499)

Indeed, the novelist Charles Dickens (Burns, 2006) could not help but record on his first visit to the USA that on one occasion a guest chewing tobacco in his hotel room and not seeing a spittoon let loose with well-directed copious stream of juice out the window. Problem was the window was closed. There trickling down the window pane, Dickens observed, the spittle resided without its depositor taking further notice.

Like its fraternal twin——alcohol, the years after 1865 saw a rise in activity to curb the spreading use of tobacco, particularly cigarettes whose popularity had grown such that by 1885 one billion were being manufactured yearly. Indeed, a total of 14 states early in the twentieth century had passed such laws but these efforts were to disappear with the advent of World War I.

The slaughter of human life had changed little since the Civil War. Frontal assaults continued to be a popular military strategy but the machine gun replaced the cannon's grape shot as the weapon of preference that segmented the line of troops worming across the open pockmarked fields of France. Between these doomed excursions, troops burrowed into the ground to hide from the death above. Again, alcohol that could numb the solider from the death encircling him was rejected in favor of the cigarette with none other than General Black Jack Pershing (Burns, 2006, p. 158) stating, "You ask me what we need to win this war? I answer tobacco as much as bullets." Indeed, he was to back these words with a demand for "tens of thousands of tons of cigarettes" from the home front which was complied with (Burns, 2006, p. 158). His endorsement of the cigarette was echoed by others on his staff, "a cigarette may make the difference between a hero and a shrinker," and even President Woodrow Wilson (a smoker himself) got into the act by endorsing the New York Sun's "Smokes for Soldier's Fund" (Burns, 2006, p. 158).

The result of these demands was the demise of antismoking measures in the USA. Well-meaning groups like the YMCA, the Salvation Army, and the Red Cross responded to these requests to support the troops overseas. With the conclusion of the war to end all wars, tobacco and the cigarette especially were an inexorable part of the American landscape. For the next 40 years, a movie could not be watched without the haze of tobacco smoke on the screen; magazine and newspapers ads touted the flavor, taste, or masculinity of tobacco products; and the new medium of radio and later television brought entertainment compliments of the tobacco companies. This advertising effort was successful with yearly production of cigarettes exceeding 80 billion in the 1920s to hundreds of billions by the 1960s.

With the return of world hostilities in 1941, it was not surprising that tobacco's importance as a necessary war item was again embraced. Replacing General Black Jack Pershing was General Douglas MacArthur (corn cob pipe smoker) who encouraged one group to use the funds it had raised to spend, "the entire amount … to buy American cigarettes," for the troops (Burns, 2006, p. 198). Franklin Roosevelt (a cigarette smoker) saw the importance of tobacco to the war effort to the extent that he instructed draft boards to provide deferments to tobacco farmers, thus ensuring an adequate supply of this once noxious weed.

It would seem that tobacco's place in American society was secured except that occasional reports would appear in the scientific literature describing the harmful effects of inhaling tobacco smoke. The first of these appeared in England in 1924 when the respected English Chemist Ernest Kennaway described a substance he called "tar" and linked this sticky substance to cancer. His study's findings were replicated over the next two decades with the findings remaining unchanged (Burns, 2006).

In 1952, a Christian Herald report of the work of the American Cancer Society was reprinted in the widely subscribed to *Reader's Digest* and the American public was made aware of the growing evidence linking tobacco to harmful health outcomes. In 1957, the UK, and in 1964, the US Government Health Services adopted formal positions linking tobacco to cancer and other diseases. Still, more than three decades would pass in the USA and it would not be until potentially bankrupting lawsuits against the makers of tobacco products were awarded that significant steps were taken to curtail tobacco use by the general public and especially youth (Burns, 2006).

Examining the data gathered from the *Monitoring the Future* (Johnston et al., 2017) study indicates that 9.4% of 8th graders, 15.9% of 10th graders, and 26.6% of 12th graders in 2017 reported trying cigarettes at least once. This compared to 74% of the graduating class of 1979. To this data must be added the % of youth who have tried Vaping—the tobacco industry's latest effort to maintain its profitability. In this regard 18.5% of 8th graders, 30.9% of 10th graders, and 35.8% of 12th graders in 2017 reported Vaping at least once. As marijuana—or as public relation firms would prefer it be known—cannabis is most often consumed via inhalation into the lungs, the rise in vaping is a disturbing trend.

Marijuana

> When I was in England I experimented with marijuana a time or two, and I didn't like it. I didn't inhale. (Candidate, Bill Clinton in Ifill, 1992, p. A15 of the *New York Times*)
>
> One reason why we appreciated pot, as y'all call it now, was the warmth it always brought forth from the other person—especially the ones that lit up a good stick of the shuzzit or gage. (Louie Armstrong cited in Sloman, 1979, p. 133)[2]

For 450 years and more another weed in the New World went relatively unnoticed. It may be that the greater calm and sense of well-being it conferred over tobacco interfered with the work to be done or that Alice B. Tokilas' recipe for

[2] It was difficult to choose a single quote to open this section so I chose two. Joining Bill and Louie in acknowledging their use are Arnold Schwarzenegger, John Kerry, Bing Crosby (his son revealed his use), Newt Gingrich, Margaret Mead, Michael Bloomberg, Carl Sagan, and Donna Shalala to name but a few (AlterNet.org, n.d.; Retrieved from www.alternet.org/dugreporter/18941).

brownies suffered by association with Gertrude Stein's often indecipherable writing. In any case, the evilness of marijuana as the entry drug into the wasteland of drug abuse dates from the late 1930s.

Marijuana or hemp had been known to civilization for thousands of years before that date. Like other substances in this chapter, it too was used as a medicinal substance for a variety of health problems. Among those uses, the Chinese mixed it with wine and administered it as an analgesic before surgery (Grinspoon & Bakalar, 1993). Others believed it to be helpful in treating malaria and venereal disease, and Robert Burton (1621/1851) in his compendium *The Anatomy of Melancholy* reported its use to treat depression.

Marijuana was raised as a cash crop in the English colonies. The fibers of the hemp plant were a valuable commodity and continue today to be turned into a variety of products including cloth and rope. Indeed, George Washington cultivated the plant. Hemp production in the USA, continued until about the time of the Civil War when other nations replaced the USA as its major producer. Its use as a medicinal substance declined in the late 1800s for two principal reasons.

The first was the uncertain effect of its psychoactive ingredient, THC (delta-9-tetra-hydrocannabinol), compared to other substances like opium and coca and their derivatives (morphine and cocaine). The second was the increased use of the hypodermic syringe after 1860, enabling soluble drugs to be injected and speed relief to the patient. In this second respect, marijuana was not soluble in water (Grinspoon & Bakalar, 1993).

Recent histories of marijuana suggest that the events that moved marijuana from being considered a relatively harmless plant to the status of "killer weed" originated in the southwest during the 1930s. Prior to that time, the substance was essentially ignored. For example, it was not regulated by the Harrison Narcotics Act of 1914. Indeed, in 1920 the US Department of Agriculture published a booklet encouraging its production as a cash crop. The circumstances surrounding marijuana's decline from relative obscurity to infamy involved the migration of Mexicans into the USA during the Great Depression and the scarcity of work.

Other than Alice and Gertrude, it appears that in the late 1920s and early 1930s the largest group of users of marijuana for recreational purposes was Mexican Americans. Recall the treatment of the Joad family in its migration from Oklahoma to California in search of work in Steinbeck's epic novel *The Grapes of Wrath* and the tensions are evident. Add to those tensions of high unemployment and ethnic prejudice and the conditions are ripe for harmful actions to be taken (Austin, 1979; Grinspoon, 1971; Sloman, 1979).

Interestingly, while legislative delegations from the southwest lobbied the federal government for action, those requests were initially ignored by Harry Anslinger then heading the Federal Bureau of Narcotics. However, neither the requests nor the depression disappeared and by 1937 Congress had enacted the Marijuana Tax Act. With marijuana now a substance of concern, legal authorities in the southwest acted quickly by deporting individuals found in possession of marijuana. In their zealousness—perhaps prejudice is the better word—against those with a Central American ancestry, individuals deported included native-born Americans with family histories extending back generations in the USA to a nation that was foreign to them—Mexico.

Since the 1930s, marijuana has been understood at various times in North American society to offer "one moment of bliss and a lifetime of regret" or to provide "a mildly intoxicating, sensory altering, view of the cosmos." Some have suggested the substance possesses no legitimate medicinal uses. Others believe marijuana has medicinal value in reducing side effects experienced in the treatment of cancer, for example. In recent years, state legislatures have passed laws allowing individuals with a variety of medical issues to possess and use marijuana for medical purposes. More recently, states such as Vermont, Colorado, California, and Massachusetts have passed recreational marijuana use acts in spite of existing federal law that prohibits its use.

The data from Johnston et al. (2017) indicate that 13.5% of 8th graders, 30.7% of 10th graders, and 45% of seniors in 2017 admitted to having tried marijuana at least once. This compared to 60.4% of the graduating class of 1979. The good news is that lifetime marijuana usage among young people is down. The questions that remained to be answered in the coming years are: What effect will Vaping have on usage? Secondly, should the legal availability of marijuana in states increase, what impact will that exert on adolescent usage?

Heroin and Other Opiates

> And now my beauties, something with poison in it, but attractive to the eye and soothing to the smell…poppies, poppies, poppies will put them to sleep. (Wicked Witch of the West, [Motion picture], 1939 cited in LeRoy et al., 1939)

> Among the remedies which has pleased the almighty God to give to man to relieve his sufferings, none is so universal and so efficacious as opium. (Sydenham, 1680/2010, p. 72)

> Edmund: We're talking about Mama…After you found out she'd.
> been made a morphine addict, why didn't you send her to a cure.
> then, at the start, when she still had a chance. (O'Neil, 1956, p. 139–140)

We begin with the poppy. From its seed pods we extract a milky white substance (opium) that as one Witch observed, "put them to sleep." Useful substance this opium in a time long before medicine had evolved to offer more than palliative care. A touch of distillation and from opium we extract a more potent substance called morphine. Not willing to leave well enough alone—remember, the pharmaceutical industry is not profitable using natural ingredients—altering nature a touch produces oxycodone and hydrocodone. But why stop there? In a plastic world, chemists create new previously unknown substances that outperform the best that nature can provide as in OxyContin and fentanyl.

But to return to the beginning, discover a "medicinal" substance like opium or its offspring morphine and watch the creative uses to which it can be put. For example, in *Dr. Chase's Recipes or Information for Everybody: An Invaluable Collection of About Eight Hundred Practical Recipes* (Chase, 1866) the good doctor offered up these helpful aids to Mom for her family:

> For Nervousness—Nervous Pill—Morphine 9 grs.; extract of stramonium and hyoseyamus, of each 18 yrs.; form into pill-mass by using solution of gum arabic and tragacanth… Dose—in case of severe pain or nervousness, 1 pill taken at bedtime will be found to give a quiet night of rest.
>
> Or for the children—Cough Candy—Tincture of squalls 2 ohs.; camphorated tincture of opium, and tincture of holy, of each 1/4 oz.; wine of impeach 1/2 oz.; oils of gaultheria 4 drops, sassafras 3 drops, and of anise seed oil 2 drops… Druggists will get confectioners to make this for a trifle on the pound over common candies. (Chase, 1866, pp. 149, 171–172)

The good Dr. Chase was not alone in his liberal use of opium and morphine. Patent medicines of the day like *Mrs. Winslow's Soothing Syrup* and *Dr. LeGear's Colic Remedy* freely mixed alcohol with opium in a concoction called laudanum. No doubt Mrs. Winslow and Dr. LeGear delivered on their promises to parents. A teaspoon or two of either elixir would reduce a child to a quiet, drooling, limp doll. As World War I approached, the federal government gradually strengthened its restrictions on the use of these substances decreasing over time the number of women like Eugene O'Neil's Mary Tyrone's addiction to opiates.

While decreasing availability reduced abuse, opiates remained a problem—particularly heroin—but this abuse was considered a problem of the lower classes and the fringe artistic community; that is until the 1990s. It was then that a new class of drugs like OxyContin was introduced to the marketplace. I use the word marketplace intentionally as this and similar substances like fentanyl were heralded by their manufacturers as superior to existing and less potent alternatives (Courtwright, 2001).

As public relations firms know, to sell a product a demand must be established and in this case that demand was pain management—pain management not just for those needing palliative care at the conclusion of their lives but those temporarily discomforted by a removed tooth, a dislocated shoulder or a broken toe. With a free dinner, a goody bag containing among other things a golf ball, and a brief lecture by a paid drug representative medical practitioners were encouraged to prescribe and prescribe they did with sales of OxyContin rising from $45 million dollars in 1996 to $1.5 billion in 2002. Despite fines for misrepresenting the potential harm of these new opiates, the drug industry continues the profitable excessive manufacturing of these substances (Deprez & Barrett, 2017; Etter, 2017).

The data from Johnston et al. (2017) indicate that less than 1% of 8th, 10th, and 12th graders admitted to having tried heroin at least once in their lifetime. The lifetime use of narcotics other than heroin (including pain medications) is 6.8% among seniors. This data point of 6.8% is indicative of a slow decline in usage by youth since 2014. That said, those youth abusing opiates may well not be represented by this study as their drug behavior may have removed them from school settings. Further, the opiate crisis facing this country is described primarily as a young adult problem and not one belonging to adolescents—yet.

Closing Thoughts

From this excursion down history's pathways what inferences can be drawn?

Whether they calmed nerves, lessened hunger, offered new insights into the cosmos, or cured illness, the initial use of each substance was regulated by the shaman or community leaders. The rules governing their use enabled the community to seemingly function successfully. Difficulties arose when these substances were taken out of their original context and placed into another, that is, from medicine or religious use to recreational use and from special circumstance or ceremonial use to continual use by those who would misuse them. With the growth of knowledge, these ancient substances lost their magical ability to answer questions, cure illness, and satisfy hunger. No longer did they open doors to insight and new information valuable to the group. Instead their usefulness became personal pleasure, and it is in this context that we find ourselves today.

As a species we seem to have evolved little from our extinct cousins who discovered that grain or fruits left in vessels fermented into an often unpleasant tasting beverage with pleasant and sought-after mood-altering characteristics or that some plants had similar qualities. It is a pity that this world does not contain enough wonderment to satisfy our needs for exploration and seeking contentment. But clearly the use of these and other substances suggest that it does not. For those who would disagree with me, consider the trouble Venezuela natives go to make the native beer—Chicha. Corn would be raised, gathered, and the women of the village would chew the corn kernels. These they would then spit into a community bowl. The process of chewing the corn splits the kernels, which mixed with the saliva in their mouths and transformed the starch found in the corn to sugar. Yeast feeds on the sugar, releasing alcohol and CO. Voilà, the end result is Chicha—alledgedly a "tasty beer" (Emboden, 1979, p. 154)! Lastly, the reality that alcohol, tobacco, and increasingly marijuana are permitted for recreational use suggests that these stepping-stone substances to other drugs will not turn to sand anytime soon.

Thus, we find ourselves in a quandary that is reflected in the circumstances described in the chapters to follow. We lament the number of youth who have traveled this well-worn path to other addictive drugs and the harm brought on them as a result, the expense to society for their addictive behavior, and the less than stellar success rate of their rehabilitation. Society speaks much of prevention but really means by that word, "please wait your time and then don't overindulge."

Perhaps, if society did not then immerse youth in a world of temptation far more enticing than Eden's one lone apple tree, they might wait but that is not the case. In our society tempting apple trees are abundant, and their luscious fruit are ever ripe for the tasting. As the reader is soon to learn, prevention approaches aimed at strengthening the will power of our young Adams and Eves (using prevention's tools of education, social competency promotion, and natural caregiving) to resist those apples are increasingly being paired with approaches that build fences around those trees like ID carding and arresting adults who serve or purchase alcohol and tobacco for minors (using the prevention tools of community organization and systems intervention). Encouragingly, this multifaceted approach has shown positive results. Discouragingly, this fencing approach has not focused attention on the manufacturing or distribution element of the equation, for example, reducing the alcoholic content of beverages or the chemical composition of pain relievers. These are "harm risk reduction" approaches—a phrase dropped from the lexicon of substance abuse prevention that deserves reinstatement if we are to be serious in our efforts to limit the use of stepping-stone substances by underage Adams and Eves.

References

AlterNet.org. (n.d.). Retrieved from http://www.alternet.org/dugreporter/18941

Anonymous. (1863). A run through the southern states. *Cornhill Magazine, 7*(4), 495–515.

Austin, G. A. (1979). *Research issues 24: Perspectives on the history of psychoactive substance use*. Washington, DC: U.S. Government Printing Office.

Brown, P. (2003). *Man walks into a pub: A sociable history of beer*. London, UK: Macmillan.

Burnham, J. C. (1993). *Bad habits: Drinking, smoking, taking drugs, gambling, sexual misbehavior, and swearing in American history*. New York, NY: University Press.

Burns, E. (2006). *The smoke of the gods: A social history of tobacco*. New York, NY: Temple University Press.

Burton, R. (1621/1851). *The anatomy of melancholy* (4th ed.). Philadelphia, PA: J. W. Moore.

Byrne, G. (1988). Nicotine likened to cocaine, heroin. *Science, 240*(4856), 1143. https://doi.org/10.1126/science.3375807

Chase, A. W. (1866). *Dr. Chase's recipes or information for everybody: An invaluable collection of about eight hundred practical recipes*. Ann Arbor, MI: Author.

Child, F. S. (1896). *The colonial parson of New England*. New York, NY: Baker & Taylor.

Courtwright, D. T. (2001). *Dark paradise: A history of opiate addiction in America*. Cambridge, MA: Harvard University Press.

Crane, S. (1895/2001). *The red badge of courage*. New York, NY: Barnes and Noble.

Deprez, E. E., & Barrett, P. (2017, October 5). The lawyer who beat big tobacco takes on the opioid industry. *Bloomberg Businessweek*, 1–14. Retrieved from https://www.bloomberg.com/news/features/2017–10-05/the-lawyer-who-beat-big-tobacco-takes-on-the-opioid-industry

Emboden, W. (1979). *Narcotic plants: Hallucinogens, stimulants, inebriants, and hypnotics, their origins and uses*. New York, NY: Macmillan.

Etter, L. (2017, October 26). Heroin and opioids. *Bloomberg*. Retrieved from https://www.bloomberg.com/quicktake/heroin

Goodman, J. (1994). *Tobacco in history: The cultures of dependence*. New York, NY: George Routledge.

Grinspoon, L. (1971). *Marijuana reconsidered*. Cambridge, MA: Harvard University Press.

Grinspoon, L., & Bakalar, J. B. (1993). *Marijuana forbidden medicine*. New Haven, CT: Yale University Press.

Ifill, G. (1992, March 30). *The 1992 campaign: New York; Clinton admits experiment with marijuana in 1960's* (p. A15). The New York Times.

James, I. (1604/1932). *A counter-blaste to tobacco*. Yellow Springs, OH: Antioch Press.

Johnston, L. D., O'Malley, P. M., Miech, R. A., Bachman, J. G., & Schulenberg, J. E. (2017). *Monitoring the Future: National survey results on drug use, 1975–2016. Overview, key findings on adolescent drug use*. Ann Arbor, MI: Institute for Social Research, The University of Michigan.

Kandel, D. B. (1981). Drug use by youth: An overview. In D. J. Lettieri & J. P. Lundford (Eds.), *Drug abuse and the American adolescent (NIDA research monograph no. 38, #ADM 81–1166)* (pp. 1–24). Washington, DC: U.S. Government Printing Office.

Kandel, D. B., & Faust, R. (1975). Sequence and stages in patterns of adolescent drug use. *Archives of General Psychiatry, 32*(8), 923–932.

Kandel, D. B., Kessler, R., & Margulies, R. (1978). Adolescent initiation into stages of drug use: A developmental analysis. In D. B. Kandel (Ed.), *Longitudinal research on drug use: Empirical findings and methodological issues* (pp. 225–252). Washington, DC: Hemisphere-Wiley.

Kandel, D. B., Yamaguchi, K., & Chen, K. (1992). Stages of progression in drug involvement from adolescence to adulthood: Further evidence for the gateway theory. *Journal of Studies on Alcohol, 53*(4), 447–457.

Kuntz, P. (1995, August 14). *Alcohol beverage industry lobbies for bill to gut substance abuse agency see as threat* (p. A12). Wall Street Journal.

LeRoy, M., Fleming, V., LeRoy, M., Vidor, K., Taurog, N., & Cukor, G. (1939). *The Wizard of Oz [Motion picture]*. Beverly Hills, CA: Metro-Goldwyn-Mayer Studios.

National Institute on Alcohol Abuse and Alcoholism (NIAAA). (2008). *Alcohol research and health, 31(4)*. Rockville, MD: U.S. Government Printing Office.

O'Neil, E. (1956). *Long day's journey into night*. New Haven, CT: Yale University Press.

Shoemaker, W. L. (1898). *La santa yerba*. Boston, MA: Copeland and Day.

Sloman, L. (1979). *The history of marijuana in America: Reefer madness*. New York, NY: Bobbs-Merrill.

Sydenham, T. (1680/2010). *The entire works of Thomas Sydenham newly made English from the originals*. Hampshire, UK: Gale ECCO.

Tannahill, R. (1973). *Food in history*. New York, NY: Stein & Day.

Wagner, S. (1971). *Cigarette country: Tobacco in American history and politics*. New York, NY: Praeger.

A Biological/Genetic Perspective: The Addicted Brain

Thomas H. Kelly, Arit Harvanko, Mark E. Pierce, Abner O. Rayapati, and Catherine A. Martin

Introduction

Exposure to medications, chemicals, infectious disease, or environmental agents (i.e., potential teratogens) presents a significant health risk during human development, particularly during critical periods of organ and system development. Risk of exposure during the critical periods of embryonic and fetal development has been well documented, but recent evidence suggests that critical periods of organ development, especially brain development, extend into childhood and adolescence. Given the extended period of brain development, risks associated with exposure to teratogens having direct effects on the brain (i.e., psychoactive drugs) may also extend into childhood and adolescence. This chapter examines the health risks associated with developmental exposure to psychoactive drugs of abuse.

Exposure to psychoactive drugs can impact normal biological development in ways that are similar to other teratogens. However, psychoactive drugs can also influence brain and behavioral functions through direct pharmacological modula-

T. H. Kelly (✉)
Department of Behavioral Science, College of Medicine, University of Kentucky, Lexington, KY, USA
e-mail: thkelly@uky.edu

A. Harvanko
Department of Psychology, College of Arts & Sciences, University of Kentucky, Lexington, KY, USA
e-mail: Arit.H@uky.edu

M. E. Pierce
College of Medicine, University of Kentucky, Lexington, KY, USA
e-mail: mark.pierce@uky.edu

A. O. Rayapati · C. A. Martin
Department of Psychiatry, College of Medicine, University of Kentucky, Lexington, KY, USA
e-mail: aora222@uky.edu; catherine.martin@uky.edu

C. G. Leukefeld, T. P. Gullotta (eds.), *Adolescent Substance Abuse*, Issues in Children's and Families' Lives, https://doi.org/10.1007/978-3-319-90611-9_3

tion of neuronal function and structure. As such, the developmental risk related to exposure to psychoactive drugs is exacerbated by the potential for adverse consequences related to the neuropharmacological effects of the drugs occurring during critical periods of development. Concerns are further heightened if one considers frequency of exposure. Some psychoactive drugs function as reinforcers and engender repeated drug-taking behavior, and increased frequency of neuropharmacological exposure exacerbates risk of developmental problems.

Risk of prenatal exposure to psychoactive drugs of abuse is substantial, given that rates of drug use in the general population are highest among individuals of reproductive age and significant drug use is reported among pregnant women (e.g., 11.5% of pregnant adolescent women report past month alcohol use, and 23% report past month use of tobacco) (Oh, Reingle Gonzalez, Salas-Wright, Vaughn, & DiNitto, 2017). Exposure to psychoactive drugs of abuse can occur postnatally through passive exposure from environmental sources (e.g., tobacco smoke, methamphetamine production). Developmental exposure to drugs of abuse among children and adolescents has escalated in the past decades as drugs have become increasingly available to younger age groups and experimentation has increased. Furthermore, genetic, developmental, and other neurobiological factors influence individual sensitivity to the reinforcing and other neuropharmacological effects of psychoactive drugs (Chambers, Taylor, & Potenza, 2003). In combination with cultural, community, peer, and family influences, enhanced sensitivity to the reinforcing and other pharmacological effects of drugs place some children and adolescents at increased vulnerability for repeated drug use (e.g., Kelly et al., 2006; Stoops et al., 2007) and for the development of heavy use, abuse, and dependence (Chaloupka & Johnston, 2007). Individual differences in sensitivity to the neuropharmacological effects of drugs can increase the risk of adverse health consequences associated with drug use, including engaging in other risky behaviors (e.g., sexual behavior, driving behavior, self-injurious behavior, and gambling), as well as adverse short- and long-term social (education, peer and family relations), medical (mental and physical health), and legal consequences. Finally, evidence links exposure to psychoactive drugs of abuse during critical periods of development to enhanced sensitivity to the reinforcing and other neuropharmacological effects of drugs, which, in turn, leads to enhanced likelihood of repeating drug use, followed by further enhancement of sensitivity (e.g., Derauf, Kekatpure, Neyzi, Lester, & Kosofsky, 2009; Glantz & Chambers, 2006).

Neurodevelopment

Substantial neuronal growth occurs during prenatal embryonic development. However, critical periods of neurogenesis and synaptic remodeling also occur in response to environmental experiences and continue after birth and throughout childhood and adolescence (e.g., Tau & Peterson, 2010). For example, maturation of the mesolimbocortical system—a pathway often implicated in the rewarding effects of drugs of abuse—continues during childhood and early adolescence, while inhibitory functions of the orbitofrontal cortex—a brain region shown to be involved in self-regulation—continue to develop into the early twenties (e.g., Galvan et al., 2006; Nigg, 2017; Steinberg, 2010). High levels of impulsiveness and risk-taking behavior among adolescents have been linked to asynchronous development of reward and inhibitory functions, with the alerting and motivating functions of the dopaminergic reward pathway emerging during early adolescence, while the inhibitory processes of the frontal cortex that hold these functions in check may not become fully mature until early adulthood (Crews, He, & Hodge, 2007). Risk associated with psychoactive drug exposure during critical periods of prenatal and postnatal human brain development has been well recognized. However, since periods of critical development continue throughout childhood and adolescence, it is important to recognize that risks to optimal brain development associated with psychoactive drug exposure extend well beyond the period of embryonic growth (Tau & Peterson, 2010).

Pharmacology

Drugs enter the body through several routes: parenteral (intravenous, intramuscular, and subcutaneous), enteral (oral, sublingual, and rectal), inhalation, intranasal, intrathecal, transdermal, and topical. Research has established that a rapid rise in plasma levels, quick entry into the brain, and relatively short-acting behavioral effects increase the reinforcing effects and abuse liability of a compound (Feldman, Meyer, & Quenzer, 1997). Drugs enter the bloodstream and reach the brain most rapidly when administered intravenously or via inhalation (i.e., smoking).

Drug action diminishes through metabolic and excretory processes. Body mass, total body water, amount of body fat, and maturity of liver enzymes involved in drug metabolism influence the rate at which a drug is metabolized and eliminated. Each of these factors varies as a function of stage of development. For example, children and adolescents are more vulnerable to some drug effects because they do not have the ability to clear drugs from the body as efficiently as adults (e.g., Holford, Heo, & Anderson, 2013). The implications of a slower metabolic transformation are that the active drug or active metabolites remain in the bloodstream for a longer period of time and often increase the duration of the drug's effects. Blood level engendered by a dose of drug is also an important determinant of the effect of a drug (e.g., blood alcohol levels and performance impairment). Body mass is an important determinant of blood levels, such that blood concentration is proportional to body mass. Because children and adolescents are typically smaller than the average adult, drug doses typically used by adults will engender relatively higher blood concentrations in children and adolescents than in adults. For example, when a 200 lb. (or 90.72 kg) adult consumes 100 mg of caffeine, a dose of 1.10 mg/kg of body weight is consumed. If a 90 lb. (or 40.82 kg) adolescent consumes the same beverage containing 100 mg of caffeine, a dose of 2.45 mg/kg, over two times the relative dose consumed by the adult man, is consumed.

Relative drug dose determined by body mass is relevant when examining the effects of drugs in the fetus and infant. Drugs pass from mother to fetus through the vasculature of the placenta and to the newborn through breast milk. Many compounds that the mother consumes during pregnancy cross the placenta and enter the bloodstream of the fetus (Myllynen, Pasanen, & Pelkonen, 2005). The total dose of the drug that reaches the fetus is dependent on the dose of the drug ingested by the mother, the manner in which the drug is excreted, and the metabolic rate and pathway of the drug (Ostrea, Mantaring, & Silvestre, 2004). Several reviews detail the effects and risks associated with placental transfer of a wide range of licit and illicit drugs (Briggs, Freeman, & Yaffe, 1998; Garland, 1998; Ostrea et al., 2004). Mothers can also expose infants to drugs through breast milk. The total dose that reaches the infant depends on the dose the mother ingested, the duration of the drug regimen (occasional vs. consistent use), the route of administration (drugs that enter the mother's system parenterally are typically less concentrated in the breast milk than those administered orally), the pharmacokinetics of the drug (drugs with longer half-lives have greater potential to collect in significant amounts in milk), and the infant's ability to absorb, metabolize, and excrete the drug, with older infants being able to process most drugs more efficiently than premature or younger infants (Ostrea et al., 2004).

Neuropharmacology

Neuronal communication in the brain occurs through an electrochemical process, with electrical impulses in a neuron modulating the release of chemicals [i.e., neurotransmitters, such as dopamine, serotonin, endogenous opiates, *N*-methyl-D-aspartate (NMDA), gamma-aminobutyric acid (GABA), and acetylcholine]. Released chemicals diffuse across small spaces (i.e., synapse) between adjacent neurons, and binding of these neurochemicals to proteins (i.e., receptors) on the membranes of the adjacent neurons leads to modulation of electrical signals and other activities in adjacent neurons. Action by neurotransmitters in the synapse is then terminated by metabolic enzymes, or reabsorption into presynaptic neurons. Psychoactive drugs capitalize on this system, modulating action at the receptor level or altering the manner in which neurons regulate neurotransmitters. Homeostatic functions keep a regular balance of neurotransmitter release and inhibition, and upset of this balance by drugs can lead to effects on hormonal action, learning, memory, mood, reward, and behavior.

Most drugs of abuse have direct or indirect effects on neurons utilizing dopamine as the neurotransmitter signal, particularly those in the dopamine-rich mesolimbocortical system (e.g., caudate/putamen, nucleus accumbens, tuberculum olfactorium, and prefrontal and frontal cortex), sometimes referred to as the dopamine reward pathway. Increased activation of dopamine release (i.e., potentiation) in this pathway is a common neuropharmacological mechanism of action of the drugs that function as reinforcers (i.e., drugs with abuse liability). The mesolimbocortical system is still undergoing development in childhood and adolescence, and it has been argued that enhanced stimulation of this pathway during development, as would occur during exposure to drugs of abuse, can cause permanent changes in the sensitivity of these regions (e.g., Andersen & Navalta, 2004).

Summary

Prenatal, childhood, and adolescent stages are times of rapid neurodevelopment with synaptic connections continually forming and brain structures constantly developing. Exposure to drugs and other teratogens during these critical periods of development has both short- and long-term health consequences. Psychoactive drugs are of particular concern, given that these compounds have direct effects on brain function and engender both short- and long-term effects on the brain and behavior, with risk of exposure elevated among psychoactive drugs of abuse.

Caffeine

Caffeine is the most widely consumed psychoactive drug among adults and children (Warzack, Evans, Floress, Gross, & Stoolman, 2011). Of increasing concern is the use of energy drinks by children, adolescents and young adults who are at particular risk for harmful effects (Seifert, Schaechter, Hershorin, & Lipshultz, 2011).

Mechanisms of Action

Caffeine (1, 3, 7-trimethylxanthine) is a purine alkaloid found in the beans, leaves, and fruits of over 60 plants (Weinberg & Bealer, 2001). Effects in the central nervous system (CNS) occur primarily through binding with and blocking the membrane proteins (i.e., receptors) that are activated by the endogenous neurotransmitter adenosine (Daly & Fredholm, 1998; Fredholm, Bättig, Holmén, Nehlig, & Zvartau, 1999). Adenosine is an inhibitory neuromodulator that increases sedation and acts as an anticonvulsant. In addition, adenosine decreases blood pressure, respiration, gastric secretions, diuresis, and lipolysis (Daly & Fredholm, 1998; Garrett & Griffiths, 1996). By blocking adenosine receptors, caffeine antagonizes the typical effects of adenosine, such as sedation, which results in the stimulant-like effects of the drug.

Caffeine also has indirect agonist effects on dopamine activity, which is related to its adenosine receptor blockade. Heavy concentrations of adenosine receptors are found in the dopamine reward pathway (Daly & Fredholm, 1998; Ferre, Euler, Johansson, Fredholm, & Fuxe, 1991; Ferre, Fuxe, von Euler, Johansson, &

Fredholm, 1992). Adenosine receptors regulate dopamine release as well as GABA neuron activation; GABA serves an inhibitory role in the dopamine reward pathway. By antagonizing adenosine, caffeine indirectly enhances dopamine release and diminishes the inhibitory functions of the GABA system (Daly & Fredholm, 1998; Ferre et al., 1992; Garrett & Griffiths, 1996).

Epidemiology and Health Consequences of Prenatal, Early Childhood, and Adolescent Caffeine Exposure

On average, a mug of drip-brewed coffee contains ~100 mg of caffeine. A similar size serving of tea contains 80 mg, and a 12 oz. serving of a caffeinated soda contains ~40 mg. The average daily amount of caffeine consumption for adults is ~230 mg/day (3.3 mg/kg/day), with 30% of adults consuming more than 500 mg/day (7.1 mg/kg/day; DSM-IV). Caffeine is the psychotropic drug most commonly consumed by pregnant and nursing women, with 60–68% of this population consuming moderate amounts (100–200 mg) of caffeine daily (Frary, Johnson, & Wang, 2005; Pirie, Lando, Curry, McBride, & Grothaus, 2000). While mean daily caffeine consumption for children and adolescents has been estimated to range from 37 to 63 mg/day (Morgan, Stults, & Zabik, 1982; Valek, Laslavić, & Laslavić, 2004), 20–25% of this population consume over 100 mg/day, with occasional reports of consumption of 290–500 mg/day or more (Leviton, 1992; Rapoport, Berg, Ismond, Zahn, & Neims, 1984). Caffeine consumption does not vary as a function of gender, but differences have been reported among racially classified groups (Arbeit et al., 1988; Leviton, 1992). It is important to point out that soft drink consumption, which is the major source of caffeine in school-aged children, has more than tripled since 1970 (Story & Neumark-Sztainer, 1998; Valek et al., 2004). Sales of caffeinated "energy" drinks, which contain 2–3 times the amount of caffeine per given volume compared to conventional caffeinated soft drinks, are increasing among adolescents and young adults (Malinauskas, Aeby, Overton, Carpenter-Aeby, & Barber-Heidal, 2007).

In the third trimester of pregnancy, caffeine's half-life (amount of time required to eliminate 50% of the drug concentration) increases from 2–6 to 10–20 h (Brazier, Ritter, Berland, Khenfer, & Faucon, 1983; Knutti, Rothweiler, & Schlatter, 1982). In utero, caffeine is passed from mother to child through the placenta, readily entering the fetal bloodstream, such that ~75% of babies are born with detectable levels of caffeine in their blood (Brazier & Salle, 1981; Dumas et al., 1982). After birth, it is also passed via breast milk to nursing infants (Benowitz, 1990; Julien, 2001). From prenatal stages to at least 3 months of age, the hepatic enzymes necessary to metabolize the drug are absent or immature, causing the drug's half-life to be anywhere from 32 to 149 h (Parsons & Neims, 1981). As such, blood levels of caffeine may be elevated in the neonate and newborn in relation to levels seen in adolescents and adults. After the metabolic enzymes develop, metabolic rates approximate that of adults (James, 1991).

The degree to which caffeine exposure affects the health and well-being of a fetus, neonate, newborn, or infant remains unclear. The research literature on this topic is vast and equivocal, with reports ranging from virtually no adverse health consequences (Giannelli, Doyle, Roman, Pelerin, & Hermon, 2003; Leviton & Cowan, 2002; Savitz, Chan, Herring, Howards, & Hartmann, 2008) to early term birth and increased risk of miscarriage (Bech, Nohr, Vaeth, Henriksen, & Olsen, 2005; George, Granath, Johansson, Olander, & Cnattingius, 2006; Rasch, 2003). More recently, Galéra et al. (2016) found that prenatal caffeine exposure was negatively associated with full scale and performance IQ at age 5.5 years. This relationship was maintained even when controlling for tobacco use. Earlier studies have not found associations between intrauterine caffeine exposure and behavioral changes in early childhood (Loomans, 2012).

A variety of studies have examined the effects of caffeine in children and adolescents. In normal children and adolescents, low doses of caffeine (3 mg/kg) have been reported to improve attention and performance of vigilance tasks, reduce reaction time, improve manual dexterity, improve memory, reduce errors of omission on continuous performance tests, and increase speech production (Castellanos & Rapoport, 2002; Elkins et al., 1981; Hughes & Hale, 1998; Leon, 2000; Leviton, 1992; Rapoport, Elkins, Neims, Zahn, & Berg, 1981; Stein, Krasowski, Leventhal, Phillips, & Bender, 1996), particularly when performance is less than optimal due to boredom or fatigue. Caffeine use is associated with later sleep times, less time in bed, and changes in sleep architecture (e.g., decreased depth of sleep, Aepli, Kurth, Tesler, & Huber, 2015), and poorer academic performance (Dimitriou, Cornu Knight, & Milton, 2015). Higher doses of caffeine can also be associated with inattentiveness, restlessness, nausea, stomachache, and dysphoria and depression—including nervousness, jitteriness, stress, and anxiety (Hughes & Hale, 1998; Orbeta, Overpeck, Ramcharran, Kogan, & Ledsky, 2006; Pollak & Bright, 2003; Richards & Smith, 2015; Sojar et al., 2015). Symptoms of caffeine withdrawal (Bernstein et al., 1998; Hughes & Hale, 1998) and caffeinism (Castellanos & Rapoport, 2002) have been noted in children and adolescents. In general, these effects are similar to those reported in adults.

There is evidence that heavy caffeine use is associated with drug use and other problem behaviors in children and adolescents (Tennant & Detels, 1976). In particular, moderate and heavy energy drink use in middle and high school predicted lifetime alcohol, tobacco, and other drug use (Polak et al., 2016). It is not known whether behavioral problems in children and adolescents who consume large amounts of caffeine are due to caffeine, or whether children and adolescents with these problems consume large amounts of caffeine in order to self-medicate their symptoms (Leviton, 1992).

Caffeine may interact with and enhance the effects of other drugs of abuse. For example, caffeine has been found to enhance the reinforcing and stimulant subjective effects of nicotine in adult cigarette smokers (Jones & Griffiths, 2003). Of particular concern is the increase in emergency room presentations related to energy drink toxicity frequently in combination with alcohol and other drugs of abuse (Substance Abuse and Mental Health Services Administration, Center for Behavioral Health Statistics and Quality, 2013a).

Implications

Levels of caffeine exposure during human development are higher than any other psychoactive drug. Caffeine levels during prenatal development and for the first several months after birth are elevated due to the absence of enzymes required for efficient caffeine metabolism. Caffeine intake in sodas and energy drinks is increasing among children and adolescents, and heavy intake has been linked to drug use and other problem behaviors. The American Academy of Pediatrics (2011) recommends that energy drinks should "never be consumed" by children or adolescents.

Nicotine

Nicotine is consumed in tobacco cigarettes, chewing tobacco, hookah, nicotine gums and patches, and electronic cigarettes. Use of tobacco cigarettes, the most widespread form of nicotine delivery, cause approximately one in five deaths in the USA every year (US Department of Health and Human Services, 2014). Nicotine has been described as one of the most addictive substances of abuse based on observations that close to 32% of individuals who "ever" smoke go on to develop nicotine dependence (Anthony, Warner, & Kessler, 1994). The next closest drug is heroin, with 23% of ever users developing dependence, followed by cocaine at 17%, and alcohol at 15%. Recent prevalence estimates of daily tobacco cigarette use among 12th graders have decreased from approximately 21% in 1980 to 7% in 2015 (Johnston, O'Malley, Miech, Bachman, & Schulenberg, 2016). There are also large gender differences in smoking rates. In 1980, it was estimated that 41.2% of men and 10.6% of women used cigarettes daily, while in 2015 an estimated 31.1% of men and 6.2% of women are daily cigarette users (Ng et al., 2014). The majority of adult smokers initiate tobacco use before age 18, and the earlier the age of smoking initiation, the greater the likelihood of lifetime use (Kopstein, 2001). Although tobacco cigarette use has decreased over time, consumption of nicotine in electronic cigarettes has rapidly increased over the past few years, with recent estimates of past month use of electronic cigarettes among emerging adults as high as 41% in 2013 (Ramo, Young-Wolff, & Prochaska, 2015). Of concern, neither the behavioral nor the health effects of electronic cigarette use are well characterized at the present time.

Mechanisms of Action

Nicotine binds to receptors widely distributed throughout the brain that are normally bound by the endogenous neurotransmitter acetylcholine. There are several subtypes of "nicotinic acetylcholine" receptors, composed of differing arrangements of alpha and beta protein subunits. Nicotinic acetylcholine receptors exert a variety of effects in the CNS, including modulation of dopamine function. As with other drugs of abuse, nicotine modulation of the dopamine reward pathway is considered a primary mechanism for its abuse liability (Picciotto & Corrigall, 2002). The alpha-4, beta-2 nicotinic acetylcholine receptor type is most closely linked with dopamine modulation and nicotine dependence (Tapper et al., 2004). Nicotine enhancement of dopamine neurotransmission is believed to be responsible for tolerance to nicotine and for the development of conditioning to environmental cues associated with smoking behavior (Liu et al., 2003; Maskos et al., 2005; Picciotto, Zoli, & Changeux, 1999; Pidoplichko et al., 2004; Salminen et al., 2004; Tapper et al., 2004).

Epidemiology and Health Consequences of Prenatal, Early Childhood, and Adolescent Nicotine Exposure

Approximately 23% of pregnant adolescents report past month use of tobacco (Oh et al., 2017). Rates of smoking identified with surveys are generally lower than those identified when quantitative measures of smoking (e.g., salivary cotinine) are used to determine smoking rates (Walsh, Redman, & Adamson, 1996), suggesting that the 23% frequency could be an underestimate of the true rate.

In utero exposure to nicotine has important implications for brain development. Nicotine receptors appear by the end of the first month of human fetal life and are critical for brain growth and neuronal connectivity, including modulation of nerve growth and formation of new synaptic connections between neurons in the brain (Hellstrom-Lindahl, Seiger, Kjaeldgaard, & Nordberg, 2001). Animal studies have found that prenatal and postnatal nicotine exposure is associated with alterations of a variety of endogenous neurotransmitter systems mediated by dopamine, norepinephrine, and serotonin (Muneoka et al., 2001; Richardson & Tizabi, 1994; Slotkin, Pinkerton, Auman, Qiaio, & Seidler, 2002; Xu, Seidler, Ali, Slikker, & Slotkin, 2001). Research has shown that the thickness of regions in the cortex (orbitofrontal, middle frontal, and parahippocampal) associated with cognition and social control is reduced in adolescents exposed to maternal smoking (Toro et al., 2008). There is also evidence that offspring of mothers who smoked cigarettes during pregnancy have children with reduced total brain volume later in childhood (El Marroun et al., 2013).

In utero exposure to nicotine has important implications for behavioral development. Prenatal nicotine exposure is associated with the development of altered patterns of behavior during early postnatal life and later in childhood (Law et al., 2003; El Marroun et al., 2013). For example, children exposed in utero are more likely to be impulsive, hyperactive, oppositional, and have lower language skills than their unexposed peers (Day, Richardson, Goldschmidt, & Cornelius, 2000; Faden & Graubard, 2000; Fried & Watkinson, 1990; Wakschlag, Leventhal, Pine, Pickett, & Carter, 2006). Multiple studies suggest that these effects continue to be expressed during adolescence. Children of mothers who smoked during pregnancy are at greater risk for a broad range of mental health problems (Goodwin et al.,

2013). Specifically, in utero exposure increases the risk of developing both internalizing and externalizing disorders (e.g., mood disorders, conduct disorder) known to be risk factors for the emergence of adolescent experimental and persistent smoking (Fried & Watkinson, 2001; Upadhyaya, Deas, Brady, & Kruesi, 2002). Postnatal environmental tobacco smoke exposure may also have an impact on child and adolescent brain and behavioral development (Okoli, Kelly, & Hahn, 2007), although disentangling postnatal and prenatal associations is methodologically difficult (Eskenazi & Castorina, 1999).

By the age of 10, nicotine-exposed offspring are more likely to have tried smoking, and smoking rates among the prenatally exposed remain higher during adolescence (Cornelius, Leech, Goldschmidt, & Day, 2000; Nichter, Nichter, Thompson, Shiffman, & Moscicki, 2002; Niemelä et al., 2017). Adult women exposed to tobacco in utero are four times more likely to be smokers than those who were not exposed (Kandel, Wu, & Davies, 1994). It is clear that there are multiple environmental, biological, and genetic factors that contribute to tobacco use, and many of these factors may also contribute to multigenerational tobacco use.

Research on the effects of nicotine use during pregnancy has focused primarily on nicotine delivered via tobacco cigarettes. Little is currently known, however, about the effects of electronic cigarette use during pregnancy. Due to the current lack of regulation on electronic cigarettes, there are a wide variety of undisclosed ingredients in their liquids, making it difficult to generalize about their health effects. Nonetheless, there is growing consensus that they typically contain fewer chemicals than tobacco cigarettes (e.g., Suter, Mastrobattista, Sachs, & Aagaard, 2015). Electronic cigarette liquids, however, usually contain nicotine, which is a known teratogen. As such, electronic cigarette use is not recommended during pregnancy.

Rates of nicotine dependence among adolescents have been difficult to determine, in part, because the criteria used to establish dependence among adults may not be as effective in assessing dependence among adolescents (Colby, Tiffany, Shiffman, & Niaura, 2000). Adolescents endorse more symptoms of dependence than do adults smoking the same number of cigarettes per day, suggesting that adolescents may be more sensitive to the effects of nicotine (Kandel & Chen, 2000). Kandel et al. (2005) found that various measures of nicotine dependence yielded different rates of dependence between adolescents and adults, especially at low levels of smoking. However, dependence rates became more consistent between adolescents and adults as the smoking rate approached one pack per day. In cross-sectional studies, withdrawal symptoms have been reported earlier in the course of tobacco use among adolescents than among adults, and may precede regular or daily use among adolescent smokers (DiFranza et al., 2007; O'Loughlin et al., 2003). It is possible that the reinforcing effects of nicotine are enhanced among adolescents, and that young smokers may develop tolerance and physical dependence more rapidly upon initiation of tobacco smoking than do adults. Based on when smoking is initiated and the associated adverse lifetime health consequences of tobacco use, nicotine addiction has been labeled a disease of adolescence (Kessler et al., 1997).

For at least some neurotransmitter systems (e.g., serotonin and acetylcholine), the CNS responses to nicotine during adolescence appear to be similar to those observed during other stages of life (Trauth, McCook, Seidler, & Slotkin, 2000; Xu et al., 2001). However, some unique nicotine effects occur during adolescence [i.e., effects that are different than those observed during either in utero or adult nicotine exposure (Slotkin, 2002)]. Laboratory experiments demonstrate differences between adolescent and adult behavioral responses to nicotine. Trauth, Seidler, and Slotkin (2000b), for example, gave nicotine to adolescent rats in a manner designed to mimic the effects of smoking over a period of days, then observed them in a novel environment while they performed a passive avoidance task. Contrary to effects seen in adult rats, nicotine decreased grooming behavior in the novel environment by adolescent females and enhanced passive avoidance behavior 24 h post-training, indicating differential effects of nicotine among adolescent rats compared to adults. Kota and Martin (2007), in a series of behavioral experiments with mice, found that adolescent mice exhibited nicotine-induced changes in receptor sensitivity and fewer withdrawal signs than did adult mice. A series of experiments by Faraday, Elliott, Phillips, and Grunberg (2003) demonstrated that behavioral sensitivity to nicotine in adult rats was increased by prior exposure to nicotine during adolescence. Timing of initial exposure also impacted rates of nicotine self-administration during adulthood, with adolescent-exposed rats self-administering more nicotine than did adult-exposed rats (Adriani et al., 2003; Levin, Rezvani, Montoya, Rose, & Swartzwelder, 2003).

Implications

There is considerable evidence indicating that risk for development of nicotine dependence is increased by nicotine exposure during early human development (Ginzel et al., 2007). Prenatal nicotine exposure engenders adverse behavioral outcomes that are associated with increased risk of adolescent smoking. Research demonstrates that adolescence is a critical time period during which nicotine exposure may permanently restructure the brain and increase lifetime risk of smoking. Environmental factors interacting with this biological vulnerability may set the stage for adult nicotine dependence and other psychopathology. Consequently, strategies and policies designed to limit exposure to nicotine during early life have the potential for prevention of significant adult morbidity and mortality.

Alcohol

Alcohol is widely used among American youth and threatens their health and safety. The Centers for Disease Control and Prevention (CDC) (2015a) reported that one in five youth between ages 12 and 17 reported past-year alcohol use. From 1996 to

2016, past month use reported by 8th, 10th and 12th graders through the Monitoring the Future (MTF) survey has shown a decline with percentage of use in 2016 noted at 7.3, 19.9 and 33.2, respectively (Johnston et al., 2016). That said, the 2015 Youth Risk Behavior Survey of high school students reported 8% drove after drinking and 22% rode in a car with someone who had been drinking alcohol (Kann et al., 2016). Motor vehicle accidents are the leading cause of death among teens. Between 2006 and 2010, average alcohol related deaths annually were greater than 4300 with more than 1500 associated with motor vehicle accidents (Centers for Disease Control and Prevention (CDC), 2013). In addition to physical injuries, adverse consequences related to excessive alcohol consumption include development of chronic diseases, including psychiatric disorders, neurologic impairment, cardiovascular disease, malignant neoplasms and fetal alcohol spectrum disorders (Cargiulo, 2007). Adverse social and cultural consequences of alcohol use are also apparent (National Institute on Alcohol Abuse and Alcoholism, 2004–2005). Early exposure to alcohol can have detrimental effects on future health. Fetal and infantile alcohol exposure is predictive of subsequent alcohol use during adolescence, and alcohol use during adolescence is associated with excessive alcohol use later in life (Spear, 2002; Spear & Molina, 2005). Onset of drinking alcohol before age 15 increases risk of abuse or dependency sixfold compared to those starting at the legal drinking age (Centers for Disease Control and Prevention (CDC), 2015a). Alcohol use during adolescence is also associated with elevated risks for liver disease and adverse endocrine and metabolic effects (National Institute on Alcohol Abuse and Alcoholism, 2004–2005).

Mechanisms of Action

Alcohol engenders multiple neurochemical effects and has a potent adverse impact on the developing brain. Changes in the integrity of the neuronal cell membrane occur during intoxication (Deitrich, Dunwiddie, Harris, & Erwin, 1989). Alcohol acts on multiple neurotransmitter systems, including NMDA, GABA, serotonin, and the endogenous opiate systems, with variability in the form and function of these neurotransmitter systems having a likely role in individual sensitivity to alcohol's effects (Charness, Hu, Edwards, & Querimit, 1993; Lesch, 2005; Wafford, Burnett, Harris, & Whiting, 1993). The NMDA and GABA systems modulate dopamine function, and alcohol modulates the dopamine reward pathway via its effects on NMDA and GABA receptors (Grobin, Matthews, Devaud, & Morrow, 1998; Verheul, van den Brink, & Geerlings, 1999; Zhang, Maldve, & Morrisett, 2006). The neurotoxic effects of acute and chronic alcohol exposure are also mediated via these mechanisms. Abstinence following heavy alcohol exposure (e.g., alcohol withdrawal) also has adverse effects on brain neurotransmitter systems and neuronal cell function (Grobin et al., 1998; Tsai et al., 1998).

Epidemiology and Health Consequences of Prenatal, Early Childhood, and Adolescent Alcohol Exposure

In utero alcohol exposure can have a profound impact on brain development. Approximately 50% of women above the age of 18 report occasional alcohol use, and 10% report continued use during pregnancy (National Institute on Alcohol Abuse and Alcoholism, 2015). Bertrand et al. (2004) estimated rates of in utero alcohol exposure at 13% of all pregnancies with 3% of pregnant women reporting frequent (seven or more drinks per week) or binge drinking (five or more drinks in one setting). The prevalence of fetal alcohol syndrome in the USA is 0.3 per 1000 children between age 7 and 9 (Centers for Disease Control and Prevention (CDC), 2015b). Even very low levels of in utero exposure have been associated with adverse cognitive and other behavioral health effects, including inattention, reduced memory, hyperactivity, impulsivity, and aggression; these effects may persist into adolescence (Sokol, Delaney-Black, & Nordstrom, 2003; Sood et al., 2001). Alcohol exposure in the developing child can have equally devastating consequences. The creation of new brain cells during adolescence (and other times) is important for the development of optimal learning and memory capacity. Crews, Mdzinarishvili, Kim, He, and Nixon (2006) demonstrated that acute alcohol interfered with the formation of new neuronal cells in adolescent rats, a process that may disrupt optimal cognitive development. Structural changes have also been identified in adolescents and adults as a function of heavy alcohol consumption over many years. DeBellis et al. (2005) found reduced prefrontal cortex volume in adolescents with early onset alcohol use and comorbid mental health conditions, although the study design was not able to differentiate acquired from preexisting volume decrements. Another study by DeBellis et al. (2000) found reduced hippocampal volumes in individuals with early onset alcohol-use disorders, and age of onset was inversely associated with total volume, suggesting that hippocampal development and associated memory processes may be particularly vulnerable to the impairing effects of alcohol during adolescence. More recently, Treit et al. (2013) compared 5–15 year olds with Fetal Alcohol Spectrum Disorders (FASD) to age-matched controls in a longitudinal study capturing serial imaging and found delayed white matter development in frontal association tracts consistent with earlier MR and functional MR imaging studies (Ewing, Sakhardande, & Blakemore, 2014; Squeglia, Jacobus, & Tapert, 2014).

Adolescents using alcohol are at risk for cognitive impairments as a consequence of the toxic effects of alcohol on brain development. Brown and Tapert (2004) found visuospatial deficits and information retrieval deficits 3 weeks after adolescents detoxified from heavy drinking patterns. Among adolescents, the presence of an alcohol-use disorder has been associated with changes in working memory task performance (Sher, 2006). Changes such as these may contribute to a dynamic negatively spiraling interaction between biological and environmental risk factors. For example, students with low school connectedness are at increased risk of problematic use of alcohol, and if cognitive impairments develop with use, then the likelihood of a negative trajectory of poor academic achievement and further disconnection with school is more likely, intensifying the risk for continued heavy alcohol use and dependence.

Environmental and biological factors may interact to influence risk. Exposure to traumatic experiences, such as violence, is a well-known risk factor for adolescent alcohol use (Vermeiren, Schwab-Stone, Deboutte, Leckman, & Ruchkin, 2003). Less dramatic, but not less important as a risk factor, the experience of stress in social interactions increases the risk for alcohol use and progression to dependence (Kreek & Koob, 1998). Animal models suggest that the effects of stress vary with age. For example, using a well-established place-preference conditioning procedure, Song et al. (2007) found that after exposure to chronic stress, adolescent mice demonstrated greater preference for an alcohol-paired environment, whereas for adult mice, the stress exposure did not change place preference.

Compared to adults, adolescent rats are less sensitive to sedation and motor impairment but more sensitive to social facilitation (Spear, 2004). Sensitivity differences have been associated with alcohol effects on NMDA receptor activity (Swartzwelder, Wilson, & Tayyeb, 1995). In humans, sensitivity to the effects of alcohol has been shown to be greater following fetal alcohol exposure and among individuals with a family history of alcohol dependence (Schuckit & Smith, 2004; Spear, 2002).

In addition to affecting the development of sensitivity and dependence, the age of initial alcohol use may also have an impact on response to treatment. Odansetron decreases alcohol craving by reducing serotonin receptor activity. Subjects with onset of alcohol dependence before the age of 25 years were found to have a more robust therapeutic response to odansetron than did those exhibiting alcohol-related problems at a later age (Johnson et al., 2000). An interesting study from Silveri (2014) using magnetic resonance spectroscopy to investigate the role of GABA in the comorbidity of impulse control, mental illness, and susceptibility to substance abuse found that a decreased GABA signal was associated with impulsivity among adolescents. This study provides a compelling rationale for considering non-benzodiazepine GABAergic medications, specifically topiramate, a well-known antiepileptic shown to be safe in the adolescent population, as a possible treatment medication (Silveri, 2014). By mimicking and replacing endogenous GABA at the level of cortex (the most likely site of antiepileptic activity), topiramate could be effective for treating adolescents prone to impulsivity and alcohol abuse.

Implications

There is a considerable body of evidence that the brain of the developing organism is at increased vulnerability to the adverse effects of alcohol from conception through adolescence, and that exposure to alcohol during this period of development may cause long-lasting or permanent neuroadaptation that may be associated with deficits in cognitive, emotional, and behavioral function during later life. These findings underscore the critical importance of early prevention and treatment of alcohol problems among children and adolescents. Given growing evidence for the critical role of social context (e.g., traumatic experience, stress) in risk for alcohol use and abuse among adolescents, along with evidence that treatment interventions developed for adults may be less effective, it will be important moving forward to consider interventions for adolescents that address a broader range of factors than modulating the reinforcing effects of alcohol (e.g., acamprosate, naltrexone; Clark, 2012), particularly given that these treatment drugs may themselves have detrimental effects on the developing adolescent brain. Adolescents often exhibit a sense of invulnerability when evaluating risk (Cohn, Macfarlane, Yanez, & Imai, 1995), and impulsivity is closely linked with alcohol use among adolescents. Perhaps adopting more holistic approaches that include social interventions, psychotherapy, and increasing home stability that also target impulsivity will be as effective for managing alcohol problems with less developmental risk for adolescents (Simantov, Schoen, & Klein, 2000).

Marijuana

Marijuana is the most commonly used illicit substance among adolescents (Johnston et al., 2016). Following a rise in use that began during the 1960s, annual marijuana prevalence peaked among 12th graders in 1979 at 51%. From 1996 to 2016, past-month marijuana use was mostly steady among 8th (5.4%), 10th (14.0%), and 12th graders (22.5%). However, perception of harm is a strong predictor of future use and 68.9% of high school seniors do not view regular marijuana smoking as harmful. Because of this, along with increasing legalization and accessibility, there are concerns that rates may rise. Early observations suggest that states where marijuana has been decriminalized have reported a dramatic increase in poison control center calls and hospital admissions regarding pediatric marijuana ingestion (Wang et al., 2014).

Mechanisms of Action

Endocannabinoid receptors are found throughout the body with cannabinoid 1 (CB1) in the brain and cannabinoid 2 (CB2) in the immune system. The endogenous cannabinoid system impacts a range of bodily functions from appetite and sleep to memory and cognition and coordination. The main psychoactive chemical in marijuana is delta-9-tetrahydrocannabinol (THC), which binds to both the CB1 and CB2 receptors. Through its effects on cannabinoid receptors, THC interacts with an array of neurotransmitters and modulators including glutamate, GABA, and opioids (for a review see Martin, 2004). The dopaminergic pathway associated with reward systems is also modulated by endocannabinoid receptor activity.

Epidemiology and Health Consequences of Prenatal, Early Childhood, and Adolescent Marijuana Exposure

Marijuana use in pregnant adolescents and young adults is increasing at a greater rate than seen in older pregnant populations (Brown et al., 2017). Prenatal marijuana exposure has been associated with future developmental problems for the exposed fetus, including hyperactivity and lower attention span (Goldschmidt, Day, & Richardson, 2000) and difficulties with visual memory, analysis, and learning (Fried, O'Connell, & Watkinson, 1992; Fried & Watkinson, 2000; Goldschmidt et al., 2000; Pope & Yurgelun-Todd, 1996). Other difficulties include academic underachievement and increased risk of future marijuana and nicotine use (Day, Goldschmidt, & Thomas, 2006; Fergusson & Boden, 2008; Silins et al., 2014).

Beyond prenatal exposure, marijuana accumulates in breast milk, and the American Academy of Pediatrics (2013) believes breastfeeding is contraindicated in active marijuana users. The American College of Obstetricians and Gynecologists Committee on Obstetric Practice (2015) recommends marijuana cessation prior to and during pregnancy.

Acute effects of marijuana use in adolescents can include mood instability, increased eating, decreased energy, and cognitive and psychomotor impairment (American Psychiatric Association, 2013). The user may experience euphoria, relaxation, heightened sensory perception and altered perception of time. Depending on the dose and the vulnerability of the user, hallucinations and panic can be experienced (National Institute on Drug Abuse (NIDA), 2017).

Several chronic health issues related to marijuana use are of concern, notably neurocognitive performance. Lane, Cherek, Tcheremissine, Steinberg, and Sharon (2007) have associated heavy use with poor performance on tasks requiring perseveration and decreases in flexible thinking and motivation. Other studies show a decrease in attention, learning, and memory (Harvey, Sellman, Porter, & Frampton, 2007; Solowij et al., 2011), and slower processing speed and verbal learning (Medina et al., 2007; Tapert, Granholm, Leedy, & Brown, 2002). Some studies suggest that when use begins before age 16 there is risk for a lower verbal IQ (Meier et al., 2012; Pope Jr., Gruber, Hudson, Huestis, & Yurgelun-Todd, 2003). That said, in prospective twin studies, Jackson et al. (2016) could not find a causal relationship between marijuana use and IQ loss but emphasized the potential importance of genetic and environmental factors.

In a review, Jacobus and Tapert (2014) highlight that in addition to the adverse performance on cognitive tasks, there may be changes in gray matter and neural functioning. Specifically, heavy use is associated with greater gray matter volume, particularly in the left hippocampal area that suggest interference with the normal developmental process of synaptic pruning of needless connections (Batalla et al., 2013; Medina et al., 2007; Nagel, Schweinsburg, Phan, & Tapert, 2005). Beyond these specific observations of cognitive changes, there are general concerns about decline in social functioning, such as performance in school and on the job and interpersonal relations (McCaffrey, Pacula, Han, & Ellickson, 2010; National

Institute on Drug Abuse (NIDA), 2017). Other concerns include the association between heavy marijuana use and the development of psychosis, specifically schizophrenia in those with genetic vulnerabilities (Caspi et al., 2005; Gage, Munafò, MacLeod, Hickman, & Smith, 2015).

Whether these neurological, psychological, and behavioral changes are singularly related to the use of marijuana is not clear. There are questions of differences in the brains of young substance abusers before drug effects. Further complicating determination of causation is that pure use of only one substance is rare, making it difficult to determine which substance (tobacco, alcohol, marijuana or other drug use) has had the greatest impact on brain changes (Jacobus et al., 2016). Finally, in adolescents, marijuana is associated with other high risk activities, such as unprotected sexual behavior resulting in unplanned pregnancies and sexually transmitted diseases; motor vehicle accidents, including those with fatal outcomes; and other violent and accidental deaths (Brady & Li, 2014; Hartman & Huestis, 2013).

Implications

In their 2014 policy statement, the American Academy of Child and Adolescent Psychiatry (2014) summarizes the implications of marijuana use for children and adolescents as: "Marijuana use is not benign, and adolescents are especially vulnerable to its many known adverse effects (Jager & Ramsey, 2008; Schneider, 2008). One in six adolescent marijuana users develop cannabis use disorder, a well characterized syndrome involving tolerance, withdrawal, and continued use despite significant associated impairments (Anthony et al., 1994; Hasin et al., 2013). Heavy use during adolescence is associated with increased incidence and worsened course of psychotic, mood, anxiety, and substance use disorders across the lifespan (Hasin et al., 2013; Hayatbakhsh et al., 2007; Moore et al., 2007; Rubino, Zamberletti, & Parolaro, 2012). Furthermore, marijuana's deleterious effects on adolescent brain development, cognition, and social functioning may have immediate and long-term implications, including increased risk of motor vehicle accidents, sexual victimization, academic failure, lasting decline in intelligence measures, psychopathology, addiction, and psychosocial and occupational impairment (Champion et al., 2004; Fergusson & Boden, 2008; Fergusson, Horwood, & Swain-Campbell, 2002; Hall & Degenhardt, 2009; Hartman & Huestis, 2013; Lynskey & Hall, 2000; Meier et al., 2012; Shapiro & Buckley-Hunter, 2010)."

Opiates

An epidemic of illicit opioid use, evidenced by dramatic increases in opioid dependency, hospitalization and death, has emerged in recent years. During 2014, 47,055 deaths from overdose occurred in the US, more than any previous year on record—61% of these deaths involved the use of opioids. Heroin related overdose deaths have more than tripled since 2010 (Rudd, Aleshire, Zibbell, & Matthew Gladden, 2016). Between 1997 and 2012, annual incidence of hospitalization for opioid poisoning among adolescents between ages 15 and 19 increased by 176%. Heroin poisoning showed an increase of 161% while methadone poisoning increased by 950% (Gaither, Leventhal, Ryan, & Camenga, 2016). Clearly, adolescent and young adult opioid use is emerging as a major public health concern.

Mechanisms of Action

Opioids belong to a chemical family of compounds that activate opioid receptors with differing affinities. The effects of these compounds on opioid receptors at different locations in the body produce the therapeutic effects of these drugs. Opium, derived from the Papaver somniverum, or poppy plant, has been used as an analgesic agent since at least 1500 BC Egypt. With minor chemical adjustments, opium can be made to permeate the blood brain barrier more effectively to calm the fussy infant, act more specifically at the level of the gastrointestinal system to reduce diarrhea, or target the pulmonary system as an antitussive. Opioid compounds that activate the μ-opioid receptor with different levels of affinity in the CNS, such as morphine, codeine, heroin, dihydromorphone, oxycodone, meperidine, fentanyl, methadone, and buprenorphine, contribute to the complex history of opiate abuse (Meyer & Quenzer, 2005).

The net result of increased opioid receptor binding is neuronal hyperpolarization which is accomplished in two main ways: (1) binding at inhibitory metabotropic G-protein coupled receptors, which decreases the activity of adenylate cyclase (AC) and open potassium channels, thereby hyperpolarizing postsynaptic cells, and (2) axo-axonically on other systems, decreasing the likelihood of calcium channel opening and, with it, the release of other families of target neurotransmitters, both excitatory and inhibitory. Of note, many endogenous neurons with opioid receptors also exhibit autoregulation, as presynaptic receptors are sensitive to the effects of endorphins. A slight variant on the opioid agonist theme is buprenorphine, which acts as a partial agonist at opioid receptors, regulating the magnitude of opioid receptor activation.

The density of opioid receptors varies across brain regions. Opioids are known for their ability to suppress respiratory drive by interfering with breathing pattern generation related to a high density of opioid receptors in the pons and medulla, making opioids among the most deadly drugs of abuse (Pattinson, 2008). As with almost all known drugs of abuse, molecular changes in dopamine function co-occur with opioid use during the process of addiction (Nestler, 2012), and such changes in dopamine function in the developing adolescent brain can have significant behavioral implications.

Epidemiology and Health Consequences of Prenatal, Early Childhood, and Adolescent Opioid Exposure

Various biopsychosocial factors have been implicated in illicit opioid use. Developmental vulnerability, stress, cultural permissiveness, substance use in the family or psychiatric illness can increase the risk of developing a substance use disorder (Sharma, Bruner, Barnett, & Fishman, 2016). Nonmedical prescription opioid users, for example, report greater psychological symptom burden compared to those that never use opioids (Boyd, Young, & McCabe, 2014). Increased availability of prescription opioids has also been identified as a factor contributing to the recent escalation of adolescent opioid abuse. Tormoehlen, Mowry, Bodle, and Rusyniak (2011) noted that increases in adolescent opioid abuse and associated medical complications increased following the 2000 Joint Commission on Accreditation of Healthcare Organizations (JCAHO) pain initiative, which highlighted importance of effective pain management for optimal health care. This initiative had a major influence on clinical practice for pain management and promoted more liberal use of opioid prescriptions, which in turn escalated the volume of prescription opioid medication being dispensed to the general population. Greater access to nonmedical prescription opioids via diversion from friends and relatives was reported by 12th graders participating in the Monitoring the Future (MTF) drug-use survey (Johnston et al., 2016). Indications of nonmedical use of prescription drugs have been detected in 2.3 of 11 million tweets on the popular Twitter platform, reflecting the potential impact of social media on drug-use behavior (Kalyanam, Katsuki, Lanckriet, & Mackey, 2017).

The highest rate of heroin use occurs between 18 and 25 years of age, with use of nonmedical prescription opioids being a strong predictor of future heroin use among adolescents, especially among those who first use between the ages of 10 and 12 (Cerdá, Santaella, Marshall, Kim, & Martins, 2015). Data from the MTF study indicate that the rate of intravenous heroin use remains low at 0.3% among high school seniors, while the rate of nonmedical prescription opioid use has been decreasing over the past 4 years (Johnston et al., 2016). Though promising, adolescents continue to be at risk for early transition to heroin. Onset of opioid use during adolescence is associated with shorter duration from first use to dependence (Clark, Kirisci, & Tarter, 1998). Early initiation of heroin use is associated with a number of adverse life events, including a greater likelihood of dropping out of school, using/sharing needles, criminal behavior and meeting diagnostic criteria for an opioid use disorder. Health risks associated with needle use include Hepatitis C and HIV (Subramaniam, Fishman, & Woody, 2009; Subramaniam & Stitzer, 2009).

Neonatal Abstinence Syndrome

Neonatal abstinence syndrome (NAS) describes a constellation of findings displayed by a newborn as a result of abrupt withdrawal from exposure to opioids due to maternal use. Substantial increases in NAS have occurred over the last decade. Following a threefold increase between 2000 and 2009, incidence continued to rise from 3.4 to 5.8 per 1000 births between 2009 and 2012. In 2012, 21,732 infants were diagnosed in the USA (Patrick, Davis, Lehman, & Cooper, 2015). First described by Dr. Loretta Finnegan in the 1970s, the syndrome is still poorly understood with factors of licit/illicit substance exposure, genetic predisposition and epigenetic modifications that, along with maternal physiology, can lead to significant morbidity (Jansson & Velez, 2012). Manifestation of NAS can be grouped into metabolic findings, such as fever and sweating, gastrointestinal (vomiting, loose watery stools) and central nervous system findings such as tremors, seizures, and increased muscle tone (McQueen & Murphy-Oikonen, 2016). Though an NAS can be produced from a variety of chemical offenders, its association with opioid exposure is common and requires early detection. Urine or meconium drug screens can assist in detecting opioids along with other substances associated with increased severity, such as benzodiazepines. Clinical observation, along with use of severity tools like the Finnegan scoring system, can direct treatment with nonpharmaceutical intervention as the preferable first option. Mothers who have been treated with methadone or buprenorphine as part of medication-assisted treatment can breastfeed, which has shown to reduce the need for pharmaceutical intervention and length of stay in the hospital (Kocherlakota, 2014).

Health consequences of NAS are significant. In the words of Anand and Campbell-Yeo (2015), "After adjusting for confounders, illicit opioid abuse was associated with increased odds of preterm labor, early onset delivery, poor fetal growth, prematurity and stillbirth... Another study found increased odds of maternal death (4.6-fold), cardiac arrest (3.6-fold), intrauterine growth restriction (2.7-fold), placental abruption (2.4-fold), preterm labor (2.1-fold), oligohydramnios (1.7-fold), stillbirth (1.5-fold) and premature rupture of membranes (1.4-fold) associated with illicit opioid abuse. Preterm birth occurred three times more commonly in primiparous mothers hospitalized for opioid abuse (other drugs), and their babies were six times more likely to require NICU admission."

An interaction of genes for opioid drug transport through the placenta, maternal metabolism, and fetal metabolism make NAS a highly variable phenomenon, difficult to predict based on amount or type of opiate ingested during pregnancy, alone. In a large cohort study of Medicaid patients who were pregnant, 23% filled an opiate prescription at some point during their pregnancy (Desai, Hernandez-Diaz, Bateman, & Huybrechts, 2014), suggesting that risk for NAS may occur in as many as one in every four patients. Recent studies have demonstrated that methadone is able to induce the synthesis of opiate transporters in the placenta, thereby increasing fetal exposure to opioid drugs. Because the factors impacting the development of NAS remain obscure, any opioid use during pregnancy should be identified as a potential health risk.

Although the exact mechanism and frequency remains unclear, opioid exposure in utero has been associated with changes in timing of myelination, dendritic growth changes, cortical pyramidal neuron growth and migration, basal ganglia volume, and lifelong behavioral changes including hyperactivity, inattention, ADHD symptoms, and impulsivity (Anand & Campbell-Yeo, 2015; Fodor, Tímár, & Zelena, 2014). In this manner, opioid addicted mothers, who often have had difficulty receiving prenatal care due to their addiction, bring children who as a result of prenatal opioid exposure are predisposed to impulsive decision-making, into an unstable home environment wherein opiates are ubiquitously available, thereby promoting an escalating cycle of opioid-related adverse health outcomes.

Implications

Across the lifespan, illicit opioid use can have a devastating impact on the neurodevelopment of a growing child. In utero exposure to opioids can lead to fetal distress and various pregnancy or birth complications. There is currently controversy over the use of medication-assisted treatment (MAT) in opioid dependent pregnant women. A meta-analysis comparing buprenorphine to methadone, both evidenced based treatments for opioid dependence, noted lower risk of preterm birth with improved birth weight and head circumference among mothers treated with buprenorphine (Zedler et al., 2016). In turn, buprenorphine has been shown to be superior to methadone in the treatment of NAS (Hall et al., 2016). Progressing through childhood, availability of opioids in the household continues to pose a risk. According to one study using data from 1996 to 2012, opioid prescriptions to children and adolescents remained low, 2.68% and 2.91%, respectively. In contrast, opioid prescriptions to family members increased during this time (Groenewald, Rabbitts, Gebert, & Palermo, 2016). Children and adolescents are being exposed to nonmedical prescription opioid through friends and family, putting them at risk of dependence or transition to heroin use. Gaither et al. (2016) observed that the largest increase in hospitalization for opioid poisoning was among 1- to 4-year-old children. The study further commented that opioid poisoning in children older than 10 were primarily associated with suicide attempts. Continued efforts in limiting access to opioids through improved prescribing practices and diversion are a priority. In addition, recognition of risk factors such as poverty, genetic predisposition, and ADHD, has received attention in the literature, as has the use of medication-assisted treatment, which has garnered support among pediatricians (Ryan et al., 2016).

Therapeutic Stimulants

Stimulants are the most frequently prescribed and thoroughly investigated medications for the management of ADHD (e.g., Barkley, 1991; Swanson et al., 2002; Zito et al., 1999), which is most commonly diagnosed and treated during childhood.

Medical use of stimulants has steadily increased in the past 20 years, and use in the USA is much greater than in other countries (Scheffler, Hinshaw, Modrek, & Levine, 2007; Zuvekas, Vitiello, & Norquist, 2006). In 2011, it was estimated that 6.1% of children 4–17 years of age were currently taking medication for ADHD in the USA (Visser et al., 2014). Associated with the rise in therapeutic stimulant use, there is increasing concern about the misuse of stimulants by students and the diversion of prescription stimulants both in college student and patient populations (McCabe, Teter, & Boyd, 2004, 2006a, 2006b; McCabe, Teter, Boyd, & Guthrie, 2004; Upadhyaya et al., 2005; Wilens, Gignac, Swezey, Monuteaux, & Biederman, 2006). Commensurate with this rise in use, emergency department visits associated with nonmedical use of prescription stimulants in the USA have been steadily increasing, with approximately 5000 visits occurring in 2004, increasing to approximately 22,000 visits in 2011 (Substance Abuse and Mental Health Services Administration, Center for Behavioral Health Statistics and Quality, 2013b).

Mechanisms of Action

Most therapeutic stimulants have two overlapping neuropharmacological effects: they inhibit monoamine reuptake and they enhance monoamine neurotransmitter release. Both these actions increase the extracellular concentrations of dopamine and norepinephrine, although magnitude of effect is greater at dopamine sites, particularly those in the dopamine reward pathway (e.g., Solanto, 1998; Volkow et al., 2001). The specific mechanisms by which these effects are produced vary among the different stimulant medications (e.g., Ritalin, Adderall, and Dexedrine). Increased extracellular dopamine and norepinephrine is associated with enhanced wakefulness, alertness, mood, initiative, confidence, concentration, motor activity, and task performance and decreased fatigue.

Epidemiology and Health Consequences of Prenatal, Early Childhood, and Adolescent Stimulant Exposure

While it had long been thought that abuse of prescription stimulant medication was low, recent evidence suggests that prescription stimulant misuse may be a growing problem. In healthy adults, stimulant medications function as potent reinforcers and have a well-established abuse liability (e.g., Henningfield, Johnson, Jasinski, & Bozarth, 1987; Jasinski, Johnson, & Henningfield, 1984; Martin, Sloan, Sapira, & Jasinski, 1971). Nonmedical prescription stimulant use (i.e., diversion of prescription medication) appears to be on the rise. For example, one study found that 61.7% of college students had diverted their ADHD medication at least once (Garnier et al., 2010). Significant numbers of college-aged individuals who have received prescriptions for stimulant medication report misusing their own or other prescription medication (Arria et al., 2008; Upadhyaya, Rose, et al., 2005). Many of those who misuse prescription medication meet the criteria for conduct disorder and substance use disorder (Wilens et al., 2006). Diversion of prescription stimulant medication in college-aged students who initiated treatment in grade school is no greater than that of the general population, but diversion escalates among college-aged students who were first prescribed stimulant medication after completing grade school (McCabe et al., 2006a).

Nonmedical stimulant use is prevalent among adolescents. Poulin (2007) reported that about 26% of junior and senior high school students who were receiving prescribed stimulants had given or sold their medication to others, though another sample including middle- and high-school students found only a 10% diversion rate (Epstein-Ngo et al., 2016). Illicit stimulant medication use among high school students has been linked with the use of other drugs, including tobacco cigarette smoking, heavy episodic drinking, marijuana and cocaine use (McCabe, Boyd, & Teter, 2009; McCabe, Teter, & Boyd, 2004; Poulin, 2007).

While there is risk for the misuse of prescription stimulants, these medications may be protective for other forms of drug abuse. Individuals with ADHD are at a higher risk for developing a substance use problem (Lee, Humphreys, Flory, Liu, & Glass, 2011). Some research, however, has suggested that treatment of ADHD with stimulant medications reduces the risk for substance use disorders (Dalsgaard, Mortensen, Frydenberg, & Thomsen, 2014; Wilens et al., 2008). A recent meta-analysis (Humphreys, Eng, & Lee, 2013) and a topical review (Zulauf, Sprich, Safren, & Wilens, 2014), however, both suggest that treatment of ADHD with a stimulant medication is neither protective nor a risk factor for the development of a substance abuse problem. Due to a lack of consensus on this topic, more research is required to determine what the effect of stimulant medications is on the development of substance use problems among individuals being treated for ADHD.

A recent report found a significant increase in the use of stimulant medications among pregnant women between 1998 (0.2%) and 2013 (1.3%) (Louik, Kerr, Kelley, & Mitchell, 2015). While research on prenatal exposure to stimulant medications in humans is scarce, several studies examining the potential teratogenic effects of nonmedical stimulant use (cocaine and methamphetamine) have been conducted and found growth restrictive effects on the fetus (Bada et al., 2002; Smith et al., 2006). Preclinical studies on stimulant medications indicate that exposure to these drugs during early brain development can cause lasting effects at the cellular level. For example, daily prenatal exposure to dl-amphetamine (0.5 mg/kg/day) induced changes in the biochemistry of the central catecholaminergic system of the adult rat (Nasello, Astrada, & Ramirez, 1974; Nasello & Ramirez, 1978a, 1978b; Ramirez & Carrer, 1983; Ramirez, Carrer, & Nasello, 1979). Nasif, Cuadra, and Ramirez (1999) did not observe any gross teratogenic effects of prenatal exposure to d-amphetamine, but did observe decreased firing rate of norepinephrine neurons in the locus ceruleus in adult rats that had received prenatal exposure to the drug. This preclinical evidence suggests that prenatal exposure to stimulant drugs might produce long-term changes in neuronal cellular function in humans. Consistent with this research, the Food and Drug Administration (FDA) has placed therapeutic stimulants in Category C (i.e., animal reproduction studies have shown an adverse effect on the fetus, or there are no adequate and well-controlled studies in humans, and/or the benefits from the use of the drug in pregnant women may be acceptable despite its potential risks), and as such, these medications should be prescribed to pregnant women only if the benefit justifies the potential risk to the fetus (Berkowitz, Coustan, & Mochizuki, 1998).

Preclinical studies suggest that exposure to stimulant medication during early childhood may have the potential to disrupt the normal sequence of gene expression in the developing brain, resulting in altered neurochemistry and behavior, and that these effects can endure into adulthood (Chase, Carrey, Brown, & Wilkinson, 2005a). Moll, Hause, Ruether, Rothenberger, and Huether (2001), for example, found that methylphenidate exposure in young rats caused a 25% decrease in the density of striatal dopamine transporters, which persisted into adulthood, even after discontinuation of the medication in the prepubertal rat. In a three-part study using adolescent gerbils, Grund et al. (2007) demonstrated that (1) early exposure to methamphetamine resulted in a 30% decrease in dopamine fiber innervations in the prefrontal cortex and amygdala complex; (2) these abnormalities were prevented by methylphenidate administration during adolescence; and (3) methylphenidate alone did not alter dopamine innervation. Researchers have also documented other effects of stimulant medications on gene expression, but the clinical implications remain to be explored (Chase, Carrey, Brown, & Wilkinson, 2005b; Chase, Carrey, Soo, & Wilkinson, 2007; Hawken, Brown, Carrey, & Wilkinson, 2004). Preclinical evidence, however, demonstrates that adolescent exposure to methylphenidate causes persistent neurobehavioral consequences including decreased sensitivity to natural and drug rewards, and long-term modulation of self-control (Adriani, Zoratto, & Laviola, 2011; Marco et al., 2011). Further research is required to determine if these effects are present in humans.

Sensitization (progressively augmented behavioral response following repetitive administration of a drug) and cross-sensitization associated with repeated or chronic stimulant administration have been commonly reported in preclinical studies (Brandon, Marinelli, Baker, & White, 2001; Gaytan, Yang, Swann, & Dafny, 2000; Guerriero, Hayes, Dhaliwal, Ren, & Kosofsky, 2006; Kuczenski & Segal, 2001, 2002; Marco et al., 2011; Torres-Reveron & Dow-Edwards, 2005; Yang, Swann, & Dafny, 2003). Valvassori et al. (2007) demonstrated that early exposure to methylphenidate in adolescent rats resulted in augmented locomotor response after amphetamine challenge as compared to controls, suggesting pretreatment with methylphenidate during adolescence elicited cross-sensitization (the behavioral augmentation that occurs when pretreatment leads to a greater sensitivity to another substance). Methylphenidate and amphetamine have also been shown to increase nicotine administration in rats, suggesting that methylphenidate and amphetamine might engender increased sensitization to the reinforcing effects of nicotine (Santos, Marin, Cruz, DeLucia, & Planeta, 2009; Wooters, Neugebauer, Rush, & Bardo, 2008). Clinical research has, however, failed to find increased rates of tobacco use among adolescents treated with methylphenidate (e.g., Hammerness et al., 2013).

Among children, the most common side effects of therapeutic stimulant use are insomnia, decreased appetite and weight loss, headache, fatigue, abdominal cramps, jitteriness, increase in heart rate and blood pressure, and emotional liability including depression, irritability, and increased frequency of crying. Delirium, psychotic symptoms with vivid hallucinations, and paranoia can be seen with higher doses. Stimulants have peripheral adrenergic effects and increase systolic and diastolic blood pressure and heart rate (Efron, Jarman, & Barker, 1998; Harvanko, Martin, Lile, Kryscio, & Kelly, 2016; Wolraich & Doffing, 2004). Amphetamine abuse is associated with increased risk of hemorrhagic stroke in young adults (Westover, McBride, & Haley, 2007). (Note: FDA requires a warning label on stimulant drugs used to treat ADHD because stimulants cause a rise in blood pressure and heart rate and may increase the risk of heart attack, stroke, or sudden death (Charatan, 2006).)

As mentioned earlier, stimulant medications have a well-documented abuse liability among healthy adults. There is also evidence suggesting that stimulant medications may have abuse liability in children and adolescents. In 1937, Bradley demonstrated that hospitalized children reported positive subjective effects, such as euphoria, following the administration of Benzedrine. Martin, Guenther, Bingcang, Rayens, and Kelly (2007) examined the behavioral effects of methylphenidate (0, 0.25 mg/kg) under randomized, double-blind conditions in 24 children with ADHD between the ages of 11 and 15 years. Methylphenidate increased measures of abuse liability adopted for use in children with ADHD (e.g., modified MBG scale of the Addiction Research Center Inventory). In a pilot study, Fredericks and Kollins (2005) observed that three of the five children and adolescents with ADHD reliably chose methylphenidate over placebo under controlled double-blind conditions, suggesting that the drug functions as a reinforcer under some conditions. In an earlier study, they found that young adults with ADHD chose methylphenidate significantly more frequently than placebo or no capsule (Fredericks & Kollins, 2004). The subjects who chose methylphenidate more reliably exhibited greater methylphenidate-induced reductions in ADHD symptoms, suggesting that the reinforcing effects of the drug may be associated with the drug's therapeutic effect. These results suggest that stimulant medications may have abuse liability in children comparable to that in adults. However, it is important to note that even given these concerns, if used as prescribed, stimulants have a high margin of safety and have been used effectively for decades in treating ADHD (Barkley, 1991; Klein-Schwartz, 2002; Swanson et al., 2002; Weyandt et al., 2014; Zito et al., 1999).

Implications

It is essential that stimulants should be prescribed only for well-documented disorders. For example, if an adolescent presents for the first time with symptoms of ADHD, the diagnosis must be made rigorously with input from the adolescent, as well as confirmation from parents and educators. Standardized and structured testing, including the Conners Rating Scale, can assist in validation of the diagnosis

(Conners, Sitarenios, Parker, & Epstein, 1998). The Achenbach, Connors, Quay behavior (ACQ) check list for parents, teachers, and youth is also useful for confirming the diagnosis of ADHD and can be used to evaluate comorbidities such as conduct disorder (Achenbach, 1991). Self-report measures and urine drug screening may be helpful in assessing whether or not the patient has a comorbid substance use disorder.

In the clinical setting the decision to use stimulants to treat ADHD may be especially challenging for parents when their adolescents are at the age when risk for experimentation with drugs is increasing. Parents are often concerned about whether the medical use of stimulants could increase the risk of future drug use in their children. The medical and scientific community has also raised concerns about ongoing psychostimulant treatment based on compelling preclinical evidence for the development and persistence of behavioral consequences following repeated exposure to psychostimulants, particularly among adolescent animals (for review see Marco et al., 2011), as well as growing numbers of reports of misuse and diversion of prescription stimulants (Benson, Flory, Humphreys, & Lee, 2015; Poulin, 2007; Upadhyaya, Deas, & Brady, 2005a; Wilens et al., 2006). Clinicians who prescribe stimulants (pediatricians, child psychiatrists, family physicians, and neurologists) should inform their patients of the risk of medication diversion. Patients and, if appropriate, their parents should be informed of potential pressures to share or sell stimulant medication. Prescription-monitoring programs should be considered (Sussman, Pentz, Spruijt-Metz, & Miller, 2006), and random urine drug screening could aid in early identification and prevention of prescription misuse and diversion. Likewise, adolescents who are not being treated for ADHD should be warned about the risks of nonmedical use of prescription medication.

Prescription stimulant misuse and diversion is more likely among individuals with ADHD who are not diagnosed or treated until entering high school. Late treatment and undertreatment of ADHD is associated with the emergence of a constellation of high-risk behaviors; drug diversion may be an element of this constellation. It is equally possible that ADHD is not easily diagnosed in some individuals until supplemental symptom clusters or associated comorbidities, such as sensation seeking or conduct disorder, emerge during the developmental process (Martin et al., 2004). It may be that this subgroup of ADHD adolescents who are engaged in a range of problem behaviors, including other drug use and poor school performance, are at increased risk for misuse and diversion of prescription stimulants (McCabe, Teter, & Boyd, 2004; McCabe, Teter, Boyd, & Guthrie, 2004). While stimulants are the first-line treatment for early-onset ADHD, it remains to be seen whether they should be used for late-onset ADHD patients with high-risk behavioral comorbidities. Interestingly, Klein et al. (1997) demonstrated that high-dose stimulants enhanced outcome of ADHD with comorbid conduct disorder, and Biederman, Wilens, Mick, Spencer, and Faraone (1999) observed that drug use did not escalate when ADHD adolescents and young adults with substance abuse disorders were treated with stimulants.

Conclusions

This chapter examines the neurobiological implications of exposure to caffeine, nicotine, alcohol, marijuana, opiates, and therapeutic stimulants, the drugs of abuse that are most frequently encountered during human development. Each of these drugs produces potent neuropharmacological effects on brain function. While it remains difficult to isolate direct causal influences and disentangle the direct effects of drug exposure from indirect effects associated with environmental, social, and cultural influences that are often closely associated with drug exposure, particularly in clinical studies, this chapter provides compelling evidence that developmental exposure to drugs of abuse can have both subtle and dramatic effects with important behavioral and societal consequences. Levels of exposure are substantial during all phases of development (i.e., prenatal, postnatal, childhood, and adolescence), and evidence indicates that exposure to these drugs during critical phases of development have both short-term and long-term consequences. Of critical importance, exposure to psychoactive drugs of abuse during critical periods of development can engender increased sensitivity to the neuropharmacological effects of drugs, which, in turn, leads to increased frequencies of drug use and further changes in sensitivity (e.g., Derauf et al., 2009; Glantz & Chambers, 2006).

References

Achenbach, T. M. (1991). *Integrative guide for the 1991 CBCL 14–18, YSR, and TRF profiles*. Burlington, VT: University of Vermont Department of Psychiatry.

Adriani, W., Spijker, S., Deroche-Gamonet, V., Laviola, G., Le Moal, M., Smit, A. B., & Piazza, P. V. (2003). Evidence for enhanced neurobehavioral vulnerability to nicotine during periadolescence in rats. *Journal of Neuroscience, 23*(11), 4712–4716.

Adriani, W., Zoratto, F., & Laviola, G. (2011). Brain processes in discounting: Consequences of adolescent methylphenidate exposure. In C. Stanford & R. Tannock (Eds.), *Behavioral neuroscience of attention deficit hyperactivity disorder and its treatment* (pp. 113–143). New York, NY: Springer.

Aepli, A., Kurth, S., Tesler, N., & Huber, R. (2015). Caffeine consuming children and adolescents show altered sleep behavior and deep sleep. *Brain Sciences, 5*(4), 441–544.

American Academy of Child & Adolescent Psychiatry. (2014). Marijuana legalization policy statement. Retrieved from https://www.aacap.org/aacap/Policy_Statements/2014/aacap_marijuana_legalization_policy.aspx

American Academy of Pediatrics. (2011). Clinical report–sports drinks and energy drinks for children and adolescents: Are they appropriate? *Pediatrics, 127*(6), 1182–1189.

American Academy of Pediatrics. (2013). Prenatal substance abuse: Short- and long-term effects on the exposed fetus. *Pediatrics, 131*(3), 1009–1024.

American College of Obstetricians and Gynecologists Committee on Obstetric Practice. (2015). Marijuana use during pregnancy and lactation. *Obstetrics & Gynecology, 126*(1), 234–238.

American Psychiatric Association. (2013). *Diagnostic and statistical manual of mental disorders* (5th ed.). Washington, DC: Author.

Anand, K. J., & Campbell-Yeo, M. (2015). Consequences of prenatal opioid use for newborns. *Acta Paediatrica, 104*(11), 1066–1069.

Andersen, S. L., & Navalta, C. P. (2004). Altering the course of neurodevelopment: A framework for understanding the enduring effects of psychotropic drugs. *International Journal of Developmental Neuroscience, 22*(5–6), 423–440.

Anthony, J. C., Warner, L. A., & Kessler, R. C. (1994). Comparative epidemiology of dependence on tobacco, alcohol, controlled substances, and inhalants: Basic findings from the National Comorbidity Survey. *Experimental and Clinical Psychopharmacology, 2*(3), 244–268.

Arbeit, M. L., Nicklas, T. A., Frank, G. C., Webber, L. S., Miner, M. H., & Berenson, G. S. (1988). Caffeine intakes of children from a biracial population: The Bogalusa heart study. *Journal of the American Dietetic Association, 88*(4), 466–471.

Arria, A. M., Caldeira, K. M., O'Grady, K. E., Vincent, K. B., Johnson, E. P., & Wish, E. D. (2008). Nonmedical use of prescription stimulants among college students: Associations with attention-deficit-hyperactivity disorder and polydrug use. *Pharmacotherapy, 28*(2), 156–169.

Bada, H. S., Das, A., Bauer, C. R., Shankaran, S., Lester, B., Wright, L. L., … Maza, P. L. (2002). Gestational cocaine exposure and intrauterine growth: Maternal lifestyle study. *Obstetrics and Gynecology, 100*(5 Pt. 1), 916–924.

Barkley, R. A. (1991). The ecological validity of laboratory and analogue assessment methods of ADHD symptoms. *Journal of Abnormal Child Psychology, 19*(2), 149–178.

Batalla, A., Bhattacharyya, S., Yücel, M., Fusar-Poli, P., Crippa, J. A., Nogué, S., … Martin-Santos, R. (2013). Structural and functional imaging studies in chronic cannabis users: A systematic review of adolescent and adult findings. *PLoS One, 8*(2), e55821.

Bech, B. H., Nohr, E. A., Vaeth, M., Henriksen, T. B., & Olsen, J. (2005). Coffee and fetal death: A cohort study with prospective data. *American Journal of Epidemiology, 162*(10), 983–990.

Benowitz, N. L. (1990). Clinical pharmacology of caffeine. *Annual Review of Medicine, 41*, 277–288.

Benson, K., Flory, K., Humphreys, K. L., & Lee, S. S. (2015). Misuse of stimulant medication among college students: A comprehensive review and meta-analysis. *Clinical Child and Family Psychology Review, 18*(1), 50–76.

Berkowitz, R. L., Coustan, D. R., & Mochizuki, T. K. (1998). *Handbook for prescribing medication during pregnancy*. Philadelphia, PA: Lippincott-Raven.

Bernstein, G. A., Carroll, M. E., Dean, N. W., Crosby, R. D., Perwien, A. R., & Benowitz, N. L. (1998). Caffeine withdrawal in normal school-age children. *Journal of the American Academy of Child and Adolescent Psychiatry, 37*(8), 858–865.

Bertrand, J., Floyd, R. L., Weber, M. K., O'Connor, M. J., Riley, E., Johnson, K. A., … Warren, K. R. (2004). *National Task Force on fetal alcohol syndrome/fetal alcohol effects. Fetal alcohol syndrome: Guidelines for referral and diagnosis. Screening and brief intervention*. Atlanta, GA: Centers for Disease Control and Prevention.

Biederman, J., Wilens, T., Mick, E., Spencer, T., & Faraone, S. V. (1999). Pharmacotherapy of attention-deficit/hyperactivity disorder reduces risk for substance use disorder. *Pediatrics, 104*(2), e20.

Boyd, C. J., Young, A., & McCabe, S. E. (2014). Psychological and drug abuse symptoms associated with nonmedical use of opioid analgesics among adolescents. *Substance Abuse, 35*(3), 284–289.

Bradley, C. (1937). The behavior of children receiving benzedrine. *American Journal of Psychiatry, 94*(3), 577–585.

Brady, J. E., & Li, G. (2014). Trends in alcohol and other drugs detected in fatally injured drivers in the United States, 1999–2010. *American Journal of Epidemiology, 179*(6), 692–699.

Brandon, C. L., Marinelli, M., Baker, L. K., & White, F. J. (2001). Enhanced reactivity and vulnerability to cocaine following methylphenidate treatment in adolescent rats. *Neuropsychopharmacology, 25*(5), 651–661.

Brazier, J. L., Ritter, J., Berland, M., Khenfer, D., & Faucon, G. (1983). Pharmacokinetics of caffeine during and after pregnancy. *Developmental Pharmacology and Therapeutics, 6*(5), 315–322.

Brazier, J. L., & Salle, B. (1981). Conversion of theophylline to caffeine by the human fetus. *Seminars in Perinatology, 5*(4), 315–320.

Briggs, G. G., Freeman, R. K., & Yaffe, S. J. (1998). *Drugs in pregnancy and lactation* (4th ed.). Baltimore, MD: Wilkins & Wilkins.

Brown, Q. L., Sarvet, A. L., Shmulewitz, D., Martins, S. S., Wall, M. M., & Hasin, D. S. (2017). Research letter: Trends in marijuana use among pregnant and nonpregnant reproductive-aged women, 2002–2014. *Journal of the American Medical Association, 317*(2), 207–208.

Brown, S. A., & Tapert, S. F. (2004). Adolescence and the trajectory of alcohol use: Basic to clinical studies. *Annals of the New York Academy of Sciences, 1021*, 234–244.

Cargiulo, T. (2007). Understanding the health impact of alcohol dependence. *American Journal of Health-System Pharmacy, 64*(5, Suppl. 3), S5–S11.

Caspi, A., Moffitt, T. E., Cannon, M., McClay, J., Murray, R., Harrington, H., … Craig, I. W. (2005). Moderation of the effect of adolescent-onset cannabis use on adult psychosis by a functional polymorphism in the catechol-O-methyltransferase gene: Longitudinal evidence of a gene X environment interaction. *Biological Psychiatry, 57*(10), 1117–1127.

Castellanos, F. X., & Rapoport, J. L. (2002). Effects of caffeine on development and behavior in infancy and childhood: A review of the published literature. *Food and Chemical Toxicology, 40*(9), 1235–1242.

Centers for Disease Control and Prevention (CDC). (2013). Alcohol and public health: Alcohol-Related Disease Impact (ARDI) application, 2013. Retrieved from https://nccd.cdc.gov/DPH_ARDI/Default/Report.aspx?T=AAM&P=f6d7eda7-036e-4553-9968-9b17ffad620e&R=d7a9b303-48e9-4440-bf47-070a4827e1fd&M=8E1C5233-5640-4EE8-9247-1ECA7DA325B9&F=AAMCauseGenderUnder21&D=H

Centers for Disease Control and Prevention (CDC). (2015a). Fact sheets – Underage drinking. Retrieved from https://www.cdc.gov/alcohol/fact-sheets/underage-drinking.htm

Centers for Disease Control and Prevention (CDC). (2015b). Fetal alcohol syndrome among children aged 7–9 years – Arizona, Colorado, and New York, 2010. *Morbidity and Mortality Weekly Report, 64*(3), 54–57.

Cerdá, M., Santaella, J., Marshall, B. D., Kim, J. H., & Martins, S. S. (2015). Nonmedical prescription opioid use in childhood and early adolescence predicts transitions to heroin use in young adulthood: A national study. *The Journal of Pediatrics, 167*(3), 605–612.

Chaloupka, F. J., & Johnston, L. D. (2007). Bridging the gap: Research informing practice and policy for healthy youth behavior. *American Journal of Preventive Medicine, 33*(Suppl. 4), S147–S161.

Chambers, R. A., Taylor, J. R., & Potenza, M. N. (2003). Developmental neurocircuitry of motivation in adolescence: A critical period of addiction vulnerability. *American Journal of Psychiatry, 160*(6), 1041–1052.

Champion, H. L., Foley, K. L., DuRant, R. H., Hensberry, R., Altman, D., & Wolfson, M. (2004). Adolescent sexual victimization, use of alcohol and other substances, and other health risk behaviors. *Journal of Adolescent Health, 35*(4), 321–328.

Charatan, F. (2006). FDA committee votes for warning labels on stimulant drugs. *British Medical Journal, 332*(7538), 380.

Charness, M. E., Hu, G., Edwards, R. H., & Querimit, L. A. (1993). Ethanol increases delta-opioid receptor gene expression in neuronal cell lines. *Molecular Pharmacology, 44*(6), 1119–1127.

Chase, T., Carrey, N., Soo, E., & Wilkinson, M. (2007). Methylphenidate regulates activity regulated cytoskeletal associated but not brain-derived neurotrophic factor gene expression in the developing rat striatum. *Neuroscience, 144*(3), 969–984.

Chase, T. D., Carrey, N., Brown, R. E., & Wilkinson, M. (2005a). Methylphenidate regulates c-fos and fosB expression in multiple regions of the immature rat brain. *Brain Research, Developmental Brain Research, 156*(1), 1–12.

Chase, T. D., Carrey, N., Brown, R. E., & Wilkinson, M. (2005b). Methylphenidate differentially regulates c-fos and fosB expression in the developing rat striatum. *Brain Research, Developmental Brain Research, 157*(2), 181–191.

Clark, D. B. (2012). Pharmacotherapy for adolescent alcohol use disorder. *CNS Drugs, 26*(7), 559–569.
Clark, D. B., Kirisci, L., & Tarter, R. E. (1998). Adolescent versus adult onset and the development of substance use disorders in males. *Drug and Alcohol Dependence, 49*(2), 115–121.
Cohn, L. D., Macfarlane, S., Yanez, C., & Imai, W. K. (1995). Risk-perception: Differences between adolescents and adults. *Health Psychology, 14*(3), 217–222.
Colby, S. M., Tiffany, S. T., Shiffman, S., & Niaura, R. S. (2000). Are adolescent smokers dependent on nicotine? A review of the evidence. *Drug and Alcohol Dependence, 59*(Suppl. 1), S83–S95.
Conners, C. K., Sitarenios, G., Parker, J. D., & Epstein, J. N. (1998). The revised Conners' parent rating scale (CPRS-R): Factor structure, reliability, and criterion validity. *Journal of Abnormal Child Psychology, 26*(4), 257–268.
Cornelius, M. D., Leech, S. L., Goldschmidt, L., & Day, N. L. (2000). Prenatal tobacco exposure: Is it a risk factor for early tobacco experimentation? *Nicotine and Tobacco Research, 2*(1), 45–52.
Crews, F., He, J., & Hodge, C. (2007). Adolescent cortical development: A critical period of vulnerability for addiction. *Pharmacology Biochemistry and Behavior, 86*(2), 189–199.
Crews, F. T., Mdzinarishvili, A., Kim, D., He, J., & Nixon, R. (2006). Neurogenesis in adolescent brain is potently inhibited by ethanol. *Neuroscience, 137*(2), 437–445.
Dalsgaard, S., Mortensen, P. B., Frydenberg, M., & Thomsen, P. H. (2014). ADHD, stimulant treatment in childhood and subsequent substance abuse in adulthood a naturalistic long-term follow-up study. *Addictive Behaviors, 39*(1), 325–328.
Daly, J. W., & Fredholm, B. B. (1998). Caffeine – An atypical drug of dependence. *Drug and Alcohol Dependence, 51*(1–2), 199–206.
Day, N. L., Goldschmidt, L., & Thomas, C. A. (2006). Prenatal marijuana exposure contributes to the prediction of marijuana use at age 14. *Addiction, 101*(9), 1313–1322.
Day, N. L., Richardson, G. A., Goldschmidt, L., & Cornelius, M. D. (2000). Effects of prenatal tobacco exposure on preschoolers' behavior. *Journal of Developmental and Behavioral Pediatrics, 21*(3), 180–188.
DeBellis, M. D., Clark, D. B., Beers, S. R., Soloff, P. H., Boring, A. M., Hall, J., … Keshavan, M. S. (2000). Hippocampal volume in adolescent-onset alcohol use disorders. *American Journal of Psychiatry, 158*(5), 820–821.
DeBellis, M. D., Narasimhan, A., Thatcher, D. L., Keshaven, M. S., Soloff, P., & Clark, D. B. (2005). Prefrontal cortex, thalamus, and cerebellar volumes in adolescents and young adults with adolescent-onset alcohol use disorders and comorbid mental disorders. *Alcoholism, Clinical and Experimental Research, 29*(9), 1590–1600.
Deitrich, R. A., Dunwiddie, T. V., Harris, R. A., & Erwin, V. G. (1989). Mechanism of action of ethanol: Initial central nervous system actions. *Pharmacological Reviews, 41*(4), 489–537.
Derauf, C., Kekatpure, M., Neyzi, N., Lester, B., & Kosofsky, B. (2009). Neuroimaging of children following prenatal drug exposure. *Seminars in Cell and Developmental Biology, 20*(4), 441–454.
Desai, R. J., Hernandez-Diaz, S., Bateman, B. T., & Huybrechts, K. F. (2014). Increase in prescription opioid use during pregnancy among medicaid-enrolled women. *Obstetrics and Gynecology, 123*(5), 997–1002.
DiFranza, J. R., Savageau, J. A., Fletcher, K., O'Loughlin, J., Pbert, L., Ockene, J., … Wellman, R. J. (2007). Symptoms of tobacco dependence after brief intermittent use: The development and assessment of nicotine dependence in youth-2 study. *Archives of Pediatric and Adolescent Medicine, 161*(7), 704–710.
Dimitriou, D., Le Cornu Knight, F., & Milton, P. (2015). The role of environmental factors on sleep patterns and school performance in adolescents. *Frontiers in Psychology, 6*, 1717. https://doi.org/10.3389/fpsyg.2015.01717

Dumas, M., Gouyon, J. B., Tenenbaum, D., Michiels, Y., Escousse, A., & Alison, M. (1982). Systematic determination of caffeine plasma concentrations at birth in preterm and full term infants. *Developmental Pharmacology and Therapeutics, 4*(Suppl. 1), 182–186.

Efron, D., Jarman, F. C., & Barker, M. J. (1998). Child and parent perceptions of stimulant medication treatment in attention deficit hyperactivity disorder. *Journal of Paediatrics and Child Health, 34*(3), 288–292.

Elkins, R. N., Rapoport, J. L., Zahn, T. P., Buchsbaum, M. S., Weingartner, H., Kopin, I. J., … Johnson, C. (1981). Acute effects of caffeine in normal prepubertal boys. *American Journal of Psychiatry, 138*(2), 178–183.

Epstein-Ngo, Q. M., McCabe, S. E., Veliz, P. T., Stoddard, S. A., Austic, E. A., & Boyd, C. J. (2016). Diversion of ADHD stimulants and victimization among adolescents. *Journal of Pediatric Psychology, 41*(7), 786–798.

Eskenazi, B., & Castorina, R. (1999). Association of prenatal maternal or postnatal environmental tobacco smoke exposure and neurodevelopmental and behavioral problems in children. *Environmental Health Perspectives, 107*(12), 991–1000.

Ewing, S. W. F., Sakhardande, A., & Blakemore, S. J. (2014). The effect of alcohol consumption on the adolescent brain: A systematic review of MRI and fMRI studies of alcohol-using youth. *NeuroImage: Clinical, 5*, 420–437.

Faden, V. B., & Graubard, B. I. (2000). Maternal substance use during pregnancy and developmental outcome at age three. *Journal of Substance Abuse, 12*(4), 329–340.

Faraday, M. M., Elliott, B. M., Phillips, J. M., & Grunberg, N. E. (2003). Adolescent and adult male rats differ in sensitivity to nicotine's activity effects. *Pharmacology, Biochemistry, and Behavior, 74*(4), 917–931.

Feldman, R. S., Meyer, J. S., & Quenzer, L. F. (1997). *Principles of neuropsychopharmacology*. Sutherland, MA: Sinauer Associates.

Fergusson, D. M., & Boden, J. M. (2008). Cannabis use and later life outcomes. *Addiction, 103*(6), 969–976.

Fergusson, D. M., Horwood, L. J., & Swain-Campbell, N. (2002). Cannabis use and psychosocial adjustment in adolescence and young adulthood. *Addiction, 97*(9), 1123–1135.

Ferre, S., von Euler, G., Johansson, B., Fredholm, B. B., & Fuxe, K. (1991). Stimulation of high-affinity adenosine A2 receptors decreases the affinity of dopamine D2 receptors in rat striatal membranes. *Proceedings of the National Academy of Sciences of the United States of America, 88*(16), 7238–7241.

Ferre, S., Fuxe, K., von Euler, G., Johansson, B., & Fredholm, B. B. (1992). Adenosine-dopamine interactions in the brain. *Neuroscience, 51*(3), 501–512.

Fodor, A., Tímár, J., & Zelena, D. (2014). Behavioral effects of perinatal opioid exposure. *Life Sciences, 104*, 1), 1–1), 8.

Frary, C. D., Johnson, R. K., & Wang, M. Q. (2005). Food sources and intakes of caffeine in the diets of persons in the United States. *Journal of the American Dietetic Association, 105*(1), 110–113.

Fredericks, E. M., & Kollins, S. H. (2004). Assessing methylphenidate preference in ADHD patients using a choice procedure. *Psychopharmacology, 175*(4), 391–398.

Fredericks, E. M., & Kollins, S. H. (2005). A pilot study of methylphenidate preference assessment in children diagnosed with ADHD. *Journal of Child and Adolescent Psychopharmacology, 15*(5), 729–741.

Fredholm, B. B., Bättig, K., Holmén, J., Nehlig, A., & Zvartau, E. E. (1999). Actions of caffeine in the brain with special reference to factors that contribute to its widespread use. *Pharmacological Reviews, 51*(1), 83–133.

Fried, P. A., O'Connell, C. M., & Watkinson, B. (1992). 60- and 72-month follow-up of children prenatally exposed to marijuana, cigarettes, and alcohol: Cognitive and language assessment. *Journal of Developmental and Behavioral Pediatrics, 13*(6), 383–391.

Fried, P. A., & Watkinson, B. (1990). 36- and 48-month neurobehavioral follow-up of children prenatally exposed to marijuana, cigarettes, and alcohol. *Journal of Developmental and Behavioral Pediatrics, 11*(2), 49–58.

Fried, P. A., & Watkinson, B. (2000). Visuoperceptual functioning differs in 9- to 12-year olds prenatally exposed to cigarettes and marihuana. *Neurotoxicology and Teratology, 22*(1), 11–20.
Fried, P. A., & Watkinson, B. (2001). Differential effects on facets of attention in adolescents prenatally exposed to cigarettes and marijuana. *Neurotoxicology and Teratology, 23*(5), 421–430.
Gage, S. H., Munafò, M. R., MacLeod, J., Hickman, M., & Smith, G. D. (2015). Cannabis and psychosis. *The Lancet Psychiatry, 2*(5), 380–381.
Gaither, J. R., Leventhal, J. M., Ryan, S. A., & Camenga, D. R. (2016). National trends in hospitalizations for opioid poisonings among children and adolescents, 1997 to 2012. *Journal of the American Medical Association Pediatrics, 170*(12), 1195–1201.
Galéra, C., Bernard, J. Y., van der Waerden, J., Bouvard, M. P., Lioret, S., Forhan, A., … Heude, B. (2016). Prenatal caffeine exposure and child IQ at age 5.5 years: The EDEN mother-child cohort. *Biological Psychiatry, 80*(9), 720–726.
Galvan, A., Hare, T. A., Parra, C. E., Penn, J., Voss, H., Glover, G., & Casey, B. J. (2006). Earlier development of the accumbens relative to orbitofrontal cortex might underlie risk-taking behavior in adolescents. *Journal of Neuroscience, 26*(25), 6885–6892.
Garland, M. (1998). Pharmacology of drug transfer across the placenta: Substance use in pregnancy. *Obstetrics and Gynecology Clinics of North America, 25*(1), 21–42.
Garnier, L. M., Arria, A. M., Caldeira, K. M., Vincent, K. B., O'Grady, K. E., & Wish, E. D. (2010). Sharing and selling of prescription medications in a college student sample. *The Journal of Clinical Psychiatry, 71*(3), 262–269.
Garrett, B. E., & Griffiths, R. R. (1996). The role of dopamine in the behavioral effects of caffeine in animals and humans. *Pharmacology, Biochemistry and Behavior, 57*(3), 533–541.
Gaytan, O., Yang, P., Swann, A., & Dafny, N. (2000). Diurnal differences in sensitization to methylphenidate. *Brain Research, 864*(1), 24–39.
George, L., Granath, F., Johansson, A. L., Olander, B., & Cnattingius, S. (2006). Risks of repeated miscarriage. *Paediatric and Perinatal Epidemiology, 20*(2), 119–126.
Giannelli, M., Doyle, P., Roman, E., Pelerin, M., & Hermon, C. (2003). The effect of caffeine consumption and nausea on the risk of miscarriage. *Paediatric and Perinatal Epidemiology, 17*(4), 316–323.
Ginzel, K. H., Maritz, G. S., Marks, D. F., Neuberger, M., Pauly, J. R., Polito, J. R., … Slotkin, T. A. (2007). Critical review: Nicotine for the fetus, the infant and the adolescent? *Journal of Health Psychology, 12*(2), 215–224.
Glantz, M. D., & Chambers, J. C. (2006). Prenatal drug exposure effects on subsequent vulnerability to drug abuse. *Development & Psychopathology, 18*(3), 893–922.
Goldschmidt, L., Day, N. L., & Richardson, G. A. (2000). Effects of prenatal marijuana exposure on child behavior problems at age 10. *Neurotoxicology and Teratology, 22*(3), 325–336.
Goodwin, R. D., Beesdo-Baum, K., Martini, J., Knappe, S., Höfler, M., Behrendt, S., … Wittchen, H. U. (2013). Maternal nicotine dependence and prenatal smoking and their association with mental disorders among offspring from the community. *Comprehensive Psychiatry, 54*(1), e4.
Grobin, A. C., Matthews, D. B., Devaud, L. L., & Morrow, A. L. (1998). The role of GABA receptors in the acute and chronic effects of ethanol. *Psychopharmacology, 139*(1–2), 2–19.
Groenewald, C. B., Rabbitts, J. A., Gebert, J. T., & Palermo, T. M. (2016). Trends in opioid prescriptions among children and adolescents in the United States: A nationally representative study from 1996 to 2012. *Pain, 157*(5), 1021–1027.
Grund, T., Teuchert-Noodt, G., Busche, A., Neddens, J., Brummelte, S., Moll, G. H., & Dawirs, R. R. (2007). Administration of oral methylphenidate during adolescence prevents suppressive development of dopamine projections into prefrontal cortex and amygdala after an early pharmacological challenge in gerbils. *Brain Research, 1176*, 124–132.
Guerriero, R. M., Hayes, M. M., Dhaliwal, S. K., Ren, J. Q., & Kosofsky, B. E. (2006). Preadolescent methylphenidate versus cocaine treatment differ in the expression of cocaine-induced locomotor sensitization during adolescence and adulthood. *Biological Psychiatry, 60*(11), 1171–1180.

Hall, E. S., Isemann, B. T., Wexelblatt, S. L., Meinzen-Derr, J., Wiles, J. R., Harvey, S., & Akinbi, H. T. (2016). A cohort comparison of buprenorphine versus methadone treatment for neonatal abstinence syndrome. *The Journal of Pediatrics, 170*, 39–44.
Hall, W., & Degenhardt, L. (2009). Adverse health effects of non-medical cannabis use. *Lancet, 374*(9698), 1383–1391.
Hammerness, P., Joshi, G., Doyle, R., Georgiopoulos, A., Geller, D., Spencer, T., … Biederman, J. (2013). Do stimulants reduce the risk for cigarette smoking in youth with attention-deficit hyperactivity disorder? A prospective, long-term, open-label study of extended-release methylphenidate. *The Journal of Pediatrics, 162*(1), 22–27.
Hartman, R. L., & Huestis, M. A. (2013). Cannabis effects on driving skills. *Clinical Chemistry, 59*(3), 478–492.
Harvanko, A., Martin, C., Lile, J., Kryscio, R., & Kelly, T. H. (2016). Individual differences in the reinforcing and subjective effects of d-amphetamine: Dimensions of impulsivity. *Experimental and Clinical Psychopharmacology, 24*(6), 436–446.
Harvey, M. A., Sellman, J. D., Porter, R. J., & Frampton, C. M. (2007). The relationship between non-acute adolescent cannabis use and cognition. *Drug and Alcohol Review, 26*(3), 309–319.
Hasin, D. S., O'Brien, C. P., Auriacombe, M., Borges, G., Bucholz, K., Budney, A., … Grant, B. F. (2013). DSM-5 criteria for substance use disorders: Recommendations and rationale. *American Journal of Psychiatry, 170*(8), 834–851.
Hawken, C. M., Brown, R. E., Carrey, N., & Wilkinson, M. (2004). Long-term methylphenidate treatment down-regulates c-fos in the striatum of male CD-1 mice. *Neuroreport, 15*(6), 1045–1048.
Hayatbakhsh, M. R., Najman, J. M., Jamrozik, K., Mamun, A. A., Alati, R., & Bor, W. (2007). Cannabis and anxiety and depression in young adults: A large prospective study. *Journal of the American Academy of Child and Adolescent Psychiatry, 46*(3), 408–417.
Hellstrom-Lindahl, E., Seiger, A., Kjaeldgaard, A., & Nordberg, A. (2001). Nicotine-induced alterations in the expression of receptors in primary culture from human prenatal brain. *Neuroscience, 105*(3), 527–534.
Henningfield, J. E., Johnson, R. E., Jasinski, D. R., & Bozarth, M. A. (1987). Clinical procedures for the assessment of abuse potential. In M. A. Bozarth (Ed.), *Methods of assessing the reinforcing properties of abused drugs* (pp. 573–590). New York, NY: Springer-Verlag.
Holford, N., Heo, Y. A., & Anderson, B. (2013). A pharmacokinetic standard for babies and adults. *Journal of Pharmaceutical Sciences, 102*(9), 2941–2952.
Hughes, J. R., & Hale, K. L. (1998). Behavioral effects of caffeine and other methylxanthines on children. *Experimental and Clinical Psychopharmacology, 6*(1), 87–95.
Humphreys, K. L., Eng, T., & Lee, S. S. (2013). Stimulant medication and substance use outcomes: A meta-analysis. *JAMA Psychiatry, 70*(7), 740–749.
Jackson, N. J., Isen, J. D., Khoddam, R., Irons, D., Tuvblad, C., Iacono, W. G., … Baker, L. A. (2016). Impact of adolescent marijuana use on intelligence: Results from two longitudinal twin studies. *Proceedings of the National Academy of Sciences, 113*(5), E500–E508.
Jacobus, J., Castro, N., Squeglia, L. M., Meloy, M. J., Brumback, T., Huestis, M. A., & Tapert, S. F. (2016). Adolescent cortical thickness pre- and post marijuana and alcohol initiation. *Neurotoxicology and Teratology, 57*, 20–29.
Jacobus, J., & Tapert, S. F. (2014). Effects of cannabis on the adolescent brain. *Current Pharmaceutical Design, 20*(13), 2186–2193.
Jager, G., & Ramsey, N. F. (2008). Long-term consequences of adolescent cannabis exposure on the development of cognition, brain structure and function: An overview of animal and human research. *Current Drug Abuse Reviews, 1*(2), 114–123.
James, J. E. (1991). *Caffeine and health*. San Diego, CA: Academic.
Jansson, L. M., & Velez, M. (2012). Neonatal abstinence syndrome. *Current Opinion in Pediatrics, 24*(2), 252–258.
Jasinski, D. R., Johnson, R. E., & Henningfield, J. E. (1984). Abuse liability assessment in human subjects. *Trends in Pharmacological Sciences, 5*, 196–200.

Johnson, B. A., Roache, J. D., Javors, M. A., DiClemente, C. C., Cloninger, C. R., Prihoda, T. J., … Hensler, J. (2000). Ondansetron for reduction of drinking among biologically predisposed alcoholic patients: A randomized controlled trial. *Journal of the American Medical Association, 284*(8), 963–971.

Johnston, L. D., O'Malley, P. M., Miech, R. A., Bachman, J. G., & Schulenberg, J. E. (2016). *Monitoring the future national survey results on drug use, 1975–2015: Overview, key findings on adolescent drug use.* Ann Arbor, MI: Institute for Social Research, The University of Michigan Retrieved from http://monitoringthefuture.org/pubs.html.

Jones, H. E., & Griffiths, R. R. (2003). Oral caffeine maintenance potentiates the reinforcing and stimulant subjective effects of intravenous nicotine in cigarette smokers. *Psychopharmacology, 165*(3), 280–290.

Julien, R. M. (2001). *A primer of drug action* (9th ed.). New York, NY: Worth Publishers.

Kalyanam, J., Katsuki, T., Lanckriet, G. R., & Mackey, T. K. (2017). Exploring trends of nonmedical use of prescription drugs and polydrug abuse in the Twittersphere using unsupervised machine learning. *Addictive Behaviors, 65*, 289–295.

Kandel, D. B., & Chen, K. (2000). Extent of smoking and nicotine dependence in the United States: 1991–1993. *Nicotine and Tobacco Research, 2*(3), 263–274.

Kandel, D. B., Schaffran, C., Griesler, P., Samuolis, J., Davies, M., & Galanti, R. (2005). On the measurement of nicotine dependence in adolescence: Comparisons of the mFTQ and a DSM IV-based scale. *Journal of Pediatric Psychology, 30*(4), 319–332.

Kandel, D. B., Wu, P., & Davies, M. (1994). Maternal smoking during pregnancy and smoking by adolescent daughters. *American Journal of Public Health, 84*(9), 1407–1413.

Kann, L., McManus, T., Harris, W. A., Shanklin, S. L., Flint, K. H., Hawkins, J., … Zaza, S. (2016). Youth risk behavior surveillance — United States, 2015. *Morbidity and Mortality Weekly Reports Surveillance Summaries, 65*(SS-6), 1–174. https://doi.org/10.15585/mmwr.ss6506a1

Kelly, T. H., Robbins, G., Martin, C. A., Fillmore, M. T., Lane, S. D., Harrington, N. G., & Rush, C. R. (2006). Individual differences in drug abuse vulnerability: D-amphetamine and sensation seeking status. *Psychopharmacology, 189*(1), 17–25.

Kessler, D. A., Natanblut, S. L., Wilkenfeld, J. P., Lorraine, C. C., Mayl, S. L., Bernstien, I. B. G., & Thompson, L. (1997). Nicotine addiction: A pediatric disease. *Journal of Pediatrics, 130*(4), 518–524.

Klein, R. G., Abikoff, H., Klass, E., Ganeles, D., Seese, L. M., & Pollack, S. (1997). Clinical efficacy of methylphenidate in conduct disorder with and without attention deficit hyperactivity disorder. *Archives of General Psychiatry, 54*(12), 1073–1080.

Klein-Schwartz, W. (2002). Abuse and toxicity of methylphenidate. *Current Opinion in Pediatrics, 14*(2), 219–223.

Knutti, R., Rothweiler, H., & Schlatter, C. (1982). The effect of pregnancy on the pharmacokinetics of caffeine. *Archives of Toxicology (Supplement), 5*, 187–192 Retrieved from https://www.ncbi.nlm.nih.gov/pubmed/6954898

Kocherlakota, P. (2014). Neonatal abstinence syndrome. *Pediatrics, 134*(2), e547–e561.

Kopstein, A. (2001). *Tobacco use in America: Findings from the 1999 National Household Survey on drug abuse.* (Analytic series: A-15, DHHS Publication No. SMA 02–3622). Rockville, MD: Substance Abuse and Mental Health Services Administration, Office of Applied Studies.

Kota, D., & Martin, B. R. (2007). Nicotine dependence and reward differ between adolescent and adult male mice. *The Journal of Pharmacology and Experimental Therapeutics, 322*(1), 399–401.

Kreek, M. J., & Koob, G. F. (1998). Drug dependence: Stress and dysregulation of reward pathways. *Drug and Alcohol Dependence, 51*(1–2), 23–47.

Kuczenski, R., & Segal, D. S. (2001). Locomotor effects of acute and repeated threshold doses of amphetamine and methylphenidate: Relative roles of dopamine and norepinephrine. *The Journal of Pharmacology and Experimental Therapeutics, 296*(3), 876–883.

Kuczenski, R., & Segal, D. S. (2002). Exposure of adolescent rats to oral methylphenidate: Preferential effects on extracellular norepinephrine and absence of sensitization and cross-sensitization to methamphetamine. *Journal of Neuroscience, 22*(16), 7264–7271.

Lane, S. D., Cherek, D. R., Tcheremissine, O. V., Steinberg, J. L., & Sharon, J. L. (2007). Response perseveration and adaptation in heavy marijuana-smoking adolescents. *Addictive Behaviors, 32*(5), 977–990.

Law, K. L., Stroud, L. R., LaGasse, L. L., Niaura, R., Liu, J., & Lester, B. M. (2003). Smoking during pregnancy and newborn neurobehavior. *Pediatrics, 111*(6 Pt. 1), 1318–1323.

Lee, S. S., Humphreys, K. L., Flory, K., Liu, R., & Glass, K. (2011). Prospective association of childhood attention-deficit/hyperactivity disorder (ADHD) and substance use and abuse/dependence: A meta-analytic review. *Clinical Psychology Review, 31*(3), 328–341.

Leon, M. R. (2000). Effects of caffeine on cognitive, psychomotor, and affective performance of children with attention-deficit/hyperactivity disorder. *Journal of Attention Disorders, 4*(1), 27–47.

Lesch, K. P. (2005). Alcohol dependence and gene x environment interaction in emotion regulation: Is serotonin the link? *European Journal of Pharmacology, 526*(1–3), 113–124.

Levin, E. D., Rezvani, A. H., Montoya, D., Rose, J. E., & Swartzwelder, H. S. (2003). Adolescent-onset nicotine self-administration modeled in female rats. *Psychopharmacology, 169*(2), 141–149.

Leviton, A. (1992). Behavioral correlates of caffeine consumption by children. *Clinical Pediatrics, 31*(12), 742–750.

Leviton, A., & Cowan, L. (2002). A review of the literature relating caffeine consumption by women to their risk of reproductive hazards. *Food and Chemical Toxicology, 40*(9), 1271–1310.

Liu, X., Koren, A. O., Yee, S. K., Pechnick, R. N., Poland, R. E., & London, E. D. (2003). Self-administration of 5-iodo-A-85380, a beta-2 selective nicotinic receptor ligand by operantly trained rats. *Neuroreport, 14*(11), 1503–1150.

Loomans, E. M., Hofland, L., van der Stelt, O., van der Wal, M. F., Koot, H. M., den Bergh BRH, V., & TGM, V. (2012). Caffeine intake during pregnancy and risk of problem behavior in 5- to 6-year-old children. *Pediatrics, 130*(2), e305–e313.

Louik, C., Kerr, S., Kelley, K. E., & Mitchell, A. A. (2015). Increasing use of ADHD medications in pregnancy. *Pharmacoepidemiology and Drug Safety, 24*(2), 218–220.

Lynskey, M. T., & Hall, W. D. (2000). The effects of adolescent cannabis use on educational attainment. *Addiction, 96*(3), 433–443.

Malinauskas, B. M., Aeby, V. G., Overton, R. F., Carpenter-Aeby, T., & Barber-Heidal, K. (2007). A survey of energy drink consumption patterns among college students. *Nutrition Journal, 6*, 35.

Marco, E. M., Adriani, W., Ruocco, L. A., Canese, R., Sadile, A. G., & Laviola, G. (2011). Neurobehavioral adaptations to methylphenidate: The issue of early adolescent exposure. *Neuroscience & Biobehavioral Reviews, 35*(8), 1722–1739.

El Marroun, H., Schmidt, M. N., Franken, I. H. A., Jaddoe, V. W. V., Hofman, A., van der Lugt, A., … White, T. (2013). Prenatal tobacco exposure and brain morphology: A prospective study in young children. *Neuropsychopharmacology, 39*(4), 792–800.

Martin, B. R. (2004). Neurobiology of marijuana. In M. Galanter & H. D. Kleber (Eds.), *Textbook of substance abuse treatment* (pp. 47–54). Washington, DC: American Psychiatric Publishing.

Martin, C. A., Guenther, G., Bingcang, C., Rayens, M. K., & Kelly, T. H. (2007). Measurement of the subjective effects of methylphenidate in 11-to-15 year old children with the attention-deficit/hyperactivity disorder. *Journal of Child and Adolescent Psychopharmacology, 17*(1), 63–73.

Martin, C. A., Kelly, T. H., Rayens, M. K., Brogli, B., Himelreich, K., Brenzel, A., … Omar, H. (2004). Sensation seeking and symptoms of disruptive disorder: Association with nicotine, alcohol and marijuana use in early-and mid-adolescents. *Psychological Reports, 94*(3 Pt. 1), 75–82.

Martin, W. R., Sloan, J. W., Sapira, J. D., & Jasinski, D. R. (1971). Physiologic, subjective, and behavioral effects of amphetamine, methamphetamine, ephedrine, phenmetrazine, and methylphenidate in man. *Clinical Pharmacology and Therapeutics, 12*(2), 245–258.
Maskos, U., Molles, B. E., Pons, S., Besson, M., Guiard, B. P., Guilloux, J. P., … Changeux, J. P. (2005). Nicotine reinforcement and cognition restored by targeted expression of nicotinic receptors. *Nature, 436*(7047), 103–107.
McCabe, S. E., Boyd, C. J., & Teter, C. J. (2009). Subtypes of nonmedical prescription drug misuse. *Drug and Alcohol Dependence, 102*(1), 63–70.
McCabe, S. E., Teter, C. J., & Boyd, C. J. (2004). The use, misuse and diversion of prescription stimulants among middle and high school students. *Substance Use & Misuse, 39*(7), 1095–1116.
McCabe, S. E., Teter, C. J., & Boyd, C. J. (2006a). Medical use, illicit use and diversion of prescription stimulant medication. *Journal of Psychoactive Drugs, 38*(1), 43–56.
McCabe, S. E., Teter, C. J., & Boyd, C. J. (2006b). Medical use, illicit use and diversion of abusable prescription drugs. *Journal of American College Health, 54*(5), 269–278.
McCabe, S. E., Teter, C. J., Boyd, C. J., & Guthrie, S. K. (2004). Prevalence and correlates of illicit methylphenidate use among 8th, 10th, and 12th grade students in the United States, 2001. *Journal of Adolescent Health, 35*(6), 501–504.
McCaffrey, D. F., Pacula, R. L., Han, B., & Ellickson, P. (2010). Marijuana use and high school dropout: The influence of unobservables. *Health Economics, 19*(11), 1281–1299.
McQueen, K., & Murphy-Oikonen, J. (2016). Neonatal abstinence syndrome. *New England Journal of Medicine, 375*(25), 2468–2479.
Medina, K. L., Hanson, K. L., Schweinsburg, A. D., Cohen-Zion, M., Nagel, B. J., & Tapert, S. F. (2007). Neuropsychological functioning in adolescent marijuana users: Subtle deficits detectable after a month of abstinence. *Journal of the International Neuropsychological Society, 13*(5), 807–820.
Meier, M. H., Caspi, A., Ambler, A., Harrington, H., Houts, R., Keefe, R. S., … Moffitt, T. E. (2012). Persistent cannabis users show neuropsychological decline from childhood to midlife. *Proceedings of the National Academy of Sciences, 109*(40), e2657–e2664.
Meyer, J. S., & Quenzer, L. F. (2005). *Psychopharmacology: Drugs, the brain, and behavior.* Sunderland, MA: Sinauer Associates.
Moll, G. H., Hause, S., Ruether, E., Rothenberger, A., & Huether, G. (2001). Early methylphenidate administration to young rats causes a persistent reduction in the density of striatal dopamine transporters. *Journal of Child and Adolescent Psychopharmacology, 11*(1), 15–24.
Moore, T. H., Zammit, S., Lingford-Hughes, A., Barnes, T. R., Jones, P. B., Burke, M., & Lewis, G. (2007). Cannabis use and risk of psychotic or affective mental health outcomes: A systematic review. *Lancet, 370*(9584), 319–328.
Morgan, K. J., Stults, V. J., & Zabik, M. E. (1982). Amount and dietary sources of caffeine and saccharin intake by individuals ages 5 to 18 years. *Regulatory Toxicology and Pharmacology, 2*(4), 296–307.
Muneoka, K., Ogawa, T., Kamei, K., Mimura, Y., Kato, H., & Takigawa, M. (2001). Nicotine exposure during pregnancy is a factor which influences serotonin transporter density in the rat brain. *European Journal of Pharmacology, 411*(3), 279–282.
Myllynen, P., Pasanen, M., & Pelkonen, O. (2005). Human placenta: A human organ for developmental toxicology research and biomonitoring. *Placenta, 26*(5), 361–371.
Nagel, B. J., Schweinsburg, A. D., Phan, V., & Tapert, S. F. (2005). Reduced hippocampal volume among adolescents with alcohol use disorders without psychiatric comorbidity. *Psychiatry Research, 139*(3), 181–190.
Nasello, A. G., Astrada, A. C., & Ramirez, O. A. (1974). Effects on the acquisition of conditioned avoidance responses and seizure threshold in the offspring of amphetamine treated gravid rats. *Psychopharmacology, 40*(1), 25–31.
Nasello, A. G., & Ramirez, O. A. (1978a). Open field and Lashley III maze behavior of the offspring of amphetamine treated rats. *Psychopharmacology, 58*(2), 171–173.

Nasello, A. G., & Ramirez, O. A. (1978b). Brain catecholamines metabolism in the offspring of amphetamine treated rats. *Pharmacology, Biochemistry and Behavior, 9*(1), 17–20.

Nasif, F. J., Cuadra, G. R., & Ramirez, O. A. (1999). Permanent alteration of central noradrenergic system by prenatally administered amphetamine. *Developmental Brain Research, 112*(2), 181–188.

National Institute on Alcohol Abuse and Alcoholism. (2004–2005). Alcohol and development in youth – A multidisciplinary overview. *Alcohol Research & Health, 28*(3), 107–108.

National Institute on Alcohol Abuse and Alcoholism. (2015). Women and alcohol. Retrieved from https://pubs.niaaa.nih.gov/publications/womensfact/womensfact.htm

National Institute on Drug Abuse (NIDA). (2017). Marijuana. Retrieved from https://www.drugabuse.gov/publications/drugfacts/marijuana

Nestler, E. J. (2012). Transcriptional mechanisms of drug addiction. *Clinical Psychopharmacology and Neuroscience, 10*(3), 136–143.

Ng, M., Freeman, M. K., Fleming, T. D., Robinson, M., Dwyer-Lindgren, L., Thomson, B., … Gakidou, E. (2014). Smoking prevalence and cigarette consumption in 187 countries, 1980–2012. *The Journal of the American Medical Association, 311*(2), 183–192.

Nichter, M., Nichter, M., Thompson, P. J., Shiffman, S., & Moscicki, A. B. (2002). Using qualitative research to inform survey development on nicotine dependence among adolescents. *Drug and Alcohol Dependence, 68*(Suppl. 1), S41–S56.

Niemelä, S., Räisänen, A., Koskela, J., Taanila, A., Miettunen, J., Ramsay, H., & Veijola, J. (2017). The effect of prenatal smoking exposure on daily smoking among teenage offspring. *Addiction, 112*(1), 134–143.

Nigg, J. T. (2017). Annual research review: On the relations among self-regulation, self-control, executive functioning, effortful control, cognitive control, impulsivity, risk-taking, and inhibition for developmental psychopathology. *Journal of Child Psychology and Psychiatry, and Allied Disciplines, 58*(4), 361–383.

O'Loughlin, J., DiFranza, J., Tyndale, R. F., Meshefedjian, G., McMillan-Davey, E., Clarke, P. B., … Paradis, G. (2003). Nicotine-dependence symptoms are associated with smoking frequency in adolescents. *American Journal of Preventive Medicine, 25*(3), 219–225.

Oh, S., Reingle Gonzalez, J. M., Salas-Wright, C. P., Vaughn, M. G., & DiNitto, D. M. (2017). Prevalence and correlates of alcohol and tobacco use among pregnant women in the United States: Evidence from the NSDUH 2005–2014. *Preventative Medicine, 97*, 93–99.

Okoli, C. T. C., Kelly, T. H., & Hahn, E. L. (2007). Secondhand smoke and nicotine exposure: A brief review. *Addictive Behaviors, 32*(10), 1977–1988.

Orbeta, R. L., Overpeck, M. D., Ramcharran, D., Kogan, M. D., & Ledsky, R. (2006). High caffeine intake in adolescents: Associations with difficulty sleeping and feeling tired in the morning. *Journal of Adolescent Health, 38*(4), 451–453.

Ostrea, E. M., Mantaring, J. B., III, & Silvestre, M. A. (2004). Drugs that affect the fetus and newborn infant via the placenta or breast milk. *Pediatric Clinics of North America, 51*(3), 539–579.

Parsons, W. D., & Neims, A. H. (1981). Prolonged half-life of caffeine in healthy term newborn infants. *Journal of Pediatrics, 98*(4), 640–641.

Patrick, S. W., Davis, M. M., Lehman, C. U., & Cooper, W. O. (2015). Increasing incidence and geographic distribution of neonatal abstinence syndrome: United States 2009–2012. *Journal of Perinatology, 35*(8), 650–655.

Pattinson, K. T. S. (2008). Opioids and the control of respiration. *British Journal of Anaesthesia, 100*(6), 747–758.

Picciotto, M. R., & Corrigall, W. A. (2002). Neuronal systems underlying behaviors related to nicotine addiction: Neural circuits and molecular genetics. *Journal of Neuroscience, 22*(9), 3338–3341.

Picciotto, M. R., Zoli, M., & Changeux, J. P. (1999). Use of knock-out mice to determine the molecular basics for the actions of nicotine. *Nicotine and Tobacco Research, 1*(Suppl. 2), S121–S125.

Pidoplichko, V. I., Noguchi, J., Areola, O. O., Liang, Y., Peterson, J., Zhang, T., & Dani, J. A. (2004). Nicotinic cholinergic synaptic mechanisms in the ventral tegmental area contribute to nicotine addiction. *Learning and Memory, 11*(1), 60–69.

Pirie, P. L., Lando, H., Curry, S. J., McBride, C., & Grothaus, L. C. (2000). Tobacco, alcohol, and caffeine use and cessation in early pregnancy. *American Journal of Preventive Medicine, 18*(1), 54–61.

Pollak, C. P., & Bright, D. (2003). Caffeine consumption and weekly sleep patterns in US seventh-, eighth-, and ninth-graders. *Pediatrics, 111*(1), 42–46.

Polak, K., Dillon, P., Koch, J. R., Miller, W. G., Jr., Thacker, L., & Svikis, D. (2016). Energy drink use is associated with alcohol and substance use in eighth, tenth, and twelfth graders. *Preventive Medicine Reports, 4*, 381–384.

Pope Jr HG, & Bright, D. (2003). Caffeine consumption and weekly sleep patterns in US seventh-, eighth-, and ninth-graders. Pediatrics, 111(1), 42–46.

Pope, H. G., Jr., & Yurgelun-Todd, D. (1996). The residual cognitive effects of heavy marijuana use in college students. *Journal of the American Medical Association., 275*(7), 521–527.

Pope, H. G., Jr., Gruber, A. J., Hudson, J. I., Huestis, M. A., & Yurgelun-Todd, D. (2003). Early-onset cannabis use and cognitive deficits: What is the nature of the association? *Drug and Alcohol Dependence, 69*(3), 303–310.

Poulin, C. (2007). From attention-deficit/hyperactivity disorder to medical stimulant use to diversion of prescribed stimulants to non-medical stimulant use: Connecting the dots. *Addiction, 102*(5), 740–752.

Ramirez, O. A., & Carrer, H. F. (1983). Noradrenergic modulation of neural transmission in the offspring of amphetamine treated rats. *Canadian Journal of Physiology and Pharmacology, 61*(7), 766–769.

Ramirez, O. A., Carrer, H. F., & Nasello, A. G. (1979). Prenatal amphetamine exposure: Ovulation, sexual behavior and hypothalamic monoamine. *Pharmacology, Biochemistry and Behavior, 11*(6), 605–609.

Ramo, D. E., Young-Wolff, K. C., & Prochaska, J. J. (2015). Prevalence and correlates of electronic-cigarette use in young adults: Findings from three studies over five years. *Addictive Behaviors, 41*, 142–147.

Rapoport, J. L., Berg, C. J., Ismond, D. R., Zahn, T. P., & Neims, A. (1984). Behavioral effects of caffeine in children. Relationship between dietary choice and effects of caffeine challenge. *Archives of General Psychiatry, 41*(11), 1073–1079.

Rapoport, J. L., Elkins, R., Neims, A., Zahn, T., & Berg, C. J. (1981). Behavioral and autonomic effects of caffeine in normal boys. *Developmental Pharmacology and Therapeutics, 3*(2), 74–82.

Rasch, V. (2003). Cigarette, alcohol, and caffeine consumption: Risk factors for spontaneous abortion. *Acta Obstetricia et Gynecologica Scandinavica, 82*(2), 182–188.

Richards, G., & Smith, A. (2015). Caffeine consumption and self-assessed stress, anxiety, and depression in secondary school children. *Journal of Psychopharmacology, 29*(12), 1236–1247.

Richardson, S. A., & Tizabi, Y. (1994). Hyperactivity in the offspring of nicotine-treated rats: Role of the mesolimbic and nigrostriatal pathways. *Pharmacology, Biochemistry and Behavior, 47*(2), 331–337.

Rubino, T., Zamberletti, E., & Parolaro, D. (2012). Adolescent exposure to cannabis as a risk factor for psychiatric disorders. *Journal of Psychopharmacology, 26*(1), 177–188.

Rudd, R. A., Aleshire, N., Zibbell, J. E., & Matthew Gladden, R. (2016). Increases in drug and opioid overdose deaths—United States, 2000–2014. *American Journal of Transplantation, 16*(4), 1323–1327.

Ryan, S. A., Gonzalez, P. K., Patrick, S. W., Quigley, J., Siqueira, L., & Walker, L. R. (2016). Medication-assisted treatment of adolescents with opioid use disorders. *Pediatrics, 138*(3), e20161893.

Salminen, O., Murphy, K. L., McIntosh, J. M., Drago, J., Marks, M. J., Collins, A. X., & Grady, S. R. (2004). Subunit composition and pharmacology of two classes of striatal presynaptic nic-

otinic acetylcholine receptors mediating dopamine release in mice. *Molecular Pharmacology, 65*(6), 1526–1535.
Santos, G. C., Marin, M. T., Cruz, F. C., DeLucia, R., & Planeta, C. S. (2009). Amphetamine- and nicotine-induced cross-sensitization in adolescent rats persists until adulthood. *Addiction Biology, 14*(3), 270–275.
Savitz, D. A., Chan, R. L., Herring, A. H., Howards, P. P., & Hartmann, K. E. (2008). Caffeine and miscarriage risk. *Epidemiology, 19*(1), 55–62.
Scheffler, R. M., Hinshaw, S. P., Modrek, S., & Levine, P. (2007). The global market for ADHD medications. *Health Affairs, 26*(2), 450–457.
Schneider, M. (2008). Puberty as a highly vulnerable developmental period for the consequences of cannabis exposure. *Addiction Biology, 13*(2), 253–263.
Schuckit, M. A., & Smith, T. L. (2004). Changes over time in the self-reported level of response to alcohol. *Alcohol and Alcoholism, 39*(5), 433–438.
Seifert, S. M., Schaechter, J. L., Hershorin, E. R., & Lipshultz, S. E. (2011). Health effects of energy drinks on children, adolescents, and young adults. *Pediatrics, 127*(3), 511–528.
Shapiro, G. K., & Buckley-Hunter, L. (2010). What every adolescent needs to know: Cannabis can cause psychosis. *Journal of Psychosomatic Research, 69*(6), 533–539.
Sharma, B., Bruner, A., Barnett, G., & Fishman, M. (2016). Opioid use disorders. *Child and Adolescent Psychiatric Clinics of North America, 25*(3), 473–487.
Sher, L. (2006). Functional magnetic resonance imaging studies of neurocognitve effects of alcohol use on adolescents and young adults. *International Journal of Adolescent Medicine and Health, 18*(1), 3–7.
Silins, E., Horwood, L. J., Patton, G. C., Fergusson, D. M., Olsson, C. A., Hutchinson, D. M., & Mattick, R. P. (2014). Young adult sequelae of adolescent cannabis use: An integrative analysis. *Lancet Psychiatry, 1*(4), 286–293.
Silveri, M. M. (2014). GABAergic contributions to alcohol responsivity during adolescence: Insights from preclinical and clinical studies. *Pharmacology & Therapeutics, 143*(2), 197–216.
Simantov, E., Schoen, C., & Klein, J. D. (2000). Health-compromising behaviors: Why do adolescents smoke or drink? Identifying underlying risk and protective factors. *Archives of Pediatrics & Adolescent Medicine, 154*(10), 1025–1033.
Slotkin, T. A. (2002). Nicotine and the adolescent brain: Insights from an animal model. *Neurotoxicology and Teratology, 24*(3), 369–384.
Slotkin, T. A., Pinkerton, K. E., Auman, J. T., Qiaio, D., & Seidler, F. J. (2002). Perinatal exposure to environmental tobacco smoke upregulates nicotinic cholinergic receptors in monkey brain. *Brain Research, Developmental Brain Research, 133*(2), 175–179.
Smith, L. M., LaGasse, L. L., Derauf, C., Grant, P., Shah, R., Arria, A., … Lester, B. M. (2006). The infant development, environment, and lifestyle study: Effects of prenatal methamphetamine exposure, polydrug exposure, and poverty on intrauterine growth. *Pediatrics, 118*(3), 1149–1156.
Sojar, S. H., Shreir, L. A., Ziemnik, R. E., Sherritt, L., Spalding, A. L., & Levy, S. (2015). Symptoms attributed to consumption of caffeinated beverages in adolescents. *Journal of Caffeine Research, 5*(4), 187–191.
Sokol, R. J., Delaney-Black, V., & Nordstrom, B. (2003). Fetal alcohol syndrome disorder. *Journal of the American Medical Association, 290*(22), 2996–2999.
Solanto, M. V. (1998). Neuropsychopharmacological mechanisms of stimulant drug action in attention-deficit hyperactivity disorder: A review and integration. *Behavioural Brain Research, 94*(1), 127–152.
Solowij, N., Jones, K. A., Rozman, M. E., Davis, S. M., Ciarrochi, J., Heaven, P. C., … Yücel, M. (2011). Verbal learning and memory in adolescent cannabis users, alcohol users and non-users. *Psychopharmacology, 216*(1), 131–144.
Song, M., Wang, X. Y., Zhao, M., Wang, X. Y., Zhai, H. F., & Lu, L. (2007). Role of stress in acquisition of alcohol-conditioned place preference in adolescent and adult mice. *Alcoholism, Clinical and Experimental Research, 31*(12), 2001–2005.

Sood, B., Delaney-Black, V., Covington, C., Nordstrom-Klee, B., Ager, J., Templin, T., … Sokol, R. J. (2001). Prenatal alcohol exposure and childhood behavior at age 6 and 7. *Pediatrics, 108*(2), e34.
Spear, L. P. (2002). The adolescent brain and the college drinker: Biological basis of propensity to use and misuse alcohol. *Journal of Studies on Alcohol, 14*(Suppl), 71–81.
Spear, L. P. (2004). Adolescence and the trajectory of alcohol use: Introduction to part VI. *Annals of the New York Academy of Sciences, 1021*, 202–205.
Spear, N. E., & Molina, J. C. (2005). Fetal or infantile exposure to ethanol promotes ethanol ingestion in adolescence and adulthood: A theoretical review. *Alcoholism, Clinical and Experimental Research, 29*(6), 909–929.
Squeglia, L. M., Jacobus, J., & Tapert, S. F. (2014). The effect of alcohol use on human adolescent brain structures and systems. *Handbook of Clinical Neurology, 125*, 501–510.
Stein, M. A., Krasowski, M., Leventhal, B. L., Phillips, W., & Bender, B. G. (1996). Behavioral and cognitive effects of methylxanthines. A meta-analysis of theophylline and caffeine. *Archives of Pediatric and Adolescent Medicine, 150*(3), 284–288.
Steinberg, L. (2010). A dual systems model of adolescent risk-taking. *Developmental Psychobiology, 52*(3), 216–224.
Stoops, W. W., Lile, J. A., Robbins, C. G., Martin, C. A., Rush, C. R., & Kelly, T. H. (2007). The reinforcing, subject-rated, performance, and cardiovascular effects of d-amphetamine: Influence of sensation-seeking status. *Addictive Behaviors, 32*(6), 1177–1188.
Story, M., & Neumark-Sztainer, D. (1998). Diet and adolescent behavior: Is there a relationship. *Adolescent Medicine, 9*(2), 283–298.
Subramaniam, G. A., Fishman, M. J., & Woody, G. (2009). Treatment of opioid-dependent adolescents and young adults with buprenorphine. *Current Psychiatry Reports, 11*(5), 360–363.
Subramaniam, G. A., & Stitzer, M. A. (2009). Clinical characteristics of treatment-seeking prescription opioid vs. heroin-using adolescents with opioid use disorder. *Drug and Alcohol Dependence, 101*(1), 13–19.
Substance Abuse and Mental Health Services Administration, Center for Behavioral Health Statistics and Quality. (2013a). *The DAWN report: Update on emergency department visits involving energy drinks: A continuing public health concern*. Rockville, MD: Substance Abuse and Mental Health Services Administration, Center for Behavioral Health Statistics and Quality Retrieved from http://archive.samhsa.gov/data/2k13/DAWN126/sr126-energy-drinks-use.htm
Substance Abuse and Mental Health Services Administration, Center for Behavioral Health Statistics and Quality. (2013b). *Drug abuse warning network, 2011: National Estimates of drug-related emergency department visits*. Rockville, MD: Substance Abuse and Mental Health Services Administration, Center for Behavioral Health Statistics and Quality Retrieved from https://www.samhsa.gov/data/sites/default/files/DAWN2k11ED/DAWN2k11ED/DAWN2k11ED.pdf.
Sussman, S., Pentz, M. A., Spruijt-Metz, D., & Miller, T. (2006). Misuse of "study drugs": Prevalence, consequences, and implications for policy. *Substance Abuse Treatment, Prevention and Policy, 1*, 15.
Suter, M. A., Mastrobattista, J., Sachs, M., & Aagaard, K. (2015). Is there evidence for potential harm of electronic cigarette use in pregnancy? *Birth Defects Research Part A: Clinical and Molecular Teratology, 103*(3), 186–195.
Swanson, J. M., Gupta, S., Williams, L., Agler, D., Lerner, M., & Wigal, S. (2002). Efficacy of a new pattern of methylphenidate for the treatment of ADHD: Effects on activity level in the classroom and on the playground. *Journal of the American Academy of Child and Adolescent Psychiatry, 41*(11), 1306–1314.
Swanson, J. M., Lerner, M., Wigal, T., Steinhoff, K., Greenhill, L., Posner, K., … Wigal, S. (2002). The use of a laboratory school protocol to evaluate concepts about efficacy and side effects of new formulations of stimulant medications. *Journal of Attention Disorders, 6*(Suppl. 1), S73–S88.

Swartzwelder, H. S., Wilson, W. A., & Tayyeb, M. I. (1995). Age-dependent inhibition of long-term potentiation by ethanol in immature versus mature hippocampus. *Alcoholism, Clinical and Experimental Research, 19*(6), 1480–1485.

Tapert, S. F., Granholm, E., Leedy, N. G., & Brown, S. A. (2002). Substance use and withdrawal: Neuropsychological functioning over 8 years in youth. *Journal of the International Neuropsychological Society, 8*(7), 873–883.

Tapper, A. E., McKinney, S. L., Nashmi, R., Schwarz, J., Deshpande, P., Labarca, C., … Lester, H. A. (2004). Nicotine activation of alpha4* receptors: Sufficient for reward, tolerance, and sensitization. *Science, 306*(5698), 1029–1032.

Tau, G. Z., & Peterson, B. S. (2010). Normal development of brain circuits. *Neuropsychopharmacology, 35*(1), 147–168.

Tennant, F. S., & Detels, R. (1976). Relationship of alcohol, cigarette, and drug abuse in adulthood with alcohol, cigarette and coffee consumption in childhood. *Preventive Medicine, 5*(1), 70–77.

Tormoehlen, L. M., Mowry, J. B., Bodle, J. D., & Rusyniak, D. E. (2011). Increased adolescent opioid use and complications reported to a poison control center following the 2000 JCAHO pain initiative. *Clinical Toxicology, 49*(6), 492–498.

Toro, R., Leonard, G., Lerner, J. V., Lerner, R. M., Perron, M., Pike, G. B., … Paus, T. (2008). Prenatal exposure to maternal cigarette smoking and the adolescent cerebral cortex. *Neuropsychopharmacology, 33*(5), 1019–1027.

Torres-Reveron, A., & Dow-Edwards, D. L. (2005). Repeated administration of methylphenidate in young, adolescent and mature rat affects the response to cocaine later in adulthood. *Psychopharmacology, 181*(1), 38–47.

Trauth, J. A., McCook, E. C., Seidler, F. J., & Slotkin, T. A. (2000). Modeling adolescent nicotine exposure: Effects on cholinergic systems in rat brain regions. *Brain Research, 873*(1), 18–25.

Trauth, J. A., Seidler, F. J., & Slotkin, T. A. (2000). Persistent and delayed behavioral changes after nicotine treatment in adolescent rats. *Brain Research, 880*(1–2), 167–172.

Treit, S., Lebel, C., Baugh, L., Rasmussen, C., Andrew, G., & Beaulieu, C. (2013). Longitudinal MRI reveals altered trajectory of brain development during childhood and adolescence in fetal alcohol spectrum disorders. *Journal of Neuroscience, 33*(24), 10098–10109.

Tsai, G. E., Ragan, P., Chang, R., Chen, S., Linnoila, M. I., & Coyle, J. T. (1998). Increased glutamatergic neurotransmission and oxidative stress after alcohol withdrawal. *American Journal of Psychiatry, 155*(6), 726–732.

U.S. Department of Health and Human Services. (2014). *The health consequences of smoking—50 years of progress: A report of the surgeon general.* Atlanta, GA: U.S. Department of Health and Human Services, Centers for Disease Control and Prevention, National Center for Chronic Disease Prevention and Health Promotion Office on Smoking and Health Retrieved from https://www.cdc.gov/tobacco/data_statistics/fact_sheets/fast_facts/

Upadhyaya, H. P., Deas, D., & Brady, K. (2005). A practical clinic approach to the treatment of nicotine dependence in adolescents. *Clinical Perspectives, 44*(9), 942–946.

Upadhyaya, H. P., Deas, D., Brady, K. T., & Kruesi, M. (2002). Cigarette smoking and psychiatric comorbidity in children and adolescents. *Journal of the American Academy of Child and Adolescent Psychiatry, 41*(11), 1294–1305.

Upadhyaya, H. P., Rose, K., Wang, W., O'Rourke, K., Sullivan, B., Deas, D., & Brady, K. T. (2005). Attention-deficit/hyperactivity disorder, medication treatment, and substance use patterns among adolescents and young adults. *Journal of Child and Adolescent Psychopharmacology, 15*(5), 799–809.

Valek, M., Laslavić, B., & Laslavić, Z. (2004). Daily caffeine intake among Osijek high school students: Questionnaire study. *Croatian Medical Journal, 45*(1), 72–75.

Valvassori, S. S., Frey, B. N., Martins, M. R., Reus, G. Z., Schimidtz, F., Inacio, C. G., … Quevedo, J. (2007). Sensitization and cross-sensitization after chronic treatment with methylphenidate in adolescent Wistar rats. *Behavioural Pharmacology, 18*(3), 205–212.

Verheul, R., van den Brink, W., & Geerlings, P. (1999). A three-pathway psychobiological model of craving for alcohol. *Alcohol and Alcoholism, 34*(2), 197–222.

Vermeiren, R., Schwab-Stone, M., Deboutte, D., Leckman, P. E., & Ruchkin, V. (2003). Violence exposure and substance use in adolescents: Findings from three countries. *Pediatrics, 111*(3), 535–540.

Visser, S. N., Danielson, M. L., Bitsko, R. H., Holbrook, J. R., Kogan, M. D., Ghandour, R. M., & Blumber, S. J. (2014). Trends in the parent-report of health care provider-diagnosed and medicated attention-deficit/hyperactivity disorder: United States, 2003–2011. *Journal of the American Academy of Child and Adolescent Psychiatry, 53*(1), 34–46.

Volkow, N. D., Wang, G., Fowler, J. S., Logan, J., Gerasimov, M., Maynard, L., … Franceschi, D. (2001). Therapeutic doses of oral methylphenidate significantly increase extracellular dopamine in the human brain. *The Journal of Neuroscience, 21*(RC121), 1–5.

Wafford, K. A., Burnett, D., Harris, R. A., & Whiting, P. J. (1993). $GABA_A$ receptor subunit expression and sensitivity to ethanol. *Alcohol and Alcoholism (Supplement), 2*, 327–330 Retrieved from https://www.ncbi.nlm.nih.gov/pubmed/7748319

Wakschlag, L. S., Leventhal, B. L., Pine, D. S., Pickett, K. E., & Carter, A. S. (2006). Elucidating early mechanisms of developmental psychopathology: The case of prenatal smoking and disruptive behavior. *Child Development, 77*(4), 893–906.

Walsh, R. A., Redman, S., & Adamson, L. (1996). The accuracy of self-report of smoking status in pregnant women. *Addictive Behaviors, 21*(5), 675–679.

Wang, G. S., Roosevelt, G., Le Lait, M. C., Martinez, E. M., Bucher-Bartelson, B., Bronstein, A. C., & Heard, K. (2014). Association of unintentional pediatric exposures with decriminalization of marijuana in the United States. *Annals of Emergency Medicine, 63*(6), 684–689.

Warzack, W. J., Evans, S., Floress, M. T., Gross, A. C., & Stoolman, S. (2011). Caffeine consumption in young children. *Journal of Pediatrics, 158*(3), 508–509.

Weinberg, B. A., & Bealer, B. K. (2001). *The world of caffeine*. New York, NY: Routledge.

Westover, A. N., McBride, S., & Haley, R. W. (2007). Stroke in young adults who abuse amphetamines or cocaine. *Archives of General Psychiatry, 64*(4), 495–502.

Weyandt, L. L., Oster, D. R., Marraccini, M. E., Gudmundsdottir, B. G., Munro, B. A., Zavras, B. M., & Kuhar, B. (2014). Pharmacological interventions for adolescents and adults with ADHD: Stimulant and nonstimulant medications and misuse of prescription stimulants. *Psychological Research and Behavioral Management, 7*, 223–249.

Wilens, T. E., Adamson, J., Monuteaux, M. C., Faraone, S. V., Schillinger, M., Westerberg, D., & Biederman, J. (2008). Effect of prior stimulant treatment for attention-deficit/hyperactivity disorder on subsequent risk for cigarette smoking and alcohol and drug use disorders in adolescents. *Archives of Pediatrics & Adolescent Medicine, 162*(10), 916–921.

Wilens, T. E., Gignac, M., Swezey, A., Monuteaux, M. C., & Biederman, J. (2006). Characteristics of adolescents and young adults with ADHD who divert or misuses their prescribed medications. *Journal of the American Academy of Child and Adolescent Psychiatry, 45*(4), 408–414.

Wolraich, M. L., & Doffing, M. A. (2004). Pharmacokinetic considerations in the treatment of attention-deficit hyperactivity disorder with methylphenidate. *CNS Drugs, 18*(4), 243–250.

Wooters, T. E., Neugebauer, N. M., Rush, C. R., & Bardo, M. T. (2008). Methylphenidate enhances the abuse-related behavioral effects of nicotine in rats: Intravenous self-administration, drug discrimination, and locomotor cross-sensitization. *Neuropsychopharmacology, 33*(5), 1137–1148.

Xu, Z., Seidler, F. J., Ali, S. F., Slikker, W., & Slotkin, T. A. (2001). Fetal and adolescent nicotine administration: Effects on CNS serotonergic systems. *Brain Research, 914*(1–2), 166–178.

Yang, P. B., Swann, A. C., & Dafny, N. (2003). Chronic pretreatment with methylphenidate induces cross-sensitization with amphetamine. *Life Sciences, 73*(22), 2899–2891.

Zedler, B. K., Mann, A. L., Kim, M. M., Amick, H. R., Joyce, A. R., Murrelle, E. L., & Jones, H. E. (2016). Buprenorphine compared with methadone to treat pregnant women with opioid use disorder: A systematic review and meta-analysis of safety in the mother, fetus and child. *Addiction, 111*(12), 2115–2128.

Zhang, T. A., Maldve, R. E., & Morrisett, R. A. (2006). Coincident signaling in mesolimbic structures underlying alcohol reinforcement. *Biochemical Pharmacology, 72*(8), 919–927.

Zito, J. M., Safer, D. J., dosReis, S., Magder, L. S., Gardner, J. F., & Zarin, D. A. (1999). Psychotherapeutic medication patterns for youths with attention-deficit hyperactivity disorder. *Archives of Pediatric and Adolescent Medicine, 153*(12), 1257–1263.

Zulauf, C. A., Sprich, S. E., Safren, S. A., & Wilens, T. E. (2014). The complicated relationship between attention deficit/hyperactivity disorder and substance use disorders. *Current Psychiatry Reports, 16*(3), 436.

Zuvekas, S. H., Vitiello, B., & Norquist, G. S. (2006). Recent trends in stimulant medication use among U.S. children. *The American Journal of Psychiatry, 163*(4), 579–585.

Needs, Services Received, and Outcomes of Adolescents and Young Adults in Substance Use Disorder (SUD) Treatment

Pamela C. Baumer, Michael L. Dennis, and Barbara Estrada

This chapter examines the characteristics and needs of substance misusing adolescents (ages 12–17) and young adults (ages 18–25), as well as implications for improving practice. The chapter begins with a review of the literature on prevalence, course, and correlates of substance misuse. It then uses a large treatment data set to provide a detailed description of the different demographics, substance use, and comorbidity characteristics of youth (ages 12–25) presenting to substance use treatment and explores how they vary by three demographic groups, type of substance problem, systems from which they could be recruited, and levels of substance use treatment. The chapter then focuses on using more detailed data on 16,361 youth from 208 Substance Abuse and Mental Health Services Administration (SAMHSA) Center for Substance Abuse Treatment (CSAT) grantee treatment programs in the USA who were interviewed with a standardized biopsychosocial assessment called the Global Appraisal of Individual Needs (GAIN; Dennis, Titus, et al., 2003). The chapter concludes with implications for assessing risk and assigning treatment.

P. C. Baumer (✉) · M. L. Dennis
Chestnut Health Systems, Normal, IL, USA
e-mail: pcbaumer@chestnut.org; pcihnes@chestnut.org; mdennis@chestnut.org

B. Estrada
Chestnut Health Systems, Normal, IL, USA
e-mail: bestrada@chestnut.org

C. G. Leukefeld, T. P. Gullotta (eds.), *Adolescent Substance Abuse*, Issues in Children's and Families' Lives, https://doi.org/10.1007/978-3-319-90611-9_4

Prevalence

Of the 24.9 million adolescents (age 12–17) in the USA in 2015, 16% report using any alcohol or other drugs, 11% have used alcohol in the past month (5.8% binge use), 8% have used marijuana, and 5% report criteria consistent with substance use disorders (SUD) in the past year (3% for alcohol use disorders and 3% for cannabis use disorders) (Substance Abuse and Mental Health Services Administration (SAMHSA) 2016a). Of the 34.9 million young adults (age 18–25), 63% used any alcohol or other drugs, 59% report using alcohol in the past 30 days (39% binge use), 21% used marijuana, and 15% report criteria consistent with substance use disorders (11% for alcohol use disorders, 5% for cannabis use disorders). However, estimates of those receiving SUD treatment in the past year are only 0.8% for adolescents and 1.8% for young adults. For the subset meeting the criteria for an SUD, this is the equivalent of 6.3% of adolescents and 7.7% of young adults.

Demographic Correlates

The age of onset is related to the long-term course of addiction. Those who initiate substance use prior to the age of 15 are significantly more likely than those who start over the age of 18 to have symptoms of dependence as an adult an average of 20 years later (Dennis, Babor, Roebuck, & Donaldson, 2002; Dennis, Scott, Funk, & Foss, 2005). The majority of youth (ages 12–25) meeting SUD criteria began using before age 16 (SAMHSA, 2016a). Therefore, understanding the distinct characteristics of adolescents is key to appropriate assessment and treatment, including their level of psychological development, relations with family and peers, and performance in school.

The period between mid-adolescence and young adulthood (ages 15–25) are a key time of intellectual development during which these youth are shifting from concrete to abstract thinking (e.g., seeing patterns, cause and effect) and gaining a future orientation (e.g., delay discounting of the value of recovery in the future, delayed gratification versus the immediate rewards of substance use) (Dennis, Dawud-Noursi, Muck, & McDermeit (Ives), 2003; Piaget, 1972; Steinberg, 2005). Similarly, adolescents suffer from poor inhibitory control due to the relative immaturity of the neurocircuitry in the ventral regions of the prefrontal cortex (Luna, Padmanabhan, & O'Hearn, 2010; Spear, 2010; Steinberg, 2010) and associated high rates of attention deficit hyperactivity disorder (ADHD) diagnoses (Chan, Dennis, & Funk, 2008; Conrad et al., 2012; Merikangas et al., 2010). Thus, assessing youth for SUD and related problems poses numerous difficulties; for example, they may not acknowledge an abstract "alcohol or drug problem" but be willing to acknowledge multiple concrete symptoms of SUD and/or the need for treatment.

The literature also emphasizes the unique characteristics of and associated complications for assessing and treating young adults; also referred to as transition age youth or emerging adults, ages typically range from 18 to 25, with some definitions including youth as young as 16 or as old as 29 (Bukstein, 2016; Coleman-Cowger, Baumer, Dennis, & Scott, 2015; Smith, Bennett, Dennis, & Funk, 2017a). Young adults are heterogeneous in terms of educational attainment, work, and living situations, presenting complications for approaching them as a single group. Additionally, a certain level of substance use is developmentally normal for young adults as they reach the age of legal majority making identifying abnormal use more complicated (Smith, Bennett, Dennis, & Funk, 2017b).

Multiple investigations have suggested that gender and race are related to the rates of initiation, prevalence, and remission from SUD (Dennis, Foss, & Scott, 2007; Grant & Dawson, 1998; Rounds-Bryant & Staab, 2001; Van Etten & Anthony, 1999). While they have similar rates of SUD as boys in the community (SAMHSA, 2016a), on average girls represent only about one-third of the people who receive publicly funded treatment (SAMHSA, 2016b). Similarly, rates of SUD are comparable by race (SAMHSA, 2016a), but minority clients made up less than 40% of those entering treatment in 2014 (SAMHSA, 2016b). Research on health disparities in behavior, system involvement, and treatment have begun to focus on not only describing what the differences between groups are, but also on whether the underlying determinants of these outcomes differ between groups, or whether similar determinants impact distinct groups differently, resulting in these observed differences (Godette, Mulatu, Leonard, Randolph, & Williams, 2011; Mulatu, Leonard, Godette, & Fulmore, 2008). Understanding not just how groups differ, but why they differ, allows for better treatment planning matched to individual needs.

Severity of Substance Use

Different substances have dramatically different effects on factors as varied as brain chemistry, physical health, and social consequences like unemployment and risk for adolescent pregnancy (Welty et al., 2016). Type of substance use can also implicate appropriate treatment options; e.g., medication-assisted treatment is more common for opioid or alcohol use disorders than other substances (Bukstein, 2016).

There have been numerous developments in the area of severity of substance use in the past decade. In 2013, the American Psychiatric Association published a new version of the Diagnostic and Statistical Manual of Mental Disorders (DSM-5) in which the symptoms for identifying SUD were changed, and significant changes were made to the criteria for diagnosis of a problem. As opposed to the previous focus on abuse vs. dependence, all problems are now identified on a continuum requiring 2–3 symptoms reported to be diagnosed as mild SUD, 4–5 symptoms for moderate SUD, and 6–11 symptoms for severe SUD. In this chapter we will look at the impact of using the old vs. the new criteria.

In a national sample of youth (ages 12–25) entering SUD treatment, the self-reported primary problem drugs at admission were 38% marijuana, 29% opioids, 19% alcohol, 10% stimulants, and 4% other drugs (SAMHSA, 2016b). These reports vary notably by gender, race, and age. In particular, young adults were more likely than adolescents to report more problems with stimulants (11% vs. 3%), opioids (37% vs. 4%), and alcohol (22% vs. 12%); they were less likely to report that their primary drug problem was marijuana (27% vs. 77%). African Americans' primary problem drug on entering treatment is marijuana (72%) at a far higher rate than other races, 50% Hispanic, 40% Mixed/other, and 27% Caucasian. Caucasian's primary problem drug is opioids (40%). Females enter treatment with significantly more problems than males with opioids (36% v. 26%) and stimulants (14% v. 6%), and less marijuana (29% v. 43%) (SAMHSA, 2016b).

Need for Screening and Intervention in Multiple Systems

Adolescent and young adult clients are referred for substance treatment by various sources. Of those entering publically funded treatment in 2014, 42% were referred by the justice system, 5% by a health care provider, 3% by the school system, less than 1% by an employer or employee assistance program, and 11% by some other community resource (e.g., religious institution, government aid agencies including child welfare) (SAMHSA, 2016b).

Numerous studies have also shown that youth in jail/detention or on community supervision (probation and parole) are disproportionately affected by behavioral health problems (Belenko et al., 2017; Welty et al., 2016). Interventions aimed at treating SUD have been reported as one of the most effective ways to interrupt the downward spiral toward a pattern of antisocial behavior and continued involvement in the justice system (Kelly, Becker, Wolff, Graves, & Spirito, 2017). As a result of the emphasis of juvenile justice reform on reducing the use of detention, community supervision, including Juvenile Drug Courts (JDC), has become the largest part of the juvenile justice system (Office of Juvenile Justice and Delinquency Prevention, 2014). While evidence for the effectiveness of JDC programs has been mixed (Dennis, Baumer, & Stevens, 2016; Marlowe, Festinger, Dugosh, Lee, & Benasutti, 2007), more rigorous studies have found that JDC using evidence based practices and those implementing the Juvenile Drug Court Strategies in Practice with more fidelity have positive outcomes for youth (Dakof et al., 2015; Henggeler et al., 2006; Ives, Chan, Modisette, & Dennis, 2010; Korchmaros, Baumer, & Valdez, 2016). In 2016, the Office of Juvenile Justice and Delinquency Prevention (OJJDP) released updated guidelines for JDC including more detailed information on appropriate implementation procedures in an attempt to bring their effectiveness in line with the more robust positive outcomes seen in Adult Drug Courts (ADC) (OJJDP, 2016).

Since the original publication of this chapter, significant research involving screening and intervention in schools has emerged. Dennis, Clark, and Huang (2014) point out that, while rates of SUD are higher among youth who drop out of school than those who stay in school, 90% of youth age 12–18 reporting criteria for an SUD remain in school, making this an important population to monitor for substance problems. Some schools offer Student Assistance Programs (SAP) with access to help with SUD. In support of previous literature indicating that providing services in school-based settings increases utilization of these services, Belur, Dennis, Ives, Vincent, and Muck (2014) and Hunter, Godley, and Godley (2014) confirmed that evidence based treatment models (Motivational Enhancement Therapy-Cognitive Behavioral Therapy, Adolescent Community Reinforcement Approach) could be implemented with equivalent, or sometimes better, effectiveness in a school-based setting compared to in a community setting, and reduced symptoms of SUD are associated with improved test scores on standardized measures of student achievement (Ratterman, 2014). Additionally, when implemented in school settings, these treatments reached youth earlier in the onset of their SUD and reduced health disparities found in community settings.

According to the Bureau of Labor Statistics, in 2016, 30% of eligible individuals between 16 and 19 were employed, and 65% of those age 20–24 were employed (USA Bureau of Labor Statistics 2017). Similar to the SAP offered by schools, some employers offer their employees Employee Assistance Programs (EAP), with access to numerous resources, including help with SUD. Based on a large, multinational data set, approximately 4% of clients accessing EAP services reported that they were seeking help with substance use (Chestnut Global Partners, 2017). Resources like EAPs may be even more valuable in times of economic recession. In a literature review across 25 years, Nagelhout et al. (2017) found evidence that recession, unemployment, and the threat of unemployment increase psychological distress, leading to increased drug use.

In the child welfare system, research suggests that 50–90% of cases involve one or more family members with an SUD (Marsh, Ryan, Choi, & Testa, 2006; McAlpine, Marshall, & Doran, 2001). Within the system, tremendous racial disparities exist, including higher likelihood of cases being opened, more case dispositions resulting in out-of-home placement, longer foster care stays, reduced likelihood of family reunification, and longer time to reunification for African Americans (Government Accountability Office [GAO], 2007; Green, Rockhill, & Furrer, 2007; Lu et al., 2004). Further, African American families in the child welfare system are less likely to have received SUD treatment and other services than Caucasian and Latino families and experience overall poorer case outcomes (Courtney et al., 1996).

It is noteworthy that most youth will be involved in multiple systems simultaneously. This provides opportunities to create interdisciplinary teams to address comorbid problems by connecting multiple systems in case management (justice, school, work, behavioral health, etc.). The Reclaiming Futures model (RF; Nissen,

Hunt, Bullman, Marmo, & Smith, 2004), and JDC and ADC approaches (National Research Council, 2012; OJJDP, 2016) have demonstrated the potential for success of such teams.

Variations by Level of Care

The American Society of Addiction Medicine (1996, 2001; Mee-Lee, Shulman, Fishman, Gastfriend, & Miller, 2013) has recommended the use of explicit patient placement criteria for determining the appropriate level of care for treating SUD, the use of which has been mandated in several states. The guidelines recommend (and studies have increasingly also found) that the severity of SUD and co-occurring problems increase with the intensity of services (i.e., early intervention, outpatient, intensive outpatient, residential) (Dennis, Dawud-Noursi, et al., 2003; Dennis, White, & Ives, 2009; Gerstein & Johnson, 1999; Hser et al., 2001; Hubbard, Cavanaugh, Craddock, & Rachal, 1985; Rounds-Bryant, Kristiansen, & Hubbard, 1999; Sells & Simpson, 1979; Simpson, Savage, & Sells, 1978). Other recent studies have indicated that it may even be detrimental to include clients with less severe problems in more intense programs, as these youth may develop new or increasingly severe symptoms (Korchmaros et al., 2016; Marlowe et al., 2007; National Research Council, 2012; Taxman & Marlowe, 2006). Based on the ASAM guidelines (1996, 2001), receipt of prior treatment makes a recommendation for more intense level of care more likely to be appropriate. Thus, it is important to recognize the heterogeneity of who is served in different types of treatment programs.

Trauma and Victimization

Trauma and victimization are among the most common problems for youth requiring SUD treatment; between 60% and 87% of adolescents in substance treatment self-report having been victimized (Shane, Diamond, Mensinger, Shera, & Wintersteen, 2006; Titus, Dennis, White, Scott, & Funk, 2003). Research has shown that adolescents and young adults who have experienced trauma and victimization are at increased risk for SUD; have greater severity of problems in terms of substance use, emotional problems, HIV risk, social risk, and recovery environment risk upon entering substance use treatment; and are at higher risk for entering the juvenile justice system (Carliner et al., 2016; Funk, McDermeit (Ives), Godley, & Adams, 2003; Garner, Hunter, Smith, Smith, & Godley, 2014; Ireland, Smith, & Walter, 2015). Youth who have experienced victimization are responsive to treatment, and have demonstrated greater reductions in substance use problems after treatment than those without a history of victimization (Funk et al., 2003; Garner et al., 2014) though the effectiveness of treatment has been shown to interact with level of care for these youth (Funk et al., 2003).

Costs to Society

The annual societal costs of SUD come to about $740 billion in the USA, including medical care spending and productivity losses, and the costs per individual are higher for certain subgroups, including those with opioid use disorders, whose higher rates of HIV and viral hepatitis require significantly more contact with the healthcare system (McCollister et al., 2017). When coupled with their frequent contacts with the justice system, these costs can soar even higher. However, the National Research Council's summary (2012) of the epidemiological literature indicates that "serious delinquents" are a very small portion of the overall population; while they commit many offenses, most are relatively minor, and there are very few chronic violent offenders. In other words, it is the few clients with the most chronic or severe problems that are responsible for a significant portion of the societal costs associated with substance use (Bickel, Johnson, Koffarnus, MacKillop, & Murphy, 2014; French et al., 2002, 2008).

Current Chapter

This chapter explores the needs, services received, and outcomes of adolescents (ages 12–17) and young adults (ages 18–25) presenting to treatment. Data were obtained from clients who were interviewed from 2002 to 2012 as part of 208 SAMHSA/CSAT adolescent and young adult treatment grants across the USA. These studies were conducted across a variety of institutional settings (e.g., addiction agencies, student assistance programs, child protective service agencies, justice agencies) and addiction treatment levels of care (e.g., early intervention, regular and intensive outpatient, short-, moderate-, and long-term residential). All data were collected as part of general clinical practice or specific research studies after voluntary consent and have been pooled for secondary analysis under the terms of data sharing agreements and the supervision of Chestnut's Institutional Review Board.

Of the 27,811 available clients age 12–25, 27,005 were due for at least one follow-up interview (97%). Of those due for a follow-up, 20,896 (77%) completed a 3-month interview, and thus were expected to have data on treatment received, and 18,695 (69%) completed a 6-month interview. In order to have a consistent number of records across analyses, follow-up data is included for both 3- and 6-month interviews, for 16,361 (59%) adolescents and young adults.

Measures

The participant characteristics, substance use, and comorbidity profiles were based on participant self-report to in-person interviews with the Global Appraisal of Individual Needs (GAIN) versions 5.1–5.6 (Dennis, Titus, White, Unsicker, &

Hodgkins, 2003). GAIN is a standardized biopsychosocial assessment that integrates clinical and research measures into one comprehensive structured interview used primarily to assess problems in order to support clinical decision-making related to diagnosis, placement, and treatment planning, to measure change, and to document service utilization. The GAIN's main scales have demonstrated excellent to good reliability (Dennis et al., 2004; Dennis, Chan, & Funk, 2006; Dennis, Dawud-Noursi, et al., 2003; Dennis, Ives, White, & Muck, 2008; Dennis, Scott, & Funk, 2003) and have been validated with time line follow-back methods, urine tests, collateral reports, treatment records, blind psychiatric diagnosis, Rasch measurement models, confirmatory factor analysis, structural equation models, and via construct or predictive validation (Conrad et al., 2010, 2012; Conrad, Conrad, Passetti, Funk, & Dennis, 2015; Conrad, Dennis, Bezruczko, Funk, & Riley, 2007; Conrad, Riley, Conrad, Chan, & Dennis, 2010; Dennis et al., 2002, 2004, 2006; Dennis, Scott, & Funk, 2003; Godley, Godley, Dennis, Funk, & Passetti, 2002, 2007; Lennox, Dennis, Ives, & White, 2006; Lennox, Dennis, Scott, & Funk, 2006; Riley, Conrad, Bezruczko, & Dennis, 2007; Riley, Dennis, & Conrad, 2010; Shane, Jasiukaitis, & Green, 2003; White, 2005; White, Funk, White, & Dennis, 2004). GAIN has also been demonstrated to be sensitive to changes in clinical diagnosis and needs by age (Chan et al., 2008; Dennis et al., 2006). A more detailed list of studies, psychometrics on over 100,000 adolescents, young adults, and adults, validations to the Rasch measurement model, and copies of the GAIN instruments and items are publicly available at www.gaincc.org.

Treatment data are from two sources: self-reported services received from the 3 month GAIN interview and clinician records. Outcomes presented in this chapter are those identified as key cross domain measures by SAMHSA, the National Outcomes Measurement System (NOMS). These outcomes are presented in a positive framework, such that endorsement indicates a better outcome (e.g., no days of substance use, no emotional problems). A summary count of positive outcomes is presented for both the period before intake and at the 6-month follow-up in order to examine change in positive life domains over time. Economic cost of health care utilization and crime for the year before intake to treatment are estimated based on self-reported frequencies from the GAIN multiplied by the most recent economic estimates of their unit costs to society (McCollister et al., 2017). The frequency of illegal activities is self-reported in the past year in the GAIN. The elements of health care utilization are reported for the 3 months before intake in the GAIN, so reported units were multiplied by 4 as an estimate of past year utilization. Costs were divided into low/moderate/high groups using all clients reporting $0 annual cost included in the low group, and the top approximately 10% making up the high group. The remainder comprises the moderate group.

Analyses

Descriptive data is presented in the tables and described overall and then by gender, race, and age, substance problem, system involvement, and level of care. The differences were tested with chi-square analysis for the mutually exclusive groups (level of care, gender, race, and age). Clients were often involved in more than one system or experienced problem use of more than one substance, thus chi-square analyses were done comparing those involved in the system or using the substance versus those who were not. For space purposes the latter is not shown. Because the large sample sizes make even small differences statistically significant, discussion of variations by subgroups focuses on differences that are both statistically significant at $p < 0.05$ and clinically meaningful based on Cohen's d effect size with an absolute value of 0.2 or greater (a small effect) when compared to the total average. Because the distributions for the cost of health care utilization and cost of crime are so deeply right skewed (with a large percentage of clients responsible for $0 of costs and the top 10% driving over half the costs), the nonparametric Mann–Whitney (dichotomous) or Kruskal–Wallis (three or more groups) rank order test was applied to test for significance, and effect sizes were calculated based on mean ranks; medians, rather than means, are reported.

Results

The results are presented in three major sections. The first section introduces the tables and overall findings across youth. The next four subsections look at how the findings vary by selected demographics, substance problem, system involvement, and level of care. The last section looks at emerging issues related to the cost of health care utilization, the cost of crime, and trauma.

Overall Findings

Demographic and environmental characteristics. As shown in the first column of Table 1, this sample of adolescents and young adults entering treatment were primarily male (73%), nonwhite (63%), and between the ages of 15 and 17 (69%). One percent was married, and 5% identified as gay, lesbian, bisexual, transgendered, or questioning (GLBTQ). Of those under the age of 18, 50% were living with a single parent. Overall, 35% reported having ever been homeless or run away from home. Twenty-two percent reported weekly alcohol use in the home, and 10% reported weekly drug use in the home. Use among social peers was more common, with 41%

Table 1 Participant demographics by gender, race group, age, substance problem, system involvement, and level of care

	Total	Male	Female	African American	White	Hispanic	Mixed/ other	12–17	18–25	Alcohol[g]	Cannabis[g]	Opioids[g]	Stimulants[g]	Other[g]
	16,361	11,904	4,449	2,465	6,090	4,865	2,934	13,989	2,372	4,456	9,680	1,066	1,685	1,183
Total %	100%	73%	27%	15%	37%	30%	18%	86%	15%	32%	66%	8%	12%	9%
Demographics														
Female	27%	–	**100%**	17%	32%	23%	32%	27%	29%	30%	23%	**37%**	**42%**	33%
Minority status	63%	65%	56%	**100%**	0%	**100%**	**100%**	63%	63%	58%	62%	38%	57%	50%
Race														
Asian	1%	1%	1%	–	–	–	**4%**	1%	1%	1%	1%	0%	1%	1%
African American\ Black	15%	17%	10%	**100%**	–	–	–	15%	17%	9%	16%	2%	4%	4%
Caucasian\White	37%	35%	44%	–	**100%**	–	–	37%	37%	42%	38%	**62%**	43%	**50%**
Hispanic	30%	32%	25%	–	–	**100%**	–	29%	32%	29%	29%	20%	34%	29%
Mixed	15%	14%	17%	–	–	–	**82%**	15%	12%	17%	15%	13%	17%	15%
Other	1%	1%	1%	–	–	–	**4%**	2%	1%	1%	1%	0%	0%	0%
Age														
<15 years	16%	15%	19%	16%	14%	18%	17%	19%	–	11%	15%	6%	8%	12%
15–17 years	69%	71%	66%	68%	71%	66%	71%	**81%**	–	70%	72%	55%	67%	67%
18–25 years	15%	14%	15%	16%	14%	15%	12%	–	**100%**	19%	13%	**39%**	**25%**	21%
Married	1%	1%	2%	1%	1%	2%	1%	0%	**7%**	1%	1%	4%	4%	2%
GLBTQ[a]	5%	1%	**16%**	5%	5%	5%	7%	5%	8%	8%	6%	**12%**	**14%**	**13%**
Family/living														
Single parent family[b]	50%	50%	49%	**61%**	43%	51%	51%	50%	49%	48%	51%	49%	48%	48%
Weekly alcohol use in home	22%	22%	25%	14%	29%	18%	24%	23%	19%	28%	24%	27%	24%	27%
Weekly drug use in home	10%	9%	14%	11%	11%	8%	12%	10%	14%	14%	13%	**20%**	17%	16%

Ever homeless/runaway	35%	30%	**46%**	26%	36%	33%	42%	33%	41%	**49%**	39%	**60%**	**65%**	**58%**
Social peers														
Regular peer alcohol use at work/school[c]	41%	41%	40%	**27%**	46%	40%	45%	44%	**25%**	**55%**	45%	45%	48%	**52%**
Regular peer alcohol use[c]	47%	46%	48%	**35%**	50%	46%	50%	48%	40%	**68%**	53%	**59%**	**63%**	**64%**
Regular peer drug use at work/school[d]	56%	57%	55%	**42%**	63%	54%	60%	61%	**27%**	61%	63%	52%	54%	61%
Regular peer drug use[d]	65%	65%	64%	56%	71%	60%	68%	67%	**50%**	**75%**	**74%**	73%	72%	**77%**
Environment														
In school[e]	84%	85%	84%	85%	84%	83%	87%	**92%**	**43%**	80%	85%	**58%**	**71%**	**75%**
Employed[e]	25%	25%	23%	**15%**	34%	19%	24%	22%	**38%**	27%	24%	32%	25%	25%
Any child welfare involvement[f]	10%	9%	14%	10%	11%	6%	16%	11%	**2%**	14%	11%	12%	17%	13%

	In school[e]	In work[e]	In welfare[f]	In jail 14+ days	Prob/parole 14+ days	Drug court	Other JSI P90[h]	Early intervention	Outpatient (OP)	Intensive outpatient	Residential	Continuing care OP
	13,775	4,027	1,665	2,575	3,999	1,325	4,661	946	11,195	1,558	1,215	1,059
Total %	84%	25%	10%	16%	25%	8%	29%	6%	70%	10%	8%	7%
Demographics												
Female	27%	25%	**38%**	**18%**	20%	**39%**	25%	26%	28%	28%	26%	24%
Minority status	63%	**49%**	59%	72%	65%	65%	58%	**77%**	60%	70%	69%	60%
Race												
Asian	1%	0%	1%	1%	1%	0%	1%	0%	1%	0%	1%	2%
African American\Black	15%	9%	14%	19%	16%	**9%**	15%	18%	14%	19%	21%	18%
Caucasian\White	37%	**51%**	41%	28%	35%	35%	42%	**23%**	40%	30%	31%	40%
Hispanic	29%	23%	**17%**	33%	31%	**42%**	27%	**43%**	30%	36%	**18%**	23%

(continued)

Table 1 (continued)

	In school[e]	In work[e]	In welfare[f]	In jail 14+ days	Prob/parole 14+ days	Drug court	Other JSI P90[h]	Early intervention	Outpatient (OP)	Intensive outpatient	Residential	Continuing care OP
Mixed	15%	15%	**23%**	17%	15%	13%	13%	16%	13%	12%	**27%**	17%
Other	1%	1%	**4%**	1%	1%	0%	1%	0%	1%	1%	1%	0%
Age												
<15 years	19%	**6%**	18%	10%	12%	15%	17%	12%	18%	14%	17%	**9%**
15–17 years	74%	72%	**80%**	68%	75%	**59%**	70%	**55%**	70%	71%	71%	71%
18–25 years	**7%**	22%	**3%**	22%	13%	**26%**	12%	**33%**	13%	15%	12%	20%
Married	0%	2%	1%	2%	1%	3%	1%	**5%**	1%	2%	2%	1%
GLBTQ[b]	5%	5%	8%	7%	4%	6%	5%	5%	5%	5%	7%	7%
Family/living												
Single parent family[c]	49%	45%	**37%**	57%	53%	51%	49%	59%	48%	56%	51%	54%
Weekly alcohol use in home	23%	27%	19%	16%	22%	22%	24%	18%	23%	19%	28%	17%
Weekly drug use in home	9%	11%	12%	12%	10%	9%	9%	12%	9%	11%	**20%**	9%
Ever homeless/ runaway	33%	33%	**58%**	**48%**	37%	33%	29%	38%	29%	39%	**56%**	**48%**
Social peers												
Regular peer alcohol use at work/school[d]	43%	46%	45%	38%	42%	40%	40%	33%	39%	42%	**52%**	41%
Regular peer alcohol use[d]	46%	51%	52%	51%	49%	47%	44%	47%	44%	46%	**64%**	50%
Regular peer drug use at work/school[e]	61%	61%	54%	**46%**	56%	53%	57%	**41%**	57%	54%	63%	49%

Regular peer drug use[e]	66%	69%	64%	60%	67%	62%	65%	61%	64%	62%	**78%**	59%
Environment												
In school[f]	**100%**	78%	87%	**<u>75%</u>**	85%	**<u>74%</u>**	86%	**<u>64%</u>**	88%	79%	79%	87%
Employed[f]	23%	**100%**	19%	17%	26%	25%	28%	27%	26%	19%	21%	17%
Any child welfare involvement[g]	11%	8%	**100%**	15%	11%	6%	8%	7%	9%	8%	**18%**	**21%**

Created by authors, Baumer, Dennis, & Estrada, 2017

Note: Values in **BOLD** indicate that relative to total, column value is significantly different ($p < 0.05$) and clinically higher (Cohen's effect size $d \geq 0.2$)

Values in **<u>BOLD and UNDERLINED</u>** indicate that relative to total, column value is significantly different ($p < 0.05$) and clinically lower (Cohen's effect size ≤ -0.2)

[a]Self-reported sexual attraction to same sex/both/unsure, self-reported identity as homosexual, bisexual, questioning, or unsure, or reported gender and sexual activity

[b]Based on data from 13,989 clients under the age of 18

[c]Spent time in the past year with 1 or more people at work/school or socially who got drunk weekly

[d]Spent time in the past year with 1 or more people work/school or socially who used drugs quarterly

[e]In the past 90 days

[f]Reports days in foster care or a group home, legal custody by the County or State, referred to treatment by social worker or DCFS/welfare, has child in foster care, group or institution

[g]Problem use is defined using the DSM5 definition of mild or more severe substance disorder problems (2+ of 11 symptoms) in the past year or weekly use of the substance

[h]Does not meet criteria for in jail 14+ days or probation/parole 14+ days but has been arrested and charged with a crime in the past 90 days, have been on probation, parole, jail, detention, house arrest, or electronic monitoring in the past 90 days, or any current justice involvement in L7

reporting weekly alcohol use among their work or school peers, and 47% reporting weekly alcohol use among their social peers. Past 90-day drug use by work or school peers was reported by 56% of clients, and drug use by social peers by 65% of clients. *Thus, many clients had one or more major environmental risk factors associated with continued use or relapse.*

Most (84%) had been in school in the past 90 days, and 25% were employed during that time. Child welfare involvement, including days in foster care or a group home, legal custody by the county or state, referred to treatment by social worker or DCFS/welfare, or having a child in foster care, group home or institution, was reported by 10% of clients. *Thus, there was clearly overlap with the populations seen by other systems of care.*

Substance use characteristics. The first column of Table 2 details the substance use history for clients entering treatment. Most clients (82%) began using alcohol or other drugs (AOD) before they were 15 years old, and more than a quarter (27%) have been using for 5 or more years. Lifetime substance severity, as defined by the DSM-IV (American Psychiatric Association, 2000), indicates that 84% of clients reported criteria consistent with an SUD (55% dependence, 29% abuse); while based on the DSM-5 definition (American Psychiatric Association, 2013) 78% of clients reported criteria consistent with an SUD (17% mild problems, 15% moderate problems, and 46% severe problems). The difference between the DSM-IV and DSM-5 criteria for substance disorders (a reduction of 6%) primarily results from clients who report only one symptom of substance abuse by the DSM-IV definition; at least two symptoms are required to meet criteria for a diagnosis in the DSM-5. Problem use in the past year, defined as reporting two or more SUD symptoms in the past year and/or use of the substance 13 or more of the past 90 days (i.e., weekly use on average), was reported by 32% for alcohol, 66% for cannabis, 8% for opioids, 12% for stimulants (including amphetamines and cocaine), and 9% for other drugs. In the past 90 days, 53% used AOD weekly or more often (another 27% used less than weekly). Clients also presented significant problems with tobacco use, with 17% reporting lifetime dependence (as defined by the DSM-IV), 66% reporting problem use in the past year (as defined above), and 48% reporting weekly use in the past 90 days (17% using less than weekly). However, 30% of clients reported spending 13 or more days in a controlled environment (e.g., treatment, jail). This time in a controlled environment likely resulted in reduced drug use for youth clients in the 90 days before their intake to treatment. More than a third (37%) had experience withdrawal in their lifetime; 19% in the past week, and 3% reported high severity withdrawal in the past week (11 or more symptoms). Approximately one-third (34%) of youth clients had received prior substance treatment, and 14% reported two or more prior treatment episodes. Most (72%) perceived a need for treatment for one or more substances, however, only 24% reported their AOD use as a problem. *While in need of treatment, this profile also suggests that the adolescents and young adults presenting to treatment are largely being seen relatively early (i.e., first 10 years) in the course of their addiction.*

Table 2 Patient substance use history at intake gender, race, age, substance problem, system involvement, and level of care

	Total	Male	Female	African American	White	Hispanic	Mixed/ other	12–17	18–25	Alcohol[c]	Cannabis[c]	Opioids[c]	Stimulants[c]	Other[c]
	16,361	11,904	4,449	2,465	6,090	4,865	2,934	13,989	2,372	4,456	9,680	1,066	1,685	1,183
Total %	100%	73%	27%	15%	37%	30%	18%	86%	15%	32%	66%	8%	12%	9%
Substance use														
Age of first use														
Under 10	9%	9%	6%	6%	9%	8%	11%	9%	8%	12%	10%	14%	15%	14%
Age 10–14	73%	72%	74%	71%	71%	76%	73%	76%	**57%**	75%	77%	71%	76%	76%
Age 15+	19%	18%	20%	23%	20%	16%	16%	16%	**35%**	13%	13%	15%	**9%**	**10%**
Years of substance use[a]														
Less than 1	5%	5%	7%	8%	5%	6%	4%	6%	**1%**	2%	3%	**1%**	**1%**	**1%**
1–2 years	37%	36%	39%	40%	37%	36%	35%	42%	**10%**	**25%**	34%	**13%**	**17%**	**19%**
3–4 years	30%	31%	29%	30%	30%	31%	30%	32%	**19%**	35%	33%	28%	32%	34%
5 or more years	27%	28%	25%	23%	28%	27%	30%	20%	**71%**	**38%**	30%	**59%**	**50%**	**46%**
Lifetime substance severity DSM-IV														
No use	1%	1%	2%	2%	1%	1%	2%	1%	1%	**0%**	**0%**	**0%**	**0%**	**0%**
Use	15%	14%	16%	**24%**	11%	14%	13%	15%	11%	**3%**	**6%**	**1%**	**1%**	**1%**
Abuse	29%	31%	23%	35%	27%	29%	27%	31%	**19%**	**19%**	27%	**3%**	**5%**	**8%**
Dependence	55%	54%	59%	**39%**	61%	55%	58%	53%	**69%**	**78%**	**67%**	**96%**	**93%**	**91%**
Lifetime substance severity DSM-5[b]														
No use	1%	1%	2%	2%	1%	1%	2%	1%	1%	**0%**	**0%**	**0%**	**0%**	**0%**
Use	21%	21%	21%	**33%**	17%	21%	19%	22%	14%	**4%**	**9%**	**1%**	**1%**	**2%**
Mild problems (2–3 symptoms)	17%	18%	14%	21%	17%	16%	16%	18%	12%	12%	17%	**2%**	**3%**	**4%**
Moderate problems (4–5 symptoms)	15%	16%	12%	17%	15%	14%	14%	15%	11%	14%	17%	**4%**	**6%**	**8%**

(continued)

Table 2 (continued)

	Total	Male	Female	African American	White	Hispanic	Mixed/ other	12–17	18–25	Alcohol[c]	Cannabis[c]	Opioids[c]	Stimulants[c]	Other[c]
Severe problems (6+ symptoms)	46%	45%	51%	**27%**	51%	48%	49%	43%	**63%**	**70%**	56%	**93%**	**90%**	**86%**
Change in any SUD diagnosis (sum of abuse/dependence minus sum of mild-severe)	6%	7%	5%	8%	5%	7%	6%	7%	3%	**1%**	3%	**0%**	**0%**	**1%**
Past year problem use (2+ symptoms or weekly use)[c]														
Alcohol	32%	31%	34%	**20%**	34%	33%	36%	30%	**43%**	**100%**	38%	**56%**	**60%**	**60%**
Cannabis	66%	70%	**55%**	71%	65%	65%	64%	67%	60%	**77%**	**100%**	**76%**	**78%**	**86%**
Opioids	8%	7%	10%	**1%**	12%	5%	7%	5%	**22%**	13%	9%	**100%**	**28%**	**43%**
Stimulants	12%	10%	19%	**3%**	13%	15%	13%	11%	**22%**	**24%**	15%	**47%**	**100%**	**47%**
Other	9%	8%	10%	**2%**	11%	9%	9%	8%	13%	**16%**	11%	**49%**	**32%**	**100%**
Past 90 day alcohol or drug use														
None (0 days)	20%	20%	21%	23%	18%	23%	20%	18%	**33%**	19%	13%	20%	26%	20%
Less than weekly (1–12 days)	27%	26%	29%	26%	28%	26%	27%	28%	21%	**16%**	**13%**	**10%**	**12%**	**11%**
Weekly (13+ days)	53%	54%	50%	51%	54%	51%	53%	54%	46%	**65%**	**74%**	**69%**	62%	**70%**
Tobacco use														
Tobacco dependence (lifetime)	17%	15%	23%	**8%**	24%	11%	20%	16%	23%	**29%**	21%	**39%**	**36%**	**38%**
Past year problem use (2+ symptoms or weekly use)[c]	66%	65%	67%	**52%**	**80%**	**51%**	68%	64%	**75%**	**81%**	74%	**91%**	**86%**	**89%**

	Total	Male	Female	African American	White	Hispanic	Mixed/ other	12–17	18–25	Alcohol[c]	Cannabis[c]	Opioids[c]	Stimulants[c]	Other[c]
Past 90 day tobacco use														
None (0 days)	35%	36%	34%	**45%**	**24%**	33%	35%	37%	**25%**	**24%**	28%	**15%**	**22%**	**18%**
Less than weekly (1–12 days)	17%	17%	15%	15%	14%	17%	17%	17%	15%	16%	17%	13%	16%	17%
Weekly (13+ days)	48%	47%	51%	40%	**62%**	50%	48%	46%	**59%**	**60%**	55%	**72%**	**62%**	**65%**
13+ Days in controlled environment[d]	30%	31%	27%	34%	27%	28%	34%	27%	**45%**	**43%**	33%	**59%**	**62%**	**54%**
Withdrawal severity														
Any lifetime	37%	34%	45%	**24%**	41%	38%	40%	36%	46%	**54%**	45%	**83%**	**73%**	**72%**
Any past week	19%	18%	21%	16%	19%	20%	21%	20%	15%	25%	25%	26%	24%	**29%**
High (11+) past week symptoms	3%	2%	4%	1%	3%	3%	3%	2%	3%	4%	3%	**12%**	**8%**	**10%**
Prior SA treatment episodes														
Any	34%	34%	35%	26%	38%	32%	37%	32%	**49%**	**46%**	37%	**65%**	**59%**	**59%**
Two or more	14%	14%	16%	**8%**	18%	12%	16%	16%	**24%**	**22%**	16%	**38%**	**34%**	**33%**
Perception														
Perceives need for treatment	72%	72%	73%	69%	74%	71%	72%	71%	**81%**	**83%**	79%	**93%**	**91%**	**88%**
Perceives AOD as a problem[e]	24%	23%	29%	**12%**	30%	21%	27%	23%	**34%**	**39%**	30%	**63%**	**57%**	**54%**

(continued)

Table 2 (continued)

	In school[f]	In work[f]	In welfare[g]	In jail 14+ days	Prob/parole 14+ days	Drug court	Other JSI P90[h]	Early intervention	Outpatient (OP)	Intensive outpatient	Residential	Continuing care OP
	13,775	4,027	1,665	2,575	3,999	1,325	4,661	946	11,195	1,558	1,215	1,059
Total %	84%	25%	10%	16%	25%	8%	29%	6%	70%	10%	8%	7%
Substance use												
Age of first use												
Under 10	8%	7%	14%	12%	11%	6%	6%	9%	7%	9%	13%	15%
Age 10–14	74%	65%	76%	77%	73%	72%	72%	67%	73%	74%	78%	75%
Age 15+	17%	**28%**	**10%**	**11%**	16%	22%	21%	24%	20%	17%	**8%**	**10%**
Years of substance use[a]												
Less than 1	6%	4%	3%	2%	3%	4%	7%	5%	7%	4%	3%	**1%**
1–2 years	41%	34%	30%	**24%**	34%	34%	41%	30%	41%	34%	**27%**	**22%**
3–4 years	31%	30%	33%	34%	32%	28%	30%	24%	30%	31%	33%	37%
5 or more years	22%	32%	34%	**40%**	31%	34%	22%	**41%**	23%	31%	**38%**	**40%**
Lifetime substance severity DSM-IV												
No use	1%	1%	1%	1%	0%	1%	1%	1%	1%	1%	1%	0%
Use	15%	13%	11%	10%	10%	14%	18%	12%	17%	11%	**4%**	**6%**
Abuse	30%	30%	21%	23%	30%	30%	32%	23%	32%	30%	**18%**	**18%**
Dependence	53%	56%	**67%**	**66%**	60%	56%	49%	65%	49%	58%	**76%**	**75%**
Lifetime substance severity DSM-5[b]												
No use	1%	1%	1%	1%	0%	1%	1%	1%	1%	1%	1%	0%
Use	22%	19%	14%	**13%**	15%	22%	25%	16%	25%	17%	**7%**	**8%**
Mild problems (2–3 symptoms)	18%	18%	13%	12%	17%	18%	18%	12%	19%	17%	10%	11%

	In school[f]	In work[f]	In welfare[g]	In jail 14+ days	Prob/parole 14+ days	Drug court	Other JSI P90[h]	Early intervention	Outpatient (OP)	Intensive outpatient	Residential	Continuing care OP
Moderate problems (4–5 symptoms)	15%	16%	13%	13%	15%	13%	15%	15%	16%	15%	11%	11%
Severe problems (6+ symptoms)	43%	46%	**60%**	**62%**	52%	47%	39%	56%	39%	51%	**71%**	**70%**
Change in any SUD diagnosis (sum of abuse/dependence minus sum of mild-severe)	7%	7%	4%	3%	5%	8%	8%	4%	8%	6%	2%	**1%**
Past year problem use (2+ symptoms or weekly use)[c]												
Alcohol	30%	34%	41%	**48%**	32%	26%	27%	34%	29%	33%	**45%**	40%
Cannabis	66%	63%	69%	**75%**	69%	59%	63%	59%	64%	67%	**78%**	65%
Opioids	5%	10%	9%	13%	7%	14%	5%	7%	7%	8%	12%	12%
Stimulants	10%	12%	**20%**	**26%**	12%	10%	8%	17%	8%	14%	**29%**	**21%**
Other	8%	9%	11%	13%	9%	11%	6%	8%	7%	9%	14%	12%
Past 90 day alcohol or drug use												
None (0 days)	20%	14%	**32%**	**38%**	21%	17%	16%	**29%**	17%	24%	15%	**50%**
Less than weekly (1–12 days)	28%	29%	25%	20%	27%	24%	29%	23%	30%	24%	**12%**	19%
Weekly (13+ days)	52%	57%	**43%**	**42%**	52%	60%	55%	48%	53%	52%	**73%**	**31%**
Tobacco use												
Tobacco dependence (lifetime)	16%	21%	**26%**	18%	20%	18%	15%	16%	16%	20%	**33%**	15%
Past year problem use (2+ symptoms or weekly use)[c]	63%	74%	**78%**	67%	73%	66%	63%	65%	62%	65%	**81%**	**78%**

(continued)

Table 2 (continued)

	In school[f]	In work[f]	In welfare[g]	In jail 14+ days	Prob/parole 14+ days	Drug court	Other JSI P90[h]	Early intervention	Outpatient (OP)	Intensive outpatient	Residential	Continuing care OP
Past 90 day tobacco use												
None (0 days)	37%	27%	29%	38%	29%	35%	36%	41%	37%	35%	<u>**21%**</u>	28%
Less than weekly (1–12 days)	17%	15%	16%	18%	14%	17%	17%	14%	17%	16%	15%	16%
Weekly (13+ days)	46%	58%	55%	43%	57%	49%	47%	45%	46%	49%	**64%**	56%
13+ days in controlled environment[d]	27%	<u>**20%**</u>	**63%**	**100%**	22%	26%	<u>**13%**</u>	**44%**	<u>**21%**</u>	36%	**51%**	**73%**
Withdrawal severity												
Any lifetime	36%	39%	44%	38%	38%	41%	34%	40%	34%	40%	**57%**	44%
Any past week	19%	22%	18%	<u>**11%**</u>	19%	20%	21%	18%	19%	18%	**34%**	<u>**10%**</u>
High (11+) past week symptoms	2%	3%	3%	2%	2%	3%	3%	2%	2%	3%	**7%**	1%
Prior SA treatment episodes												
Any	32%	35%	**51%**	**48%**	**45%**	36%	25%	31%	27%	41%	**55%**	**71%**
Two or more	13%	15%	**27%**	**23%**	21%	14%	9%	12%	10%	19%	**28%**	**39%**
Perception												
Perceives need for treatment	70%	71%	76%	75%	73%	74%	69%	74%	68%	80%	**87%**	**83%**
Perceives AOD as a problem[e]	22%	26%	33%	33%	25%	23%	20%	26%	19%	30%	**48%**	**34%**

Created by authors, Baumer, Dennis, & Estrada, 2017

Note: Values in **BOLD** indicate that relative to total, column value is significantly different ($p < 0.05$) and clinically higher (Cohen's effect size $d \geq 0.2$)

Values in <u>**BOLD and UNDERLINED**</u> indicate that relative to total, column value is significantly different ($p < 0.05$) and clinically lower (Cohen's effect sizes ≤0.2)

[a]Computed as age minus years used

[b]Estimate of DSM5 diagnosis based on 11 substance disorder symtpoms; missing data for 'craving' per DSM5 definition, but including item for problems with the law

[c]Problem use is defined using the DSM5 definition of mild or more severe substance disorder problems (2+ of 11 symptoms) in the past year or weekly use of the substance

[d]Hospital, treatment, detention, or jail (where not free to come and go as you please)

[e]"Do you currently feel that you have any problems related to alcohol or drug use?"

[f]In the past 90 days

[g]Reports days in foster care or a group home, legal custody by the County or State, referred to treatment by social worker or DCFS/welfare, has child in foster care, group or institution

[h]Does not meet criteria for in jail 14+ days or probation/parole 14+ days but has been arrested and charged with a crime in the past 90 days, have been on probation, parole, jail, detention, house arrest, or electronic monitoring in the past 90 days, or any current justice involvement in L7

Co-occurring psychiatric, victimization, HIV risk, and crime problems. Clients presented to these treatment programs with numerous co-occurring problems, as detailed in the first column of Table 3. Co-occurring mental health problems were the norm, with 41% of clients reporting symptoms consistent with an internalizing disorder in the past year, including 34% with a mood disorder, 12% with anxiety disorder, 24% with traumatic distress disorder, and 19% reporting suicidal thoughts or actions. Additionally, 55% reported symptoms consistent with any past year externalizing disorder, including 45% with conduct disorder, and 38% with ADHD. Only 38% of clients reported neither internalizing nor externalizing disorders, 22% reported only internalizing disorders, 8% reported only externalizing disorders, and 33% reported having both internalizing and externalizing disorders concurrently. Forty percent of clients had received prior mental health treatment. *Thus, co-occurring psychiatric problems are the norm and often have not been treated.*

Physical health problems were also typical for clients entering treatment. While 53% of clients reported low levels of physical health problems, 39% had moderate health problems, and 8% had high health problems. Nearly all (92%) reported receiving prior physical health treatment. They also engaged in numerous risky behaviors in the past 90 days, including needle use (2%), sexual activity (63%), unprotected sex (29%), and sex with multiple partners (29%). Victimization was very common for these clients. Overall, 61% of clients have a history of victimization in their lifetime, and 43% reported high levels of victimization. In the past year, 34% experienced victimization, and 18% had been victimized in the past 90 days. Sixteen percent expressed current worries about victimization. *Thus, victimization is widespread as both a past problem and present concern for clients entering substance treatment.*

Violence and illegal activity are frequently co-occurring problems for youth clients. Overall, 65% engaged in any acts of physical violence toward others in the past year, and 62% engaged in illegal activity, including property crimes (46%), violent/interpersonal crimes (40%), and other/drug related crimes (42%). Seventy-four percent were involved in the justice system. Sixteen percent had been in jail 14 or more days out of the past 90, 25% had been on probation or parole for 14 or more of the past 90 days with 1 or more drug screens, 8% were in a drug court, and 29% had been arrested and charged with a crime in the past 90 days, been on probation, parole, jail, detention, house arrest, electronic monitoring in the past 90 days, or other current justice involvement. *Thus, the majority of youth clients have recently engaged in illegal activity and had corresponding contact with the justice system.*

Figure 1 shows the number of past year problems endorsed in 16 areas: alcohol problems, cannabis problems, opioid problems, stimulant problems, other drug problems, tobacco problems, mood disorder, anxiety, traumatic distress, suicide, conduct disorder, ADHD, physical health problems, victimization, physical violence, and illegal activities. Most (97%) reported at least one problem, with the majority reporting multiple problems, and 59% reporting five or more problems. *Thus, multiple co-occurring problems are the norm for people entering treatment.*

Table 3 Co-occurring problems by gender, race, age, substance problem, system involvement, and level of care

	Total	Male	Female	African American	White	Hispanic	Mixed/ other	12–17	18–25	Alcohol[i]	Cannabis[i]	Opioids[i]	Stimulants[i]	Other[i]
	16,361	11,904	4,449	2,465	6,090	4,865	2,934	13,989	2,372	4,456	9,680	1,066	1,685	1,183
Total %	100%	73%	27%	15%	37%	30%	18%	86%	15%	32%	66%	8%	12%	9%
Past year psychiatric problems														
Past year internalizing problems														
Any past year internal disorder	41%	34%	**60%**	27%	45%	38%	49%	39%	44%	**56%**	45%	**74%**	**73%**	**72%**
Mood disorder	34%	27%	**53%**	21%	38%	32%	40%	32%	37%	**48%**	38%	**66%**	**65%**	**64%**
Generalized anxiety disorder	12%	9%	**21%**	6%	14%	11%	15%	10%	19%	18%	13%	**32%**	**28%**	**28%**
Suicidal thoughts or actions	19%	17%	25%	14%	21%	16%	24%	19%	16%	**27%**	22%	**31%**	**34%**	**36%**
Traumatic distress disorder[a]	24%	18%	**40%**	16%	26%	22%	31%	23%	29%	**36%**	27%	**51%**	**49%**	**47%**
Past year externalizing problems														
Any past year external disorder	55%	52%	62%	40%	62%	50%	60%	56%	39%	**70%**	62%	**75%**	**76%**	**78%**
Conduct disorder	45%	43%	50%	34%	50%	41%	51%	47%	28%	**60%**	53%	**65%**	**66%**	**70%**
ADHD	38%	35%	47%	25%	46%	33%	44%	39%	29%	**51%**	44%	**58%**	**59%**	**61%**
Pattern of psychiatric problems														
Neither	38%	42%	27%	**52%**	32%	41%	31%	37%	46%	23%	31%	13%	14%	13%
Internalizing only	22%	25%	13%	21%	23%	21%	20%	24%	10%	22%	24%	13%	13%	16%
Externalizing only	8%	7%	11%	8%	7%	9%	8%	7%	**15%**	8%	7%	11%	10%	9%
Both internalizing and externalizing	33%	27%	**49%**	19%	38%	29%	40%	32%	29%	**48%**	38%	**63%**	**63%**	**63%**

(continued)

Table 3 (continued)

	Total	Male	Female	African American	White	Hispanic	Mixed/ other	12–17	18–25	Alcohol[i]	Cannabis[i]	Opioids[i]	Stimulants[i]	Other[i]
Any prior mental health treatment	40%	37%	49%	**27%**	**55%**	**25%**	45%	39%	43%	48%	43%	**66%**	**58%**	**62%**
Physical health problems														
Past 90 day health problems[b]														
Low	53%	56%	43%	**65%**	46%	57%	48%	52%	56%	49%	51%	**37%**	44%	**38%**
Moderate	39%	37%	44%	30%	44%	37%	41%	40%	34%	41%	40%	47%	43%	47%
High	8%	7%	13%	5%	10%	7%	10%	8%	9%	10%	9%	**16%**	13%	**15%**
Any prior physical health treatment	92%	91%	93%	87%	95%	89%	93%	91%	94%	93%	92%	96%	94%	94%
Physical, sexual, or emotional victimization														
Any history of victim. or current worries	62%	61%	64%	**51%**	63%	62%	69%	60%	71%	**75%**	67%	**81%**	**84%**	**81%**
Lifetime history of victimization	61%	60%	63%	**50%**	62%	60%	68%	59%	**70%**	**74%**	66%	**80%**	**83%**	**81%**
High levels of victimization[c]	43%	39%	52%	**32%**	44%	41%	51%	42%	51%	**57%**	47%	**65%**	**70%**	**66%**
Past year	34%	33%	37%	25%	34%	36%	39%	35%	27%	**46%**	39%	**48%**	**52%**	**53%**
Past 90 days	18%	16%	21%	13%	18%	18%	20%	18%	11%	24%	20%	22%	24%	**28%**
Current worry about victimization	16%	14%	23%	12%	14%	18%	20%	16%	17%	22%	18%	23%	**27%**	**26%**
HIV risks														
Any past 90 day needle use	2%	2%	3%	1%	3%	2%	2%	1%	**7%**	2%	2%	**20%**	**7%**	**7%**
Any past 90 day sexual experience	63%	64%	62%	72%	60%	63%	61%	62%	71%	69%	68%	**73%**	69%	72%

Any past 90 day unprotected sex	29%	27%	35%	26%	28%	31%	29%	27%	**42%**	38%	32%	**46%**	**46%**	**45%**
Multiple sexual partners in past 90 days	29%	31%	23%	**39%**	25%	30%	27%	29%	27%	37%	33%	36%	37%	37%
Violence and illegal activity (other than possession/use)														
Any violence or illegal activity	79%	79%	76%	75%	78%	79%	81%	79%	72%	**88%**	84%	**89%**	**89%**	**92%**
Acts of physical violence[d]	65%	66%	63%	64%	62%	66%	70%	67%	**<u>54%</u>**	**76%**	71%	**74%**	**78%**	**84%**
Any illegal activity	62%	65%	56%	57%	63%	64%	63%	63%	**<u>52%</u>**	**73%**	70%	**79%**	**76%**	**81%**
Property crimes[e]	46%	48%	41%	39%	48%	46%	49%	47%	**<u>32%</u>**	**59%**	55%	**67%**	**65%**	**72%**
Violent crimes[f]	40%	43%	32%	39%	37%	42%	44%	43%	**<u>25%</u>**	**52%**	47%	**53%**	**55%**	**64%**
Other/drug related crimes[g]	42%	45%	32%	35%	42%	43%	43%	42%	40%	**55%**	49%	**67%**	**63%**	**68%**
Justice system involvement														
Current justice system involvement	74%	78%	**<u>63%</u>**	75%	72%	77%	71%	73%	81%	77%	75%	80%	78%	78%
Intensity of Justice System Involvement														
In jail 14+ days	16%	18%	11%	20%	12%	17%	18%	14%	**24%**	**24%**	19%	**27%**	**33%**	**24%**
Prob/parole 14+ days	25%	27%	18%	26%	23%	26%	24%	25%	21%	24%	25%	21%	23%	25%
Drug Court	8%	7%	12%	5%	8%	11%	7%	7%	**14%**	7%	7%	**15%**	7%	11%
Other JSI P90[h]	29%	30%	26%	29%	32%	26%	26%	29%	25%	24%	27%	**<u>19%</u>**	**<u>18%</u>**	20%

(continued)

Table 3 (continued)

	In school[j]	In work[j]	In welfare[k]	In jail 14+ days	Prob/ parole 14+ days	Drug court	Other JSI P90[h]	Early intervention	Outpatient (OP)	Intensive outpatient	Residential	Continuing care OP
	13,775	4,027	1,665	2,575	3,999	1,325	4,661	946	11,195	1,558	1,215	1,059
Total %	84%	25%	10%	16%	25%	8%	29%	6%	70%	10%	8%	7%
Past year psychiatric problems												
Past year internalizing problems												
Any past year internal disorder	40%	41%	**54%**	43%	39%	41%	36%	40%	37%	41%	**62%**	49%
Mood disorder	33%	34%	**46%**	36%	32%	34%	29%	33%	31%	35%	**54%**	42%
Generalized anxiety disorder	11%	13%	16%	13%	11%	12%	10%	14%	11%	13%	**21%**	13%
Suicidal thoughts or actions	19%	19%	26%	18%	18%	14%	18%	19%	17%	19%	**30%**	25%
Traumatic distress disorder[a]	23%	25%	**34%**	26%	23%	23%	21%	23%	21%	24%	**39%**	31%
Past year externalizing problems												
Any past year external disorder	56%	53%	**68%**	57%	56%	49%	51%	49%	51%	53%	**74%**	**65%**
Conduct disorder	46%	44%	**59%**	50%	47%	41%	42%	40%	41%	44%	**68%**	55%
ADHD	39%	38%	**50%**	39%	37%	36%	36%	33%	36%	37%	**55%**	47%
Pattern of psychiatric problems												
Neither	37%	38%	**<u>24%</u>**	35%	37%	40%	42%	39%	41%	38%	**<u>19%</u>**	**<u>27%</u>**
Internalizing only	23%	21%	22%	22%	24%	19%	23%	21%	22%	21%	19%	23%
Externalizing only	7%	9%	8%	8%	7%	11%	7%	12%	8%	9%	7%	8%
Both internalizing and externalizing	33%	32%	**46%**	36%	32%	30%	29%	28%	30%	32%	**55%**	42%

Any prior mental health treatment	39%	41%	**61%**	44%	42%	34%	36%	37%	38%	37%	**52%**	**54%**
Physical health problems												
Past 90 day health problems[b]												
Low	52%	50%	52%	59%	50%	57%	52%	**63%**	52%	54%	54%	48%
Moderate	40%	41%	39%	34%	41%	36%	40%	30%	40%	38%	35%	42%
High	8%	9%	9%	7%	9%	7%	8%	6%	8%	8%	11%	10%
Any prior physical health treatment	92%	94%	93%	90%	93%	88%	92%	88%	92%	87%	90%	94%
Physical, sexual, or emotional victimization												
Any history of victim. or current worries	60%	63%	**74%**	**73%**	65%	58%	57%	70%	58%	62%	**76%**	**73%**
Lifetime history of victimization	59%	62%	**73%**	**72%**	64%	57%	56%	69%	57%	61%	**75%**	**73%**
High levels of victimization[c]	41%	44%	**56%**	**53%**	45%	40%	37%	51%	38%	42%	**60%**	**56%**
Past year	34%	34%	40%	39%	36%	33%	31%	35%	31%	35%	**49%**	39%
Past 90 days	18%	19%	18%	15%	18%	16%	17%	16%	17%	17%	25%	15%
Current worry about victimization	16%	16%	20%	16%	15%	16%	15%	19%	15%	15%	21%	19%
HIV risks												
Any past 90 day needle use	1%	3%	2%	2%	2%	5%	2%	3%	2%	2%	5%	2%
Any past 90 day sexual experience	61%	72%	59%	60%	71%	71%	62%	64%	62%	66%	**73%**	59%

(continued)

Table 3 (continued)

	In school[j]	In work[j]	In welfare[k]	In jail 14+ days	Prob/ parole 14+ days	Drug court	Other JSI P90[h]	Early intervention	Outpatient (OP)	Intensive outpatient	Residential	Continuing care OP
Any past 90 day unprotected sex	27%	35%	29%	32%	33%	33%	27%	31%	28%	30%	38%	30%
Multiple sexual partners in past 90 days	28%	31%	29%	30%	34%	28%	27%	26%	27%	31%	**40%**	25%
Violence and illegal activity (other than possession/use)												
Any violence or illegal activity	79%	79%	85%	**89%**	83%	79%	79%	84%	76%	78%	**90%**	81%
Acts of physical violence[d]	65%	61%	**76%**	**78%**	70%	59%	62%	69%	62%	63%	**80%**	74%
Any illegal activity	62%	64%	67%	**74%**	69%	67%	66%	69%	59%	65%	**77%**	63%
Property crimes[e]	47%	45%	55%	**59%**	51%	42%	45%	46%	42%	48%	**63%**	54%
Violent crimes[f]	41%	37%	**51%**	**54%**	46%	36%	38%	45%	36%	41%	**58%**	47%
Other/drug related crimes[g]	41%	47%	45%	51%	45%	50%	45%	50%	37%	43%	**60%**	47%
Justice system involvement												
Current justice system involvement	72%	74%	74%	**98%**	**98%**	**96%**	**92%**	**89%**	69%	**86%**	77%	82%
Intensity of justice system involvement												
In jail 14+ days	14%	11%	24%	**100%**	–	–	–	**32%**	11%	15%	**33%**	**29%**
Prob/parole 14+ days	25%	25%	27%	–	**100%**	–	–	17%	23%	32%	25%	**42%**
Drug court	7%	8%	5%	–	–	**100%**	–	12%	8%	**17%**	**0%**	**1%**
Other JSI P90[h]	29%	33%	22%	–	–	–	**100%**	31%	31%	23%	21%	**16%**

Created by authors, Baumer, Dennis, & Estrada, 2017

Note: Values in **BOLD** indicate that relative to total, column value is significantly different ($p < 0.05$) and clinically higher (Cohen's effect size $d \geq 0.2$)

Values in **<u>BOLD and UNDERLINED</u>** indicate that relative to total, column value is significantly different ($p < 0.05$) and clinically lower (Cohen's effect sizes ≤ -0.2)

[a]Post traumatic distress, acute traumatic distress or disorders of extreme stress not otherwise specified

[b]Average of items (divided by their range) related to being bothered by physical/medical problems including days these problems kept client from meeting his/her responsibilities, and the recency of problems

[c]Reporting 4 or more of the following: types of victimization, traumagenic factors (e.g., multiple people, someone they trusted, fearing for life, sexual penetration, people didn't believe them) or continuing fear it will reoccur)

[d]Physical assault of another person within the past year

[e]Self report of or arrests related to vandalism, forgery, bad checks, shoplifting, theft, robbery, auto theft

[f]Self report of or arrests related to assault, aggravated assault with a weapon, rape, murder, and arson

[g]Self report of or arrests related to driving under the influence, manufacture or distribution, prostitution, gang involvement

[h]Does not meet criteria for in jail 14+ days or probation/parole 14+ days but has been arrested and charged with a crime in the past 90 days, have been on probation, parole, jail, detention, house arrest, or electronic monitoring in the past 90 days, or any current justice involvement in L7

[i]Problem use is defined using the DSM5 definition of mild or more severe substance disorder problems (2+ of 11 symptoms) in the past year or weekly use of the substance

[j]In the past 90 days

[k]Reports days in foster care or a group home, legal custody by the County or State, referred to treatment by social worker or DCFS/welfare, has child in foster care, group or institution

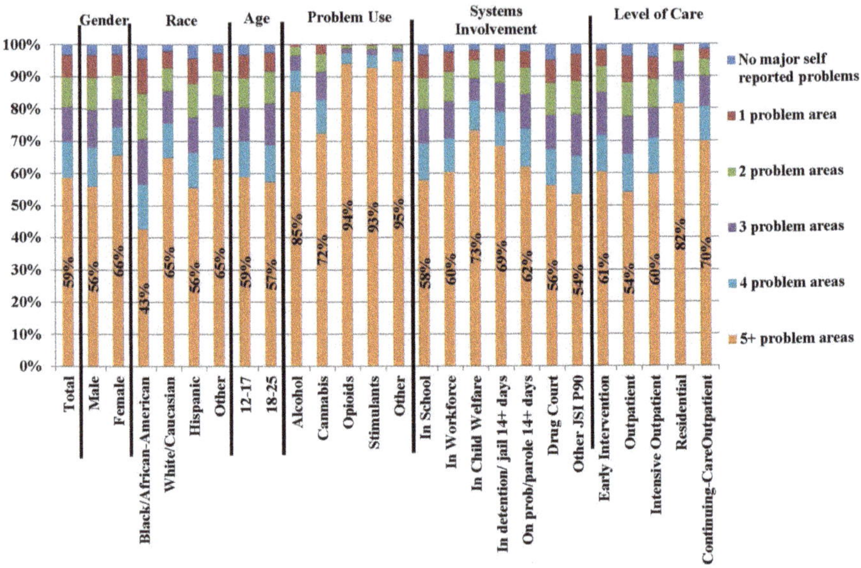

Fig. 1 Number of major clinical problems areas. (Based on a count of self-reported criteria to suggest problem use of alcohol, cannabis, opioids, stimulants, tobacco, or other drugs; depression, avxiety; trauma; suicide; ADHD; conduct disorder; physicaly health problems; victimization; violence; and illegal activity.) Created by authors, Baumer, Dennis, & Estrada, 2017

Treatment received in the first 3 months. The first column of Table 4 summarizes treatment received in the first 3 months after intake. Involvement in substance use treatment as reported by treatment providers included 81% of clients reaching initiation (i.e., entered treatment within 14 days of assessment), 66% engagement, 72% receiving continuing care, and 83% were positively discharged from treatment. While most clients received regular outpatient (OP) treatment (70%), they were receiving other levels of care including early intervention (EI, 6%), intensive outpatient (IOP, 10%), residential (8%), and continuing care outpatient (CC-OP, 7%). Overall, clients were satisfied with their treatment, with 89% reporting high satisfaction at 3 months. Less than one-quarter of clients (21%) attended self-help groups, and the average attendance in days in the past 90 days was 4.2. The average number of days in the past 90 spent in substance treatment was 14.7, including 0.4 days in detox, 4.9 nights in residential treatment, 3.3 days in an intensive outpatient program, 5.6 times in a regular outpatient program, and 0.3 days on medication. *Thus, numerous clients are not staying in treatment.*

Clients also reported days of mental health treatment in the past 90 days (mean 12.4 days), consisting mainly of vising a doctor in an office or clinic (0.8) and days on medication (12.0). In the past 90 days, clients spent an average of 6.8 days receiving physical health treatment. Most of these days were spent either visiting a doctor at an office or clinic (mean 0.7) or on medication (6.1 days). On average, clients spent

Table 4 Treatment received at 3 months by gender, race, age, substance problem, system involvement, and level of care

	Total	Male	Female	African American	White	Hispanic	Mixed/ other	12–17	18–25	Alcohol[g]	Cannabis[g]	Opioids[g]	Stimulants[g]	Other[g]
	16,361	11,904	4,449	2,465	6,090	4,865	2,934	13,989	2,372	4,456	9,680	1,066	1,685	1,183
Total %	100%	73%	27%	15%	37%	30%	18%	86%	15%	32%	66%	8%	12%	9%
Substance use disorder treatment														
System involvement														
Initiation[a]	81%	80%	82%	81%	80%	82%	82%	81%	85%	82%	80%	85%	86%	81%
Engaged[b]	66%	67%	64%	58%	70%	66%	65%	69%	62%	67%	68%	68%	65%	68%
Continuing care[c]	72%	72%	72%	72%	68%	75%	74%	64%	**83%**	75%	73%	**81%**	76%	78%
Positive system discharge status[d]	83%	83%	83%	77%	85%	85%	81%	79%	81%	80%	81%	81%	78%	84%
Level of care														
Early intervention	6%	6%	6%	7%	4%	8%	6%	5%	**13%**	7%	6%	6%	9%	6%
Outpatient	70%	70%	71%	63%	75%	70%	66%	72%	61%	62%	68%	**59%**	**47%**	**59%**
Intensive outpatient	10%	10%	10%	12%	8%	12%	8%	10%	10%	10%	10%	11%	11%	11%
Residential	8%	8%	7%	11%	6%	5%	13%	8%	6%	12%	10%	13%	**20%**	**14%**
CC-OP	7%	7%	6%	8%	7%	5%	7%	6%	9%	9%	7%	12%	**13%**	11%
Alliance														
Mean treatment satisfaction at 3 months	12.46	12.46	12.47	12.15	12.32	12.96	12.20	12.40	12.86	12.18	12.30	12.23	**11.66**	12.13
High satisfaction at 3 months[e]	89%	90%	89%	86%	89%	93%	88%	89%	93%	88%	88%	88%	84%	87%

(continued)

Table 4 (continued)

	Total	Male	Female	African American	White	Hispanic	Mixed/ other	12–17	18–25	Alcohol[g]	Cannabis[g]	Opioids[g]	Stimulants[g]	Other[g]
Type of treatment received (mean)														
Direct service at 3 months	4.62	4.62	4.62	4.16	4.87	4.62	4.48	4.62	4.58	4.76	4.72	4.93	4.69	4.84
Family services at 3 months	1.28	1.33	1.17	1.15	1.21	1.50	1.19	1.34	**0.93**	1.31	1.37	1.39	1.39	1.53
External services at 3 months	3.30	3.37	3.13	3.20	3.22	3.51	3.22	3.29	3.39	3.47	3.44	3.68	3.53	3.64
Total SUD treatment services at 3 months	9.21	9.32	8.93	8.51	9.30	9.63	8.89	9.26	8.90	9.55	9.53	10.00	9.61	10.00
Mean days attended Self-Help groups	4.18	3.67	5.55	3.16	5.90	2.06	4.99	3.26	**9.66**	6.15	4.71	**14.38**	**11.56**	**10.09**
Any self-help group attendance	21%	19%	26%	17%	26%	14%	25%	18%	**35%**	**30%**	24%	**53%**	**48%**	**41%**
Mean days in any SUD treatment	14.67	14.81	14.29	16.30	14.54	12.96	16.37	14.26	17.05	17.84	16.49	**24.32**	**22.34**	**21.43**
How many days in detox	0.35	0.35	0.35	0.48	0.36	0.24	0.42	0.32	0.55	0.41	0.44	0.78	0.67	0.48
Times in ER for AOD	0.02	0.01	0.04	0.00	0.04	0.01	0.01	0.01	0.06	0.02	0.01	0.06	0.03	0.04
Nights in residential for AOD use	4.89	5.05	4.46	6.11	4.46	3.38	7.21	4.71	5.94	7.17	6.03	**10.14**	**12.04**	**9.54**
Days in Intensive outpatient program	3.31	3.48	2.89	5.35	2.86	3.02	3.05	3.45	2.53	3.50	3.85	4.35	3.50	4.28

Times in regular outpatient program	5.62	5.50	5.93	4.31	6.26	5.92	4.88	5.39	6.98	5.84	5.74	6.81	5.08	6.17
Days on medication	0.27	0.23	0.39	0.00	0.51	0.09	0.29	0.03	**1.68**	0.25	0.16	**3.09**	0.47	0.57
Other treatment services														
Mean days in mental health treatment	12.35	10.73	16.66	6.37	**18.85**	**5.34**	15.42	12.64	10.62	15.15	13.04	**23.97**	**20.48**	**22.11**
Nights spent in MH hospital	0.11	0.09	0.15	0.05	0.15	0.05	0.16	0.12	0.03	0.15	0.10	0.07	0.18	0.15
Times gone to MH emergency room	0.02	0.01	0.03	0.01	0.02	0.01	0.02	0.02	0.01	0.02	0.02	0.02	0.03	0.02
Times seen MD in office or clinic	0.83	0.63	1.35	0.43	1.19	0.41	1.11	0.87	0.58	1.07	0.93	1.52	**1.56**	**1.72**
Days on medication	11.99	10.47	16.03	6.19	**18.35**	**5.09**	15.01	12.25	10.44	14.63	12.64	**23.54**	**19.87**	**21.57**
Mean days in physical health treatment	6.79	5.81	9.42	5.21	9.09	4.23	7.59	6.79	6.80	7.98	6.90	9.82	8.84	9.87
PH inpatient hospital day	0.05	0.04	0.08	0.08	0.05	0.04	0.07	0.05	0.11	0.05	0.05	0.13	0.06	0.12
PH emergency room visit	0.12	0.10	0.18	0.11	0.13	0.09	0.15	0.11	0.16	0.14	0.12	0.18	0.18	0.15
PH outpatient clinic/doctor's office visit	0.72	0.58	1.12	0.54	0.93	0.50	0.81	0.74	0.66	0.91	0.77	1.15	1.14	1.11
Days on medication	6.06	5.22	8.30	4.62	8.20	3.67	6.77	6.07	6.00	7.06	6.15	8.63	7.71	8.88

(continued)

Table 4 (continued)

	Total	Male	Female	African American	White	Hispanic	Mixed/ other	12–17	18–25	Alcohol[g]	Cannabis[g]	Opioids[g]	Stimulants[g]	Other[g]
Surgical procedures	0.02	0.02	0.02	0.01	0.03	0.02	0.02	0.02	0.03	0.02	0.02	0.04	0.03	0.03
Other system involvement														
Mean days involved in justice system	51.30	55.30	**40.59**	55.78	45.92	56.48	50.18	50.75	54.58	54.81	53.38	56.64	58.39	54.55
Mean days in a controlled environment[f]	14.71	15.32	13.06	**21.68**	12.49	12.03	17.89	14.16	17.94	18.37	16.95	**25.06**	**28.49**	**22.52**

	In school[h]	In work[h]	In welfare[i]	In jail 14+ days	Prob/ parole 14+ days	Drug court	Other JSI P90[j]	Early intervention	Outpatient (OP)	Intensive outpatient	Residential	Continuing care OP
	13,775	4,027	1,665	2,575	3,999	1,325	4,661	946	11,195	1,558	1,215	1,059
Total %	84%	25%	10%	16%	25%	8%	29%	6%	70%	10	8	7
Substance use disorder treatment												
Sytsemt involvement												
Initiation[a]	80%	81%	80%	85%	80%	76%	81%	**97%**	76%	87%	**89%**	**92%**
Engaged[b]	67%	67%	69%	64%	68%	58%	68%	61%	69%	65%	**55%**	62%
Continuing care[c]	70%	69%	76%	76%	77%	**84%**	66%	73%	69%	**82%**	75%	**83%**
Positive system discharge status[d]	84%	84%	82%	**75%**	83%	83%	87%	86%	85%	79%	76%	76%
Level of care												
Early intervention	4%	7%	4%	**12%**	4%	9%	6%	**100%**	–	–	–	–
Outpatient	73%	75%	**60%**	**49%**	64%	69%	76%	–	**100%**	–	–	–
Intensive outpatient	9%	8%	8%	10%	12%	**21%**	8%	–	–	**100%**	–	–

Residential	7%	7%	**14%**	**17%**	8%	**0%**	6%	–	–	–	**100%**	–
CC-OP	7%	5%	**14%**	**13%**	11%	**1%**	4%	–	–	–	–	**100%**
Alliance												
Mean treatment satisfaction at 3 months	12.43	12.45	**11.70**	12.03	12.23	**13.30**	12.56	12.74	13.03	12.71	**9.66**	**10.28**
High satisfaction at 3 months[e]	89%	90%	83%	85%	88%	**95%**	91%	92%	94%	90%	**67%**	**72%**
Type of treatment received (mean)												
Direct service at 3 months	4.64	4.74	4.62	4.47	4.73	4.60	4.70	**3.99**	4.65	4.65	4.60	4.62
Family services at 3 months	1.31	1.17	1.37	1.32	1.38	1.46	1.22	1.08	1.23	1.38	1.47	1.52
External services at 3 months	3.28	3.18	3.35	3.67	**3.86**	3.77	3.16	3.04	3.21	3.81	3.27	3.69
Total SUD treatment services at 3 months	9.24	9.09	9.34	9.46	9.97	9.83	9.09	8.11	9.11	9.85	9.34	9.83
Mean days attended self-help groups	3.27	5.00	6.15	6.36	4.22	**9.76**	2.66	**8.68**	1.94	6.10	**16.93**	6.38
Any self-help group attendance	18%	23%	**32%**	**32%**	22%	**39%**	15%	**43%**	**11%**	**30%**	**66%**	**37%**
Mean days in any SUD treatment	13.84	13.61	18.71	**21.49**	15.91	17.00	12.29	15.53	**8.86**	**26.35**	**42.53**	**22.67**
How many days in detox	0.30	0.36	0.46	0.27	0.50	0.68	0.23	0.38	0.17	0.34	**2.14**	0.22

(continued)

Table 4 (continued)

	In school[h]	In work[h]	In welfare[i]	In jail 14+ days	Prob/ parole 14+ days	Drug court	Other JSI P90[j]	Early intervention	Outpatient (OP)	Intensive outpatient	Residential	Continuing care OP
Times in ER for AOD	0.01	0.02	0.02	0.01	0.02	0.09	0.01	0.01	0.02	0.02	0.01	0.02
Nights in residential for AOD use	4.37	4.19	**8.80**	**10.91**	4.94	3.52	3.43	5.29	**1.18**	3.41	**36.18**	6.79
Days in intensive outpatient program	3.23	2.41	3.04	4.76	4.61	2.99	2.80	2.46	0.80	**18.82**	4.43	**7.96**
Times in regular outpatient program	5.51	6.00	5.58	4.73	5.57	**8.78**	5.51	4.75	6.44	**3.80**	**1.27**	5.82
Days on medication	0.10	0.49	0.07	0.11	0.08	**2.00**	0.13	0.31	0.32	0.06	0.22	0.10
Other treatment services												
Mean days in mental health treatment	12.37	12.12	**24.35**	14.98	12.83	9.32	9.96	9.89	10.61	12.00	**22.11**	17.10
Nights spent in MH hospital	0.11	0.08	0.26	0.05	0.13	0.02	0.10	0.08	0.09	0.09	0.25	0.18
Times gone to MH emergency room	0.02	0.01	0.03	0.01	0.02	0.02	0.02	0.01	0.02	0.01	0.02	0.02
Times seen MD in office or clinic	0.83	0.78	**2.22**	0.93	0.83	0.43	0.73	0.57	0.77	0.91	1.36	0.88
Days on medication	12.02	11.80	**23.34**	14.58	12.49	9.09	9.59	9.53	10.28	11.74	**21.52**	16.69
Mean days in physical health treatment	6.82	7.66	9.26	6.60	6.57	7.54	6.27	6.55	6.40	6.53	**11.36**	5.88
PH inpatient hospital day	0.05	0.04	0.05	0.06	0.04	0.12	0.05	0.09	0.05	0.04	0.06	0.03

PH emergency room visit	0.11	0.12	0.17	0.12	0.13	0.16	0.11	0.12	0.12	0.10	0.18	0.11
PH outpatient clinic/doctor's office visit	0.74	0.80	1.13	0.85	0.65	0.78	0.68	0.57	0.65	0.63	**1.46**	0.79
Days on medication	6.09	6.84	8.31	5.81	5.87	6.73	5.59	5.89	5.72	5.91	**10.12**	5.02
Surgical procedures	0.02	0.03	0.03	0.02	0.02	0.02	0.02	0.02	0.02	0.02	0.02	0.02
Other system involvement												
Mean days involved in justice system	49.67	47.03	54.45	**81.54**	**79.10**	**62.70**	45.06	58.38	46.56	**65.54**	57.65	**63.67**
Mean days in a controlled environment[f]	13.60	10.87	**27.93**	**33.79**	14.01	10.22	11.78	**21.54**	**<u>8.18</u>**	13.50	**60.31**	**23.74**

Created by authors, Baumer, Dennis, & Estrada, 2017

Note: Values in **BOLD** indicate that relative to total column value is significantly different (p <0.05) and clinically higher (Cohen's effect size $d \geq 0.2$)

Values in **BOLD and UNDERLINED** indicate that relative to total, column value is significantly different ($p < 0.05$) and clinically lower Cohen's effect size ≤−0.2)

[a]Entered treatment in under 14 days from assessment

[b]In treatment for 30 days and 3 sessions

[c]Treatment 90–180 days post admission

[d]Still in treatment, completed and discharged to the community, transferred for further SA or MH tx

[e]Treatment Satisfaction Scale at 3 months >9

[f]Day in a hospital, treatment, detention, or jail (where not free to come and go as you please)

[g]Problem use is defined using the DSM5 definition of mild or more severe substance disorder problems (2+ of 11 symptoms) in the past year or weekly use of the substance

[h]In the past 90 days

[i]Reports days in foster care or a group home, legal custody by the County or State, referred to treatment by social worker or DCFS/welfare, has child in foster care, group or institution

[j]Does not meet criteria for in jail 14+ days or probation/parole 14+ days but has been arrested and charged with a crime in the past 90 days, have been on probation, parole, jail, detention, house arrest, or electronic monitoring in the past 90 days, or any current justice involvement in L7

51.3 days involved in the justice system (parole, probation, prison/jail, detention, house arrest, or electronic monitoring), and an average of 14.7 days in any controlled environment where they were not free to come and go as they pleased. *Thus clients continued to be involved in multiple systems of care during their SUD treatment.*

National outcome measures: positive outcomes at intake and 6 months. The first column of Table 5 gives NOMS measures at baseline and 6 month follow-up, as well as a count of the number of positive outcomes at each time and the change in the count (6 month count minus intake count). In the 90 days *prior to intake* to treatment, very few clients were free of substance use problems (20%), emotional problems (11%), or social support problems (1%). Almost no clients (4%) had zero costs to society estimated based on reported use of tangible services as well as days of problems multiplied by unit costs as reported by McCollister et al. (2017). Alternatively, the majority of clients were free of past 90-day problems with nights in a psychiatric inpatient unit (98%), illegal activity (61%), arrests (78%), housing (50%), and vocational problems (79%). Overall, only 44% of clients had no substance problems in the past month, 33% had no health problems in the past 90 days, 41% had no family problems, 36% had no trouble at work or school, and 40% had no recovery environment risk. The average number of these positive measures at intake was 5.9. *Thus, there is significant variation in pervasiveness of problems at intake to treatment, with some nearly omnipresent (e.g., social support problems) and others almost never seen (e.g., nights in psychiatric inpatient).*

At *6 months after intake* to treatment, there was improvement compared to intake across all outcomes. There were very few clients who reported no or reduced problems with social support in the past 90 days (10%). Most clients reported no or reduced problems by 50% or more for substance use (68%), past month substance problems (77%), nights in psychiatric outpatient (99%), illegal activity (79%), arrests (91%), housing (73%), family (71%), recovery environment risk (52%), and vocational problems (90%). Forty-five percent of clients reported no cost to society or reduction in cost to society of 50% or more. There were also improvements in health problems (38%), emotional problems (42%), and trouble at work or school (48%). The mean count of positive outcomes at 6 months was 8.74, an increase of nearly three positive outcomes on average. *Thus, 6 months after entering treatment, youth experienced improvement across life domains, al though more so in some areas (e.g., substance problems) than others (e.g., emotional problems).*

Variation by Demographic Groups

Gender (n = 11,904 males and 4,449 females). As shown in Tables 1, 2, 3, 4, and 5, females were significantly more likely than males to report being GLBTQ (16%) and ever being homeless or runaway (46%). They were also less likely to report problem marijuana use (55%). Females were more likely to experience any internalizing disorder (60%), particularly mood disorders (53%), generalized anxiety (21%), and traumatic distress (40%). They were also more likely to report having

Table 5 National Outcome Measurement System (NOMS) positive outcomes at intake and 6 months by gender, race, age, substance problem, system involvement, and level of care

	Total	Male	Female	African American	White	Hispanic	Mixed/ other	12–17	18–25	Alcohol[c]	Cannabis[c]	Opioids[c]	Stimulants[c]	Other[c]
	16,361	11,904	4,449	2,465	6,090	4,865	2,934	13,989	2,372	4,456	9,680	1,066	1,685	1,183
Total %	100%	73%	27%	15%	37%	30%	18%	86%	15%	32%	66%	8%	12%	9%
NOMS positive outcomes: problems in past 90 days at intake														
No substance use	20%	20%	21%	23%	18%	20%	23%	18%	**33%**	19%	13%	20%	26%	20%
No substance problems (past month)	44%	45%	44%	49%	43%	44%	46%	43%	**56%**	36%	**33%**	38%	43%	**34%**
No health problems	33%	35%	29%	40%	29%	35%	31%	34%	25%	29%	32%	**18%**	25%	**22%**
No emotional problems	11%	12%	9%	17%	9%	13%	8%	12%	9%	6%	9%	**2%**	**3%**	**3%**
No nights in psychiatric inpatient unit	98%	98%	96%	99%	97%	99%	97%	98%	99%	96%	97%	95%	95%	94%
No illegal activity	61%	60%	65%	66%	60%	61%	60%	59%	**72%**	52%	55%	52%	53%	**45%**
No arrests	78%	77%	82%	78%	81%	77%	80%	77%	84%	77%	75%	71%	76%	73%
No housing problems (housed in the community)	50%	49%	52%	42%	53%	51%	47%	53%	**32%**	**36%**	44%	**21%**	**20%**	**25%**
No family problems	41%	43%	36%	**55%**	33%	44%	40%	36%	**68%**	39%	37%	42%	45%	38%
No trouble at school or work	36%	37%	34%	43%	32%	38%	34%	30%	**68%**	39%	34%	**51%**	**48%**	41%
No social support/ engagement problems	1%	1%	1%	2%	1%	1%	1%	1%	4%	1%	1%	1%	2%	1%
No recovery environment risk	40%	43%	32%	48%	35%	45%	37%	39%	49%	31%	34%	**29%**	33%	**25%**
No costs to society[a]	4%	5%	4%	6%	3%	5%	4%	4%	5%	3%	3%	2%	2%	1%

(continued)

Table 5 (continued)

	Total	Male	Female	African American	White	Hispanic	Mixed/ other	12–17	18–25	Alcohol[c]	Cannabis[c]	Opioids[c]	Stimulants[c]	Other[c]
No vocational problems (in work or school)	79%	78%	81%	75%	80%	78%	80%	84%	**46%**	74%	77%	**56%**	**62%**	**67%**
Summary count of positive outcomes	5.92	5.97	5.82	**6.40**	5.66	6.07	5.83	5.84	**6.44**	**5.33**	**5.41**	**4.94**	**5.29**	**4.86**
S.D.	2.178	2.175	2.182	2.159	2.089	2.254	2.159	2.155	2.170	2.098	2.024	2.081	2.182	2.050
Problems in the past 90 days at 6 months[b]														
No substance use or use reduced 50% or more	68%	66%	72%	71%	67%	67%	68%	67%	69%	66%	67%	69%	68%	69%
No substance problems (past month) or problems reduced 50% or more	77%	76%	80%	81%	77%	77%	76%	76%	82%	73%	74%	75%	74%	74%
No health problems or problems reduced 50% or more	38%	39%	36%	44%	36%	38%	37%	39%	36%	34%	37%	34%	32%	36%
No emotional problems or problems reduced 50% or more	42%	42%	42%	45%	39%	45%	40%	42%	43%	39%	40%	36%	38%	38%
No nights in psychiatric inpatient unit or at least 50% fewer nights	99%	99%	99%	99%	99%	100%	99%	99%	99%	99%	99%	98%	99%	99%
No illegal activity or illegal activity reduced 50% or more	79%	78%	84%	81%	78%	81%	78%	78%	86%	76%	76%	76%	76%	74%

No arrests or at least 50% fewer arrests	91%	90%	94%	91%	92%	90%	90%	90%	93%	88%	89%	88%	87%	88%
No housing problems (housed in the community) or problems reduced 50% or more	73%	72%	75%	65%	74%	78%	70%	73%	72%	70%	70%	**<u>63%</u>**	65%	65%
No family problems or problems reduced 50% or more	71%	71%	71%	78%	69%	71%	70%	69%	**86%**	70%	70%	75%	70%	70%
No trouble at school or work or trouble reduced 50% or more	48%	48%	46%	52%	44%	51%	46%	43%	**73%**	49%	47%	**62%**	55%	53%
No social support/ engagement problems or problems reduced 50% or more	10%	10%	12%	8%	11%	10%	13%	10%	11%	14%	12%	**17%**	**20%**	**17%**
No recovery environment risk or problems reduced 50% or more	52%	54%	47%	60%	48%	56%	49%	50%	**63%**	44%	48%	46%	44%	**<u>41%</u>**
No costs to society or costs reduced 50% or more[a]	45%	45%	46%	39%	47%	46%	46%	45%	49%	48%	45%	49%	47%	48%
No vocational problems (in work/ school) or problems reduced 50% or more	90%	90%	92%	87%	91%	91%	91%	91%	89%	90%	90%	87%	88%	88%

Table 5 (continued)

	Total	Male	Female	African American	White	Hispanic	Mixed/other	12–17	18–25	Alcohol[c]	Cannabis[c]	Opioids[c]	Stimulants[c]	Other[c]
Summary count of positive outcomes	8.74	8.70	8.87	8.91	8.61	8.91	8.61	8.63	**9.40**	8.51	8.54	8.66	8.55	8.48
S.D.	2.373	2.385	2.335	2.278	2.361	2.378	2.440	2.407	2.180	2.443	2.417	2.525	2.454	2.506
Change in summary count of positive outcomes (6 months–intake)	2.82	2.73	3.06	2.51	2.95	2.83	2.78	2.80	2.95	3.18	3.14	**3.72**	3.26	**3.62**
S.D.	2.965	2.988	2.889	2.861	2.931	3.042	2.977	2.955	2.896	3.053	3.001	3.236	3.176	3.229

	In School[d]	In Work[d]	In Welfare[e]	In jail 14+ days	Prob/parole 14+ days	Drug Court	Other JSI P90[f]	Early Intervention	Outpatient (OP)	Intensive Outpatient	Residential	Continuing Care OP
	13,775	4,027	1,665	2,575	3,999	1,325	4,661	946	11,195	1,558	1,215	1,059
Total %	84%	25%	10%	16%	25%	8%	29%	6%	70%	10%	8%	7%
NOMS positive outcomes: problems in past 90 days at intake												
No substance use	20%	14%	**32%**	**38%**	21%	16%	16%	**29%**	17%	24%	15%	**50%**
No substance problems (past month)	44%	40%	**54%**	**63%**	47%	44%	42%	52%	43%	44%	**32%**	**65%**
No health problems	33%	32%	33%	33%	30%	38%	33%	37%	33%	34%	36%	27%
No emotional problems	11%	11%	**6%**	9%	10%	14%	13%	11%	12%	12%	**6%**	**6%**
No nights in psychiatric inpatient unit	98%	98%	94%	98%	98%	99%	98%	98%	98%	98%	95%	98%
No illegal activity	61%	58%	63%	60%	59%	64%	57%	61%	63%	62%	**45%**	69%
No arrests	79%	77%	82%	**67%**	78%	**65%**	71%	76%	80%	78%	**68%**	**86%**

No housing problems (housed in the community)	53%	56%	**17%**	**0%**	49%	41%	58%	**28%**	59%	42%	**26%**	**16%**
No family problems	37%	37%	42%	**59%**	43%	48%	36%	**52%**	39%	47%	35%	**57%**
No trouble at school or work	**27%**	28%	40%	**56%**	36%	39%	33%	**53%**	32%	43%	39%	**48%**
No social support/ engagement problems	1%	1%	2%	2%	1%	1%	1%	1%	1%	1%	1%	**7%**
No recovery environment risk	39%	38%	38%	46%	39%	43%	41%	46%	41%	42%	**26%**	48%
No costs to society[a]	4%	4%	3%	**0%**	**0%**	3%	5%	5%	5%	3%	2%	2%
No vocational problems (in work or school)	86%	84%	79%	**55%**	81%	77%	82%	**56%**	83%	77%	75%	**68%**
Summary count of positive outcomes	5.88	5.74	5.94	5.82	5.89	5.87	5.83	6.01	6.01	6.02	**4.94**	**6.44**
S.D.	2.161	2.162	2.193	2.286	2.157	2.286	2.204	2.242	2.105	2.256	2.104	2.360
Problems in the past 90 days at 6 months[b]												
No substance use or use reduced 50% or more	67%	67%	67%	66%	65%	**79%**	68%	69%	67%	71%	**78%**	63%
No substance problems (past month) or problems reduced 50% or more	77%	77%	78%	76%	77%	82%	78%	78%	77%	80%	80%	76%
No health problems or problems reduced 50% or more	39%	38%	36%	36%	37%	38%	39%	34%	39%	43%	37%	36%
No emotional problems or problems reduced 50% or more	42%	44%	35%	36%	42%	44%	44%	45%	43%	42%	33%	38%

(continued)

Table 5 (continued)

	In School[d]	In Work[d]	In Welfare[e]	In jail 14+ days	Prob/ parole 14+ days	Drug Court	Other JSI P90[f]	Early Intervention	Outpatient (OP)	Intensive Outpatient	Residential	Continuing Care OP
No nights in psychiatric inpatient unit or at least 50% fewer nights	99%	99%	98%	99%	99%	100%	99%	99%	99%	100%	98%	99%
No illegal activity or illegal activity reduced 50% or more	79%	80%	76%	76%	78%	83%	80%	80%	80%	79%	78%	76%
No arrests or at least 50% fewer arrests	91%	92%	91%	85%	88%	91%	92%	89%	92%	91%	89%	88%
No housing problems (housed in the community) or problems reduced 50% or more	74%	77%	**<u>62%</u>**	**<u>59%</u>**	71%	73%	75%	71%	77%	71%	**<u>47%</u>**	68%
No family problems or problems reduced 50% or more	69%	73%	66%	72%	71%	74%	71%	72%	71%	74%	75%	64%
No trouble at school or work or trouble reduced 50% or more	44%	47%	44%	**58%**	48%	51%	46%	56%	46%	52%	49%	50%
No social support/ engagement problems or problems reduced 50% or more	10%	10%	15%	15%	11%	13%	9%	13%	8%	12%	**26%**	13%
No recovery environment risk or problems reduced 50% or more	51%	52%	46%	51%	52%	55%	54%	58%	53%	57%	49%	45%

No costs to society or costs reduced 50% or more[a]	45%	47%	47%	49%	44%	43%	47%	48%	44%	42%	42%	**61%**
No vocational problems (in work/school) or problems reduced 50% or more	91%	93%	89%	**<u>81%</u>**	91%	91%	91%	**<u>83%</u>**	91%	92%	91%	85%
Summary count of positive outcomes	8.68	8.86	8.38	8.48	8.64	9.03	8.81	8.84	8.77	8.95	8.64	8.55
S.D.	2.384	2.319	2.287	2.495	2.395	2.426	2.295	2.476	2.346	2.423	2.317	2.492
Change in summary count of positive outcomes (6 months–intake)	2.80	3.12	2.59	2.66	2.75	3.16	2.98	2.84	2.76	2.93	**3.69**	**<u>2.11</u>**
S.D.	2.959	2.975	3.001	3.179	3.036	2.889	2.963	3.368	2.920	2.904	3.003	2.925

Created by authors, Baumer, Dennis, & Estrada, 2017

NOTE: Values in **BOLD** indicate that relative to total, column value is significantly different ($p < 0.05$) and clinically higher (Cohen's effect size $d \geq 0.2$)

Values in **<u>BOLD and UNDERLINED</u>** indicate that relative to total, column value is significantly different ($p < 0.05$) and clinically lower (Cohen's effect size ≤ -0.2)

Higher values in this table represent fewer people with problems (i.e., higher values are better outcomes)

[c]Problem use is defined using the DSM5 definition of mild or more severe substance disorder problems (2+ of 11 symptoms) in the past year or weekly use of the substance

[a]Overall quarterly cost to society is a measure of the economics of substance use treatment and consquences. It is calculated by multiplying the frequency of using tangible services (e.g., health care utilization; days in detention, on probation, on parole) in the past 90 days and days of problems (e.g., days of missed school, days bothered by health problems or days bothered by psychiatric problems) in the past 90 days by the unit cost as estimated by McCollister et al. (2017)

[b]Outcomes from the follow-up interview at 6 months after intake

[d]In the past 90 days

[e]Reports days in foster care or a group home, legal custody by the County or State, referred to treatment by social worker or DCFS/welfare, has child in foster care, group or institution

[f]Does not meet criteria for in jail 14+ days or probation/parole 14+ days but has been arrested and charged with a crime in the past 90 days, have been on probation, parole, jail, detention, house arrest, or electronic monitoring in the past 90 days, or any current justice involvement in L7

both internalizing and externalizing disorders concurrently (49%), and relatedly less likely to report having only internalizing problems (13%) or neither type of psychiatric problem (27%). Finally, females had fewer problems with the justice system; they were less likely to be currently involved in the justice system (63%), and had spent fewer days involved in the justice system at 3 months (mean of 40.6). Females were more likely to report five or more co-occurring problems at intake (Odds Ratio (OR) = 1.35). The number of NOMS positive outcomes at intake, 6 months, and rates of change were similar. *Thus, female clients tend to be more severe on average at intake to treatment, but reported different issues (more mental health, less illegal activity) than do male clients.*

Race (n = 2,465 African American, 6,090 Caucasian, 4,865 Hispanic, and 2,934 mixed/other). In Table 1, African American clients were less likely than the average across race to be female (17%) and were the least likely of all race groups to experience numerous problems with substance use by those around them, including weekly alcohol use in the home (14%), weekly alcohol use by peers at work or school (27%) or socially (35%), and past 90-day drug use by peers at work or school (42%). They were also the least likely to be employed (15%). Table 2 shows that African Americans were less likely to report symptoms of lifetime substance dependence (DSM-IV; 39%) or lifetime severe substance problems (27%), and more likely to report only lifetime use (24% with DSM-IV and 33% with DSM-5 definition). African Americans are the least likely to report problem use of alcohol (20%), opioids (1%), stimulants (3%) and other drugs (2%). African American youth were significantly less likely to have problem use of tobacco (52%), tobacco dependence (8%), and more likely to report no days of tobacco use in the past 90 days (45%). Hispanic clients were also less likely to report past year problem use of tobacco (51%), while Caucasians are significantly more likely to report tobacco problem use (80%), weekly tobacco use (62%), and less likely to report no days of tobacco use in the past 90 (24%). African American clients were less likely to have experienced any lifetime withdrawal (24%), two or more prior substance use treatment episodes (8%), and to perceive their substance use as a problem (12%).

In Table 3, African Americans were significantly different on many co-occurring problems. They are significantly less likely to report any internalizing disorder (27%), including mood disorder (21%), generalized anxiety disorder (6%), and traumatic distress disorder (16%). They are less likely to have any externalizing disorder (40%), including conduct disorder (34%) and ADHD (25%). African Americans are the most likely to report no psychiatric problems (52%), and least likely to report having both internalizing and externalizing problems (19%). Along with Hispanics, African Americans were less likely than average to have received any prior mental health treatment (25% and 27%, respectively), while Caucasians were more likely than average to have received prior mental health treatment (55%). African Americans were significantly more likely to have low levels of physical health problems (65%), a lifetime history of victimization (50%), or high levels of victimization (32%). They were more likely to have had multiple sexual partners in the past 90 days (39%). Figure 1 shows that African Americans were less likely than the total of all clients to report five or more co-occurring problems at intake (OR = 0.52).

Unsurprisingly, given their reporting of fewer mental health problems and less previous mental health treatment, African Americans also reported fewer mean days of mental health treatment received at 3 months after intake (6.4), as did Hispanics (5.3), while Caucasians received significantly more days of treatment (18.9), primarily due to more days on medication for mental health problems (18.4). Hispanics reported significantly fewer, with only 5.1 days taking medication. African Americans experienced an average of 21.7 days in a controlled environment, significantly higher than the average. In the 90 days prior to entering treatment, African Americans were more likely to report having no family problems (55%) and reported more criteria for more positive outcomes on average (6.4). At 6 months after intake, there were no significant differences in NOMS by race.

Age (n = 13,989 adolescents ages 12–17 and 2,372 young adults ages 18–25). Young adults were more likely than adolescents to be married (7%) and employed (38%), but less likely than average to be in school (43%) or involved in the welfare system (2%). They were also less likely to experience substance problems with peers, including alcohol use with peers at work or school (25%) and drug use with peers at work or school (27%) or socially (50%). Table 2 shows that young adults were more likely to have started using at age 15 or older (35%) and to have used for 5 or more years (71%). They were more likely than average to report criteria of dependence (DSM-IV; 69%) and severe substance problems (DSM-5; 63%), but less likely to report abuse criteria (DSM-IV; 19%). They are more likely to report problem use of alcohol (43%), opioids (22%), stimulants (22%), and tobacco (75%). Young adults were more likely to report no days using AOD in the past 90 days (33%), but more likely to report weekly use of tobacco (59%). This may be related to spending 13 or more days of the past 90 in a controlled environment (45%). They report more prior substance treatment (49%), reported more need for treatment (81%), and perceive their substance use as a problem (34%). Table 3 shows that young adults were less likely to experience any externalizing disorder (39%), including conduct disorder (28%) and ADHD (29%), but are more likely to experience only externalizing disorders (15%), and less likely to experience only internalizing disorders (10%). They are more likely to report a lifetime history of victimization (70%), past 90-day needle use (7%), and unprotected sex in the past 90 days (42%). Young adults reported fewer problems with illegal activity and violence, including fewer reporting past year physical violence (54%), any illegal activity (52%), property crimes (32%), and violent crimes (25%). In terms of justice system involvement in the past 90 days, young adults were more likely to have been in jail 14 or more days (24%) or be in drug court (14%). Despite differences, Fig. 1 shows that there was no significant difference in the number of co-occurring problems reported by age. *Thus, severity and mix of clinical conditions shift with age.*

Regarding substance use treatment, Table 4 shows that young adults were more likely than adolescents to receive continuing care (83%) and be assigned to EI services (13%). They were more likely to attend self-help (35%) and received more days of self-help (mean 9.7). They spent more days of the past 90 on medication for the treatment of substance use problems (1.68). Table 5, shows that young adults reported significantly fewer problems at intake to treatment, including being more likely to have no substance use (33%), no past month substance problems (56%), no illegal activity (72%), no family problems (68%), and no trouble at work or school (68%). They were however less likely to be housed in the community (32%), which coincides with their reports of spending more time in a controlled environment at intake, and less likely to be in work or school (46%). On average, young adults met 6.4 positive outcomes at intake, significantly more than average. There were fewer differences at 6 months after intake to treatment, but young adults were more likely to report no or reduced problems by 50% or more with family (88%), work or school (76%), and recovery environment risk (64%). Young adults continued to meet more than the average number of positive outcomes at follow-up (9.6), and the rates of change were similar.

Past Year Substance Problem

Alcohol (n = 4,456). Youth clients with problem alcohol use in the past year were more likely than average to have ever been homeless or runaway (49%) and to experience weekly alcohol use among peers (55% for peers at work or school and 68% for social peers) and past 90-day drug use among social peers (75%). Table 2 shows that problem alcohol users were more likely than average to have used for 5 or more years (38%), to report lifetime criteria of dependence (DSM-IV; 78%) or severe substance problems (DSM-5; 70%), and to report problem use of cannabis (77%), stimulants (24%), other drugs (16%) and tobacco (81%). They were also more likely to report tobacco dependence (29%). They were also more likely to report weekly use of AOD (65%) and tobacco (60%), and to have spent 13 or more of the past 90 days in a controlled environment (43%). Lifetime withdrawal was more frequent for this group (54%), as is having received any prior substance treatment (46%). Those with problem alcohol use were more likely to recognize their need for substance treatment (83%) and to perceive their substance use as a problem (39%). Those with an alcohol use problem also reported numerous co-occurring problems (Table 3). They were more likely to experience any internalizing disorder (56%), including mood disorder (48%), suicidal thoughts or actions (27%), and traumatic distress (36%), as well as any externalizing disorder (70%), including conduct disorder (60%) and ADHD (51%). They were also more likely to report having both internalizing and externalizing disorders simultaneously (48%), having a history of victimization (75%), high levels of victimization (57%), and victimization in the past year (46%). These youth had numerous problems with violence and illegal activity, including any past year physical violence against others (76%), past year illegal activity (73%), property crimes (59%), violent/interpersonal crimes (52%), and other/drug related crimes (55%). Those with problem alcohol use were more likely to have spent 14 or more of the past 90 days in jail than average (24%). Per Fig. 1, they were also more likely than the average to report five or more co-occurring problems at intake (OR = 4.11).

There were few significant differences in treatment or outcomes for this group. Self-help attendance was more common for problem alcohol users (30%). In the 90 days prior to intake, they were less likely to report being housed in the community (36%). They met fewer positive outcomes at intake (mean 5.3) than average, but their number of positive outcomes and amount of change in outcomes were similar at 6 months. *Thus, despite numerous problems at intake to treatment, these clients did not receive more treatment than the average client.*

Cannabis (n = 9,680). Clients with problem cannabis use do not differ significantly from the average client in most ways. They were more likely to spend time with social peers who used drugs in the past 90 days (74%) and more likely to report symptoms of substance dependence (DSM-IV; 67%) and weekly AOD in the past 90 days (74%). At intake, they were less likely to report having no past month substance problems (33%), and have fewer positive outcomes than average (mean 5.4). However, their number of positive outcomes and amount of change in outcomes were similar at 6 months.

Opioids (n = 1,066), stimulants (n = 1,685), and other drugs (n = 1,183). Across all categories, opioid, stimulant, and other drug problem users have a very similar pattern of characteristics, services, and outcomes; therefore all three are presented simultaneously. Table 1, indicates that problem users of opioids (37%) and stimulants (42%) were more likely to be female and older, with 39% and 25% age 18–25 respectively. Both stimulant and other drug problem users were less likely to be nonwhite (38% and 50%). Each of these problem users were more likely to report being GLBTQ (12%, 14%, and 13%) and ever homeless or runaway (60%, 65%, 58%). Opioid users experienced more weekly drug use in the home (20%), and other drug users were more likely to experience weekly work/school peer alcohol use (52%) and past 90-day social peer drug use (77%). All three groups reported significantly more frequent weekly social peer alcohol use (59%, 63%, and 64%). They were also all less likely to be in school (58%, 71%, and 75%).

In terms of substance use, all three groups were more likely to have used for 5 or more years (59%, 59%, and 46%), and stimulant and other drug problem users were less likely to have begun substance use after the age of 14 (9% and 10% respectively). Each group of users was more likely to report substance dependence criteria (DSM-IV; 96%, 90%, and 91%) and criteria of severe substance problems (DSM-5; 93%, 90%, and 88%), and to have problem use of other substances, including alcohol (56%, 60%, 60%), cannabis (76%, 78%, 86%), opioids (100%, 28%, 43%), stimulants (47%, 100%, 47%), and other drugs (9%, 32%, 100%). This also includes problem use of tobacco (91%, 86%, 89%) and tobacco dependence (39%, 36%, 38%). Problem opioid (69%) and other drug users (70%) used AOD weekly more than average in the past 90 days, and all three groups reported weekly tobacco use (72%, 62%, and 65%). They were also more likely to have spent 13 or more of the past 90 days in a controlled environment (59%, 62%, 54%). They experienced more lifetime withdrawal (83%, 73%, 72%) and more high levels of withdrawal (12%, 8%, 10%), with stimulant problem users also reporting more past week withdrawal (29%). Opioid, stimulant, and other drug problem users all experienced more prior substance treatment (65%, 59%, and 59% respectively with any treatment) and were more likely to perceive the need for treatment (72%, 91%, 88%) and perceive their substance use as a problem (63%, 54%, 54%).

Problem opioid, stimulant, and other drug users were more likely to experience nearly all of the co-occurring problems (Table 3). They were more likely to have any past year internalizing disorder (74%, 73%, 72%), including mood disorder (66%, 65%, 64%), generalized anxiety disorder (32%, 28%, 28%), suicidal thoughts or actions (31%, 34%, 36%), and traumatic distress (51%, 49%, 47%), as well as any externalizing disorders (75%, 76%, 78%) including conduct disorder (65%, 66%, 70%) and ADHD (58%, 59%, 61%). They were more likely to report both internalizing and externalizing disorders simultaneously (63% for each group). They were also more likely to have received prior mental health treatment (66%, 58%, and 62%). Opioid and other drug problem users reported more physical health problems (16% and 15% respectively with high problems). All three groups had severe problems with victimization. Opioid (80%), stimulant (83%), and other drug users (81%) reported more problems with lifetime victimization, high levels of victimization (65%, 70%, 66%), and past year victimization (48%, 52%, 53%), while stimulant (27%) and other drug users (26%) also reported more current worries about victimization, and other drug users experienced more past 90-day victimization (28%). They engaged in more risky behaviors in the past 90 days, including needle use (20%, 7%, 7%) and unprotected sex (46%, 46%, 45%). All three also had the same pattern of increased problems with violence and illegal activity, including past year physical violence (74%, 78%, 84%), illegal activity (79%, 76%, 81%), property crimes (67%, 65%, 72%), violent/interpersonal crimes (53%, 55%, 64%), and other/drug related crimes (67%, 63%, 68%). They were each more likely to have been in jail for 14 or more days of the past 90 (27%, 33%, and 24%), with opioid users also more likely to be in drug court (15%). Per Fig. 1, opioid (OR = 11.4), stimulant (OR = 9.1), and other drug problem users (OR = 13.4) are the most likely to report five or more co-occurring problems at intake.

Table 4 shows that problem opioid users were more likely to receive continuing care (81%), and opioid, stimulant, and other drug problem users were each less likely to be in regular OP treatment (59%, 47%, and 59% respectively), while stimulant (20%) and other drug users (14%) were more likely to be in a residential treatment program. All three were more likely to attend self-help groups (53%, 48%, and 41%) and spent more days in self-help (mean 14.4, 11.6, and 10.1 days respectively). Stimulant problem users reported lower satisfaction with SUD treatment (mean 11.7). Each group also spent more days in substance treatment overall (24.3, 22.3, 21.4), specifically nights in residential treatment (10.1, 12.0, 9.5) with problem opioid users also reporting more days on medication (3.1). All three groups also received more days of mental health treatment (24.0, 20.5, 22.1), driven primarily by days on medication (23.5, 19.9, 21.6). Stimulant and other drug problem users also saw a doctor in an office or clinic for mental health treatment more often (1.6 and 1.7 times respectively). Significantly more days in a controlled environment than average were also reported for problem opioid users (25.1), stimulant users (28.5) and other drug users (22.5).

As shown in Table 5, at intake, opioid, stimulant, and other drug problem users were each less likely to be free of emotional problems (2%, 3%, 3%), housing problems (21%, 20%, 25%), and vocational problems (56%, 62%, 67%). Opioid and other drug problem users had more health problems (18% and 22% reporting no problems respectively) and recovery environment risk (29% and 25% with no problems), with other drug users reporting additional problems with past month SUD symptoms and illegal activity (34% and 45% with no problems). The only significant positive outcome at intake was no trouble at work or school for opioid users (51%) and stimulant users (48%). All three groups of problem users had met significantly fewer positive outcomes than the average at intake, with means of 4.9, 5.3, and 4.9 respectively. At 6 months after intake, all three groups had significantly more clients with no or reduced social support problems (17%, 20%, 17%), and opioid users also reported significantly more instances of no or reduced trouble at work or school (62%). Opioid users continued to be less likely to be housed in the community (63%), while other drug users still reported more recovery environment risk more than average (only 41% with no or reduced 50% or more problems). The number of positive outcomes at 6 months was not significantly higher for any of these three groups of users. However, for opioid and other drug problem users who had more severe problems at intake, their "change from intake to follow-up" was significantly greater (mean change of 3.7 and 3.6 outcomes met respectively). *Thus problem opioid, stimulant, and other drug users are among the most severe youth clients entering SUD treatment and receive significantly more treatment, raising serious concerns about the rising number of problem users of these classes of drugs.*

System Involvement

In school (n = 13,775). Since 84% of the youth clients were in school, the characteristics of those in school were generally within 3 percentage points of the total as noted in Tables 1, 2, 3, 4, and 5 (see overview above). However, students were less likely to be of ages 18–25 (7%) compared to those who were not in school. At intake to treatment, clients in school had more trouble at school or work, with only 27% reporting no trouble.

In the workforce (n = 4,027). Employed clients were less likely to be nonwhite (49%), and less likely to be under the age of 15 (6%). Relatedly, they were significantly more likely to have first used substances over the age of 14 (28%). Working clients were also less likely to report 13 or more days in a controlled environment (20%). No other significant differences emerged.

In child welfare (n = 1,665). Table 1 shows that youth clients in the welfare system were more likely to be female (38%), of mixed/other race (27%), and between the ages of 15 and 17 (80%). They were less likely to be Hispanic (17%) and over the age of 18 (3%). These clients were less likely to come from a single parent family (37%) and more likely to have ever been homeless or runaway (58%). They were less likely to begin using substances after the age of 14 (10%), and more likely to report dependence criteria (DSM-IV; 67%) and severe substance problems (DMS5; 60%). They were more likely to report problem use of stimulants (20%) and tobacco (78%), as well as tobacco dependence criteria (26%). However, they were less likely to have used AOD weekly in the past 90 days (13%). Clients involved in welfare were more likely to have spent 13 or more days in a controlled environment (63%) and to have received prior substance use treatment (51% with any). Table 3 details the numerous co-occurring problems for youth clients in the welfare system. They were more likely to experience any internalizing disorder (54%), including mood disorder (46%) and traumatic distress disorder (34%). They were also more likely to have any externalizing disorder (68%) including both conduct disorder (59%) and ADHD (50%). They were more likely than average to report having both internal and external problems concurrently (46%), and also to report having received any prior mental health treatment (61%). They were more likely to have a lifetime history of victimization (73%) and high levels of victimization (56%), and to have committed past year acts of physical violence (76%) and committed violent crimes (51%). Figure 1 shows that at intake, these clients were significantly more likely than the average client to report having five or more co-occurring problems (OR = 1.9).

Youth clients in the child welfare system were more likely to receive residential treatment (14%) and CC-OP (14%) and less likely to receive regular OP treatment (60%). They were also more likely to attend self-help groups (32%), and to spend more nights in residential treatment (mean of 8.8). Clients in welfare reported lower levels of satisfaction with the substance treatment they received (11.7). They reported more days of mental health treatment (23.5) primarily driven by more days on medication (23.3) and more times seen by a doctor in an office or clinic (2.2) than average. These clients also spent more days in a controlled environment (27.9). At intake to treatment, those involved in the welfare system were more likely to report having no substance problems (32% with no past 90-day substance use and 54% with no past month substance problems), but reported more emotional problems (only 6% reported having no emotional problems) and were less likely to be housed in the community (17%). At 6 months, they continued to be less likely to be housed in the community (62%), but no longer differed significantly from average in the other problem areas measured by NOMS. *Thus, clients in the welfare system were more severe and at high risk of long-term substance misuse.*

In detention/jail 14+ days of the past 90 days (n = 2,575). Table 1 shows that these clients were less likely to be female (18%) and were more likely to have ever been homeless or run away (48%). They were less likely to have social peers at work or school who used drugs in the past 90 days (46%), and, consistent with their incarceration status, were also less likely to be in school in the past 90 days (75%). Individuals detained for 14+ days were less likely to have begun their substance use over the age of 14 (11%), and were more likely to have used substances for 5 or more years (40%). They were also more likely to report lifetime substance dependence criteria (DSM-IV; 66%) and severe substance problems (DSM-5; 62%), and meeting criteria for problem use of alcohol (48%), cannabis (75%), and stimulants (26%) at higher rates than average. They were significantly less likely to have used AOD for 13 or more of the past 90 days (42%), since all of these clients were in a controlled environment for 13 or more days. Being in a controlled environment also contributed to their reduced likelihood of having past week withdrawal symptoms (11%). These clients were also more likely to have previously received substance treatment (48%). In Table 3, we see that these clients are more likely to have a lifetime history of victimization, and to have experienced high levels of victimization (53%). As expected, they reported more problems with violence and illegal activity, including past year acts of physical violence (78%), past year illegal activity (74%) property crimes (59%) and violent/interpersonal crimes (54%). As seen in Fig. 1, at intake to treatment, this group was significantly more likely to have five or more co-occurring problems (OR = 1.53).

Youth clients who had been detained 14 or more of the past 90 days were less likely to achieve positive discharge status from treatment (75%), and were more likely to receive EI (12%), residential treatment (17%), or CC-OP (13%), but less likely to receive standard OP treatment (49%). They were also more likely to attend self-help groups (32%), and received more days of substance treatment overall (mean 21.5), driven mainly by more nights in residential treatment (10.9). As expected, they spent more days involved with the justice system in the 3 months after intake to treatment (81.5) and more days in a controlled environment (33.8) than average. As shown in Table 5, this group was significantly more likely to report no past 90-day substance use and no past month substance problems at intake (38% and 63% respectively). They were also more likely to have no family problems (59%) or trouble at work or school at this time (56%). However, they were arrested more, with only 67% reporting no past 90-day arrest, and were less likely to be in work or school (55%); and, by definition, no clients reported being housed in the community or having no cost to society the past 90 days. At 6 months after intake, these clients were less likely to be housed in the community (59% with no problems) or be in work or school (81% with no problems), and continued to be more likely to have no problems at work or school (58%). *Thus, incarcerated youth reported some of the most severe problems and also received the most intense forms of substance treatment, but unlike those reporting the most severe substance use (problem opioid, stimulant, and other drug users), these clients did not achieve a significantly greater improvement in outcomes from intake to 6 months.*

On probation or parole 14+ days of the past 90 days (n = 3,999). Clients under intense community supervision were significantly more likely to have received prior substance use treatment (45%) and to spend more days involved in the justice system (mean 79.1). By definition, none had zero cost to society at intake. No other significant differences emerged.

Drug court (n = 1,325). As seen in Table 1, clients in drug courts were significantly more likely to be female (39%), to be Hispanic (42%), and to be over the age of 17 (26%). They were significantly less likely to be African American (9%) or between 15 and 17 years old (59%) and less likely to be in school (74%). Drug court clients did not differ significantly from the average client on any substance use or other co-occurring characteristics (Tables 2 and 3).

As noted in Table 4, drug court clients received more continuing care (84%) and more IOP treatment (21%), but almost no residential (0%) or CC-OP (1%) treatment. They were more likely to attend self-help groups (39%) and spent more days in self-help (mean 9.8). They were more satisfied with their treatment, reporting an average of 13.3 on the treatment satisfaction scale, and 95% with a score of 14 or higher (i.e., high satisfaction). While they did not report significantly more days of substance treatment overall, they did report more times attending a regular outpatient program (8.8) and more days on medication (2.0) for substance treatment. They also reported more days involved in the justice system (62.7). In terms of positive outcomes, drug court clients mostly reflect the average at both intake and 6 months, with the exception that they are less likely to report no past 90-day arrests at intake (65%), and they were more likely to report no substance use at follow-up (79%).

Other justice system involvement in the past 90 days (n = 4,661). These clients were largely nonsignificantly different from the average with a couple of exceptions. They were less likely to have spent 13 or more days in a controlled environment before intake to treatment (13%), and they were more likely to report current justice system involvement (92%). No other differences in demographics, substance use, co-occurring disorders, treatment, or outcomes were of note.

Level of Care

Early intervention (n = 946). Table 1 details the demographic and environmental characteristics for youth clients in EI. They were more likely to be nonwhite (77%), especially Hispanic (43%), and to be over the age of 17 (33%). They were also more likely than average to be married (5%), less likely to be in school (64%), and less likely to report past 90-day drug use among their work or school peers (41%). They were more likely to have used for 5 or more years, and more likely to report no days of AOD use in the past 90 days (29%). They also had a higher likelihood of having spent 13 or more days in a controlled environment in the past 90 days (44%). They reported very few co-occurring problems (see Table 3). They were more likely to report fewer past 90-day health problems (63%), and current justice system involvement (89%) than average, and were more likely to have been in detention or jail 14 or more of the past 90 days (32%). They reported average levels of co-occurring problems shown in Fig. 1.

Table 4 shows that clients in EI were more likely to reach initiation (97%), and more likely to attend self-help groups (43%), and to attend more days of self-help (mean 8.7). Similar to other clients who spent extensive time in a controlled environment before intake, clients in EI were more likely to have no problems with substance use (29%), family (52%), and trouble at work or school (53%), but were less likely to be housed in the community (28%) or to be in work or school (56%). At their last follow-up interview, they were less likely to be in work or school (82%), though this was an improvement over their intake rates. *Thus, rather than reaching lower severity youth, EI is reaching youth who are appropriatefor regular outpatient treatment.*

Outpatient (n = 11,195). Since 70% of youth clients participated in standard OP treatment, there were few differences between this group and the average client in terms of most demographics, substance use, clinical correlates, number of problems, treatment experience, and outcomes. However, Outpatient clients were less likely to report 13 or more days in a controlled environment before entering treatment (21%), and also fewer days in a controlled environment at 3 months (mean 8.2 days). This includes significantly fewer nights in residential substance treatment (1.2). They received fewer days of substance treatment overall (8.9), and were less likely to attend self-help groups (11%).

Intensive outpatient (n = 1,558). Youth clients in IOP treatment were similar to the average on most demographic, environmental, substance, co-occurring characteristics, and number of problems. However, they were more likely to report current justice system involvement (86%), and specifically to be in drug court (17%). As seen in Table 4, they were more likely to receive continuing care (82%), and to attend self-help groups (30%). They received more days of substance treatment overall (mean 26.4), particularly days in an intensive outpatient program (18.8). At the same time they reported significantly fewer days in regular outpatient treatment (3.8). IOP clients also reported more days involved with the justice system at 3 months (65.5). They did not differ significantly from the average client in terms of positive outcomes at baseline, 6-month follow-up, or the change in positive outcomes.

Residential (n = 1,215). Table 1 shows that youth clients in residential treatment were less likely to be Hispanic (18%) and more likely to be of mixed race (27%). They were more likely to be involved in the child welfare system (18%) to have ever been homeless or runaway (56%), and to experience substance use problems in their environments, with more common weekly drug use in the home (20%) and past 90-day use among social peers (78%), as well as more weekly alcohol use among work/school peers (52%) and social peers (64%). Residential clients were also less likely to have begun using after the age of 14 (8%) and more likely to have been using substances for 5 or more years (38%). They were more likely to report criteria of lifetime substance dependence (DSM-IV; 76%) or severe substance problems (DSM-5; 71%), and less likely to report abuse criteria (DSM-IV; 18%). They reported meeting the criteria for problems use of alcohol (45%), cannabis (78%), stimulants (29%), and tobacco (81%) more frequently than average, and were more likely to report weekly use of AOD (73%) and tobacco (64%). They were also more likely to report tobacco dependence (33%). Residential clients reported these severe substance problems although they were also more likely to report 13 or more of the 90 days before intake to treatment in a controlled environment (51%). They experienced more lifetime withdrawal (57%), past week withdrawal (34%), and severe past week withdrawal (7%) than the average client, and attended prior treatment more (55%). These clients were much more likely to perceive the need for substance treatment (87%) and to perceive their substance use as a problem (48%).

Table 3 details a number of co-occurring problems reported by residential youth clients. They were more likely to have any past year internalizing disorder (62%), including mood disorder (54%), generalized anxiety disorder (21%), suicidal thoughts or actions (30%), and traumatic distress (39%), as well as any externalizing disorder (74%), including conduct disorder (68%) and ADHD (55%). Significantly more residential clients reported concurrent internalizing and externalizing disorders (55%) and having attended prior mental health treatment (52%). They were more likely to have a lifetime history of victimization (75%), high levels of victimization (60%), and for that victimization to have occurred in the past year (49%). They were more likely to have had sex in the past 90 days (73%), and to have had multiple sexual partners during that same time (40%). They also reported significantly more problems with violence and illegal activity, including past year physical violence (80%), past year illegal activity (77%), property crimes (63%), violent/interpersonal crimes (58%), and other/drug related crimes (60%). They were significantly more likely to report 14 or more of the past 90 days in jail or detention (33%). As seen in Fig. 1, they were more likely to report five or more co-occurring problems at intake (OR = 3.1).

Given the large number of co-occurring problems, it is unsurprising that residential clients also reported numerous differences in treatment received in Table 4. They were more likely to reach initiation (89%), but less likely to become engaged (55%). They reported significantly lower levels of satisfaction with treatment (mean 9.7) and were significantly less likely to report high satisfaction (67%). They were significantly more likely to attend self-help groups (66%) and attended more days of self-help (mean 16.9). Residential clients reported more days in substance treatment overall (mean 42.5), including days in detox (2.1) and nights in residential (36.2). At the same time they spent fewer days in regular outpatient treatment (1.3). Residential clients also received more mental health treatment (22.1 days), particularly days on medication for mental health problems (21.5), and more physical health treatment (11.4 days), including both days on medication (10.1) and outpatient visits to a doctor's office or clinic (1.5). Residential clients spent significantly more days in a controlled environment (60.3).

Table 5 shows the status of residential clients on NOMS positive outcome measures at intake and 6-month follow-up. These clients were less likely to report no problems in numerous areas, including no past month substance problems (32%), no past 90-day emotional problems (6%), no illegal activity (45%), no arrests (68%), no housing problems (26%), and no recovery environment risk (26%). In total at intake, residential clients reported an average of only 4.9 positive outcomes met, significantly lower than the average. At follow-up, most differences were resolved, though residential clients were still less likely to report being housed in the community (47%). They also were more likely to report having no or reduced problems with substance use (78%) and social support problems (26%). While the total number of positive outcomes at follow-up was not significantly different, the improvement in outcomes from intake to follow-up was significantly better for this group (mean of 3.7 more outcomes met). *Thus, as expected given existing treatment guidelines (ASAM,* 1996, 2001*), youth in residential treatment had the most* *and the most severe problems across levels of care, as well as some of the highest rates of previous treatment.*

Continuing care outpatient (n = 1,059). These youth clients are unique in having been in a controlled environment (residential treatment or correctional) for some period of time prior to their current treatment. They fall between those in IOP and residential treatment in most characteristics. As seen in Table 1, these clients were less likely to be under the age of 15 (9%), and more likely to ever be homeless or runaway (48%). They also had a higher rate of child welfare involvement (21%) and were less likely to begin using substances over the age of 14 (10%), and more likely to have used for 5 or more years (40%). They had higher rates of substance dependence citeria (DSM-IV; 75%) and severe substance problems (70%), and were less likely to meet substance abuse criteria (18%). They were more likely to meet criteria for problem use of stimulants (21%) and tobacco (78%), but were less likely to report weekly use of AOD in the past 90 days (31%). They were also more likely to report 13 or more of those 90 days in a controlled environment (73%). This time in a controlled environment may have contributed to reduced rates of past week withdrawal (10%). They reported more prior substance treatment (71%), and were more likely to believe they were in need of substance treatment (83%) and to perceive their substance use as a problem (34%). Table 3 shows that these clients were more likely to report any past year externalizing disorder (65%), were less likely to report having neither an internalizing nor an externalizing disorder than average (27%), and also more likely to have received prior mental health treatment (54%). They have higher rates of lifetime victimization (73%) and high levels of victimization (56%). They reported more severe involvement with the criminal justice system (29% and 42% with 14 or more days in detention/jail or probation/parole respectively), despite average levels of illegal activity and violence. This pattern is continued in Table 4 which shows a higher than average number of days in the justice system (mean 63.7) and days in a controlled environment (23.74) at 3 months. Figure 1 shows that they were more likely than average to report five or more co-occurring problems at intake (OR = 1.6).

They were more likely to intitiate treatment within 14 days of assessment (92%) and to receive continuing care at least 90 days after entering treatment (83%). They were less satisfied with their treatment (mean 10.3) with only 72% indicating high satisfaction. They were more likely than average to attend self-help groups (37%) and received more days of substance treatment overall (mean 22.7), particularly days in intensive outpatient treatment (8.0). Numerous significant variations in outcomes met appear in Table 5. These clients, like many with significant time in a controlled environment at intake, were more likely to report no problems with substance use (50%), past month substance problems (65%), family (57%), and trouble at work or school (48%), but less likely to report being housed in the community (16%) and being in school or work (68%). Additionally they reported more emotional problems, with only 6% reporting no problems, and more likely to report no arrests (86%) and no social support problems (7%). At intake, this group met significantly more positive NOMS outcomes on average (mean 6.4). While much closer to the average at 6-month follow-up, they are much more likely to report zero cost to society (61%). While the total number of outcomes met at follow-up is not significantly different from the average, the change in outcomes from intake to follow-up is significantly lower than average (change of 2.1 outcomes met). *Thus, while having high severity in the past year, CC-OP serves clients characterized by high levels of service and recent reductions in problems.*

Emerging Topics

Health care costs. In the year before entering treatment for substance use, the youth clients in the current analyses utilized over $143 million in services including emergency room visits, doctor appointments, visits to mental health professionals, detoxification programs, and substance treatment; the average client received $9074 in services in that year. Figure 2 shows that the most costly clients (i.e., the top 10%) accounted for nearly 70% of the total cost of health care services in the year prior to intake. For youth clients entering treatment, Table 6 shows those with significantly higher treatment costs than average include problem users of opioids (27% with high costs; median cost of $4,852), stimulants (24% with high costs),

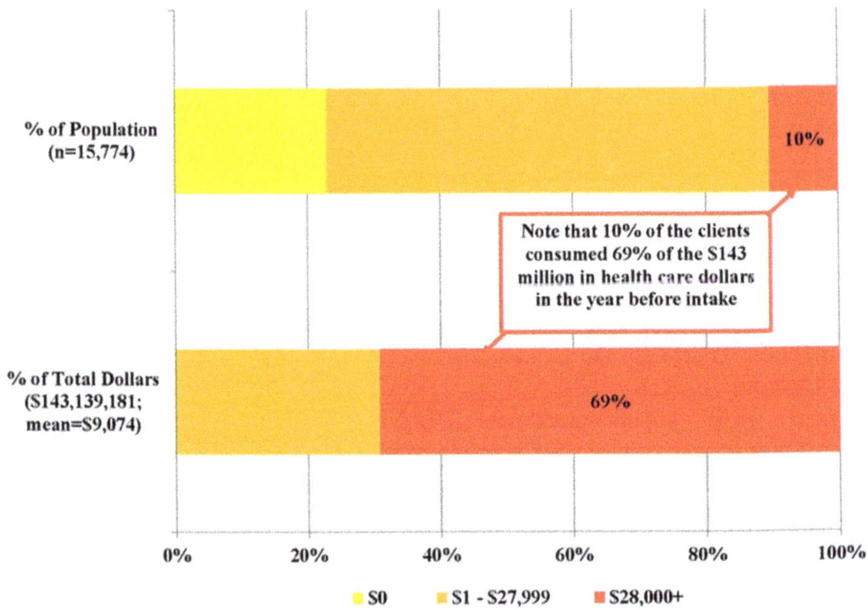

Fig. 2 Cost of health care utilization. (Costs of health care utilization are reported for the quarter before intake, then multiplied by 40 to represent the full year. Monetary conversion factors for physical health, mental health, and substance abuse treatment services came from McCollister et al. (2017) in 2016 dollars.) Created by authors, Baumer, Dennis, & Estrada, 2017

Table 6 Costs of health care utilization and crime by gender, race, age, substance problem, system involvement, and level of care

	Total	Male	Female	African American	White	Hispanic	Mixed/ other	12–17	18–25	Alcohol[c]	Cannabis[c]	Opioids[c]	Stimulants[c]	Other[c]
	16,361	11,904	4,449	2,465	6,090	4,865	2,934	13,989	2,372	4,456	9,680	1,066	1,685	1,183
Total %	100%	73%	27%	15%	37%	30%	18%	86%	15%	32	66%	8%	12%	9%
Cost of health care utilization[a]														
Low ($0)	23%	24%	21%	29%	18%	28%	21%	23%	24%	17%	20%	**11%**	**13%**	**11%**
Moderate ($1–$27,999)	67%	67%	65%	63%	70%	65%	67%	67%	63%	67%	68%	62%	62%	63%
High ($28,000+)	10%	9%	14%	8%	13%	7%	12%	10%	13%	16%	11%	**27%**	**24%**	**25%**
Median	$780	$780	$1,449	**$520**	$1,300	$,520	$1,040	$855	$1,003	$1,449	$1,003	**$ 4,852**	$2,752	$3,504
Cost of crime[b]														
Low ($0)	56%	53%	64%	62%	56%	55%	52%	54%	**68%**	**42%**	48%	**35%**	**36%**	**30%**
Moderate ($1–$499,999)	34%	36%	30%	30%	36%	34%	36%	36%	26%	40%	39%	41%	39%	43%
High ($450,000+)	10%	11%	6%	8%	9%	11%	12%	11%	6%	**17%**	13%	**24%**	**24%**	**27%**
Median	$ –	$–	$–	$–	$–	$–	$–	$–	**$–**	$14,880	$5457	$41,565	$42,096	**$89,530**

	In school[d]	In work[d]	In welfare[e]	In jail 14+ days	Prob/parole 14+ days	Drug court	Other JSI P90[f]	Early intervention	Outpatient (OP)	Intensive outpatient	Residential	Continuing care OP
	13,775	4,027	1,665	2,575	3,999	1,325	4,661	946	11,195	1,558	1,215	1,059
Total %	84%	25%	10%	16%	25%	8%	29%	6%	70%	10%	8%	7%
Cost of health care utilization[a]												
Low ($0)	23%	20%	**12%**	19%	**1%**	15%	**38%**	**32%**	26%	18%	**11%**	**12%**
Moderate ($1–$27,999)	67%	71%	62%	72%	**84%**	**76%**	**55%**	62%	67%	72%	73%	**48%**

Table 6 (continued)

	In school[d]	In work[d]	In welfare[e]	In jail 14+ days	Prob/parole 14+ days	Drug court	Other JSI P90[f]	Early intervention	Outpatient (OP)	Intensive outpatient	Residential	Continuing care OP
High ($28,000+)	10%	9%	**26%**	9%	16%	8%	7%	6%	7%	10%	16%	**40%**
Median	$780	$966	**$3,199**	$1,040	**$1,623**	$1,746	**<u>$483</u>**	**<u>$520</u>**	$743	$1300	**$2,229**	**$3,900**
Cost of crime[b]												
Low ($0)	56%	58%	47%	**<u>42%</u>**	50%	60%	58%	53%	60%	54%	**<u>36%</u>**	47%
Moderate ($1–$499,999)	35%	33%	38%	40%	38%	32%	34%	35%	32%	35%	42%	38%
High ($450,000+)	10%	9%	15%	**18%**	12%	8%	8%	11%	7%	10%	**22%**	15%
Median	$–	$–	**$5,457**	**$14,512**	$–	$–	$–	$5,457	$–	$–	**$28,920**	$5,805

Created by authors, Baumer, Dennis, & Estrada, 2017

Note: Values in **BOLD** indicate that relative to total, column value is significantly different ($p < 0.05$) and clinically higher (Cohen's effect size $d \geq 0.2$)

Values in **<u>BOLD and UNDERLINED</u>** indicate that relative to total, column value is significantly different ($p < 0.051$ and clinically lower (Cohen's effect size ≤ -0.21

[a]Costs of health care utilization are reported for the quarter before intake, then multiplied by 4 to represent the full year. Monetary conversion factors for physical health, mental health, and substance abuse treatment services came from McCollister et al. (2017) in 2016 dollars for unit costs of $2206.67 per PH hospital day; $2996 per emergency room visit; $120.75 per PH physician visit; $999 per psychiatric inpatient day; $121 per MH physician visit; $414 per day of detoxification; $177 per day of residential SUD treatment; $83 per IOP visit; $31 per standard OP visit; $24 per day using Methadone/disulfiram; and $65 per test for AOD use (urinalysis)

[b]Crime costs are reported in the past year. Monetary conversion factors for crime categories came from McCollister et al. (2017) in 2016 dollars for uint costs of $5457 per incidence of vandalism; $8953 per incidence of stolen property; $6153 per incidence of fraud, embezzlement, or forgery/counterfeiting; $7256 per household burglary; $12,095 per motor vehicle theft; $47,507 per robbery; $23,695 per arson; $120,166 per aggravated assault; $270,352 per rape/sexual assault; and $10,086,337 per murder

[c]Problem use is defined using the DSM5 definition of mild or more severe substance disorder problems (2+ of 11 symptoms) in the past year or weekly use of the substance

[d]In the past 90 days

[e]Reports days in foster care or a group home, legal custody by the County or State, referred to treatment by social worker or DCFS/welfare, has child in foster care, group or institution

[f]Does not meet criteria for in jail 14+ days or probation/parole 14+ days but has been arrested and charged with a crime in the past 90 days, have been on probation, parole, jail, detention, house arrest, or electronic monitoring in the past 90 days, or any current justice involvement in L7

and other drugs (25% with high costs), those involved in the welfare system (26% with high costs; median cost of $3,199), those on probation or parole 14 or more of the past 90 days (median cost of $1623), and those in residential (median cost of $2,229) and CC-OP treatments (40% with high costs; median cost of $3,900). Lower than average costs were associated with African Americans (median cost of $520), those with other (less severe) justice system involvement in the past 90 days (38% with low costs; median cost of $483), and those in EI treatments (32% with low costs; median cost of $520). *Thus, to effectively reduce the costs to society of accessing the health care system, these intense utilizers should be targeted for services.*

Cost of crime. The connection between substance use and criminal activity has been broadly established (National Research Council, 2012; Welty et al., 2016). But as seen with the costs of health care utilization, the larger part of the costs associated with criminal activity can be accounted for by a small portion of those with the most severe problems. Figure 3 shows that of the $7 billion of criminal costs for these clients ($446,113 per youth on average), 10% of the 15,890 individuals were responsible for 92% of the cost of crime to society. For youth clients entering treatment,

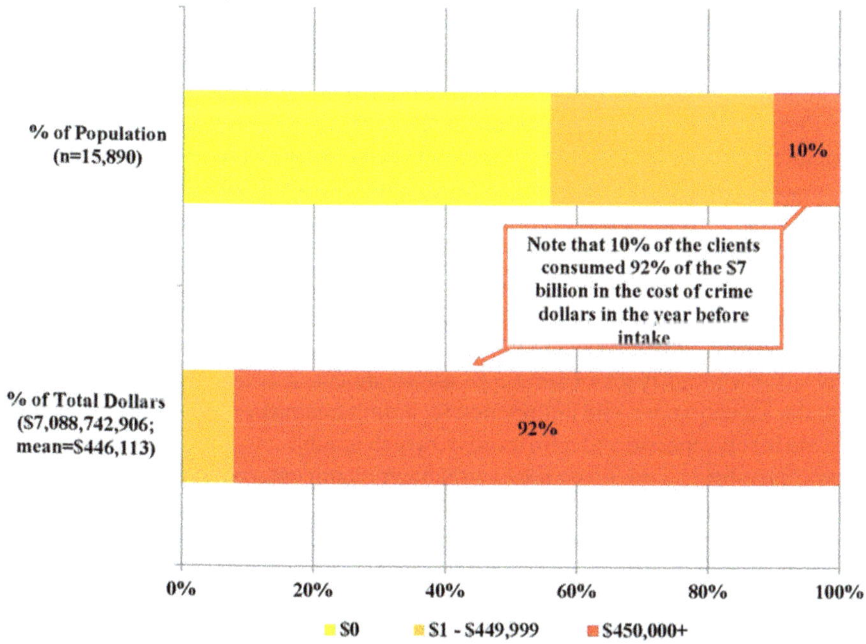

Fig. 3 Cost of crime. (Cost of crime are reported in the past year. Monetary conversion factors for crime categories came from McCollister et al. (2017) in 2016 dollars.) Created by authors, Baumer, Dennis, & Estrada, 2017

Table 6 shows that those with significantly higher costs of crime than average include problem alcohol users (17% with high costs; median cost of $14,880), problem opioid users (24% with high cost), problem stimulant users (24% with high cost), and problem other drug users (27% with high cost; median cost of $89,530). Clients in the child welfare system also have higher costs of crime, with a median cost of $5,457, along with youth who have been in jail or detention for 14 or more of the past 90 days at intake (18% with high cost; median cost of $14,512). Clients who enter residential treatment also follow this pattern, with 22% in the high cost category and a median cost of $28,920. Consistent with previous research, clients age 18–25 have lower crime costs than the average client, with 68% in the low cost category. *Thus, to effectively reduce the costs of crime, the more severe offenders need to be targeted for services.*

Trauma: The river that runs through it. As Table 3 shows, a lifetime history of physical, mental, or sexual victimization is common among youth clients entering substance use treatment (62%). Using the GAIN General Victimization Scale (Titus et al., 2003), based on types of victimization, traumagenic factors, and current worries about continued victimization, clients can be divided into groups of low (no problems), moderate (1–4 problems), and high (5–16 problems) severity victimization. More than 40% of these youth clients met the criteria for high victimization. Table 7 shows that these youth experience significantly more co-occurring problems at intake to treatment, with a mean of 7.55 out of 16 problems, and 84% reporting five or more problems. Their costs to society are significantly higher in the year before intake for both health care utilization (median of $1,524) and crime (median of $17,552 with 18% in the high cost category). Clients with high victimization have met fewer positive NOMS outcomes at intake (mean 5.3), but were similar at follow-up and in terms of the change in the count. *Thus, the experience of significant trauma is among the most strongly related characteristics to the number of problems reported by youth at intake to treatment, and to higher than average costs to society for both healthcare and crime.*

Limitations. While the data presented in this chapter has the benefits of representing a large, diverse, nation-wide sample of adolescents and young adults involved in various types of substance use treatment, it is not without limitations. With the exception of some information regarding treatment provided by clinicians, the data is self-reported and retrospective, which is subject to reporting and memory biases. That being said, given the environment, youth entering substance use treatment may be more forthcoming about their problem thoughts and behaviors than youth in the community. A second limitation is the rate of missing data available for consideration of treatment received at 3 months and outcomes at 6 months. Only 59% of those eligible for a follow-up interview had data for both the 3- and 6-month interviews, raising the possibility of incomplete or biased information available for treatment and outcomes discussed.

Table 7 Demographics, substance problem, system involvement, level of care, co-occurring problems, costs, and NOMS by victimization

	Total	Low (0)[h]	Moderate (1–3)[h]	High (4–15)[h]
	16,361	6,229	3,136	6,961
Total %	100%	38%	19%	43%
Gender				
Male	73%	75%	**83%**	67%
Female	27%	25%	**17%**	33%
Race				
African American	15%	19%	15%	11%
White	37%	36%	36%	38%
Hispanic	30%	30%	32%	29%
Mixed/other	18%	15%	17%	21%
Age				
12–17	86%	89%	85%	83%
18–25	15%	11%	15%	17%
Past year problem use (overlapping)[a]				
Alcohol	32%	**22%**	30%	41%
Cannabis	66%	60%	68%	70%
Opioids	8%	4%	7%	11%
Stimulants	12%	**6%**	9%	19%
Other	9%	4%	7%	13%
System involvement (overlapping)				
In school[b]	84%	88%	84%	82%
In work[c]	25%	24%	25%	25%
In welfare[c]	10%	7%	9%	13%
In jail 14+ days	16%	11%	16%	20%
Prob/parole 14+ days	25%	23%	26%	26%
Drug court	8%	9%	8%	8%
Other JSI P90[d]	29%	32%	30%	25%
Level of care				
Early intervention	6%	5%	6%	7%
Outpatient	70%	77%	72%	64%
Intensive outpatient	10%	10%	10%	10%
Residential	8%	5%	6%	11%
CC-OP	7%	5%	6%	9%
Count of major clinic al problems[e]				
None (0 problems)	3%	8%	**0%**	**0%**
1	7%	**16%**	3%	**1%**
2	9%	**18%**	7%	**3%**
3	11%	17%	12%	**5%**
4	11%	13%	14%	8%

(continued)

Table 7 (continued)

	Total	Low (0)[h]	Moderate (1–3)[h]	High (4–15)[h]
5 through 16	59%	**<u>28%</u>**	64%	**84%**
Mean	5.59	**<u>3.38</u>**	5.67	**7.55**
Cost of health-care utilization[f]				
Low ($0)	23%	30%	23%	17%
Moderate ($1–7,599)	67%	65%	69%	68%
High ($7,600+)	10%	6%	9%	15%
Median	$780	**<u>$520</u>**	$780	**$1,524**
Cost of crime[g]				
Low ($0)	56%	72%	54%	**<u>42%</u>**
Moderate ($1–409,000)	34%	26%	38%	40%
High ($410,000+)	10%	2%	8%	**18%**
Median	$–	$–	$–	**$17,552**
NOMS outcomes				
No problems at intake	5.92	**6.72**	5.78	**<u>5.29</u>**
No or reduced (50% or more) problems at 6 months	8.74	9.13	8.66	8.44
Change in summary count of outcomes (6 months—intake)	2.82	2.41	2.88	3.16

Created by authors, Baumer, Dennis, & Estrada, 2017

Note: Values in **BOLD** indicate that relative to total, column value is significantly different ($p < 0.05$) and clinically higher (Cohen's effect sized $d \geq 0.2$

Values in **<u>BOLD and UNDERLINED</u>** indicate that relative to total, column value is significantly different ($p < 0.05$) and clinically lower (Cohen's effect size ≤ -0.2)

[a]Problem use is defined using the DSM5 definition of mild or more severe substance disorder problems (2+ of 11 symptoms) in the past year or weekly use of the substance

[b]In the past 90 days

[c]Reports days in foster care or a group home, legal custody by the County or State, referred to treatment by social worker or DCFS/welfare, has child in foster care, group or institution

[d]Does not meet criteria for in jail 14+ days or probation/parole 14+ days but has been arrested and charged with a crime in the past 90 days, have been on probation, parole, jail, detention, house arrest, or electronic monitoring in the past 90 days, or any current justice involvement in L7

[e]Based on count of self reporting criteria to suggest tobacco, alcohol, cannabis, opioid, stimulant, or other drug disorder, depression, anxiety, trauma, suicide, ADHD, CD, physical health problems, victimization, violence/illegal activity

[f]Costs of health care utilization are reported for the quarter before intake, then multiplied by 4 to represent the full year

[g]Crime costs are reported in the past year

[h]General Victimization Scale is a count of types of victimization experienced by the respondent in his/her lifetime (including physical, emotional and sexual), plus the number of traumagenic factors involved in the victimization (including origination and duration, type and relation of perpetrator, etc.), and on-going fear of abuse happening again

Discussion

Multimorbidity and Its Implications

Consistent with the literature, this chapter demonstrates that multimorbidity is the norm for youth presenting to SUD treatment. With a median of 5 of 16 major clinical problems, we found that the number and severity of clinical problems increases with age, the degree of service system involvement, severity of substance problems, and the level of care. From a developmental perspective, this suggests the advantages of early identification at younger ages and while youth are still in school when there are fewer problems. At the same time, it provides a cautionary picture of the growing number of youth presenting for opioid or stimulant problems—they typically present with more and a wider range of problems that makes for a complicated diagnosis.

Consistent with the treatment literature reviewed earlier, it is important to recognize that different levels of care target clients with different needs and that these needs are sometimes different than expected. For instance, the severity of clients in early intervention in school settings was very similar to those in regular outpatient settings. Rather than reaching a lower severity client, these programs appear to be more assertive in reaching adolescents without removing them from their home environments. Alternatively, intensive outpatient and residential programs are reaching youth with higher rates of multimorbidity and greater justice system involvement. Residential programs in particular were differentiated by the degree of prior service utilization; i.e., prior treatment having been insufficient. Youth entering continuing care outpatient programs reported fewer and less severe problems than those entering residential treatment, but were more severe than youth entering lower levels of care, suggesting their recent treatment was beneficial, but not sufficient to eliminate the multiple, severe problems which existed when they began treatment.

A key implication of these findings is the need for better and more comprehensive clinical assessment, particularly for youth entering higher levels of care. Missing anger or suicide issues, ignoring ADHD or health problems, or failure to recognize victimization or violence toward others have critical clinical implications. In addition, having identified these problems, programs need plans to address them directly or through referral. Each of the 16 problems identified in Fig. 1 was common in all groups, service settings, and levels of care. *Thus, at a minimum all programs should develop a specific plan for youth who present with one or more of these problems.* On the other hand, most of the other problems in Tables 1, 2, and 3 occurred for less than half the youth, suggesting that there is also a need for programs to individualize services to the needs presented by each youth.

Service Utilization and Costs to Society

Using the most recent unit cost estimates (McCollister et al., 2017) this chapter has shown that in youth presenting to SUD treatment, 69% of the costs of health care service utilization are being driven by a subset of 10% of the youth. Any serious attempt to reduce these health care cost must address this issue. Similarly, 92% of the costs of crime to society were being driven by 10% of the youth. Any serious attempt to reduce violent crime and the cost of crime to society has to target this group. It is also important to note that it is not the same youth who generate the moderate/high costs of service utilization and moderate/high costs of crime.

To the extent that funders in many systems are increasingly looking at value based costs and contracting, it would be advisable for them and the collaborating programs to consider these cost risk groups. An increased understanding of these patterns of system contact would be beneficial in determining appropriate points of contact for earlier brief interventions, which may disrupt the cycle of repeated costly incidents (Tanner-Smith & Lipsey, 2015; Winters, Tanner-Smith, Bresani, & Meyers, 2014). While past costs of health care and crime are frequently predictive of future costs, they do fluctuate. Thus they are not a substitute of assessing multimorbidity, and the best prediction is likely to be made from combining these factors.

Trauma and Its Implications

The chapter delineates the high rates of victimization, factors that make victimization more traumatic, and how these factors vary by gender, race, age, substance problems, system involvement, and level of care. Specifically, severe substance problems, system involvement, and levels of care were associated with higher levels of victimization. Moreover, the degree of victimization was shown to be one of the strongest predictors of multimorbidity, health care utilization and costs of crime. In summary, trauma is the river that runs through the severity and complexity problems of youth presenting to treatment.

The key implication is the need for all youth treatment to be trauma "informed." Staff in youth SUD treatment needs to recognize these issues and avoide doing further harm. There are multiple low-cost and free trainings available through organizations like the National Children's Traumatic Stress Network (http://www.nctsn.org/) and the National Addiction Technology Transfer Center Network (http://www.nattc.org/). These trainings and associated networks include adaptations for working in schools, justice systems, and child welfare systems. Ideally, for more severe cases, systems of care should also have access to more advanced trauma "focused" programs. The networks above provide reviews and connections to such programs. Programs should also link youth to crisis lines related to trauma and suicide prevention.

Importance of Standardized Screening and Assessment

As noted in the first section of the chapter, adolescence and young adulthood are key periods of brain development. This and the high rates of ADHD make the use of standardized screening and assessment even more important than with adults. Standardization helps assure that the terms used and the language is more concrete, that specific questions are well defined, and that answers are both reliable and valid. Using screeners related to longer measures also helps make the process more efficient when further assessment is needed. Standardized reports and electronic data transfer improve communication across multiple systems in case–planning (across justice, school, work, behavioral health, etc.), across treatment episodes, as well as assisting with clinical decision-making. Pooling assessment data also helps to identify variation in needs and any mismatch between needs and the services received for different subgroups (i.e., health disparities), so programs can identify and remedy service gaps.

Integrated care, interdisciplinary teams, and connecting multiple systems for case planning are most likely to be effective ways to address multimorbidity and health disparities (Dennis et al., 2016; Korchmaros et al., 2016; Nissen et al., 2004). However, variation in staff training, technical terms, program criteria, and electronic systems can make this challenging. Automating the process can help address these barriers to providing the best possible support to youth clients during and after their SUD treatment.

Acknowledgement This chapter using data provided by the following grants and contracts from the Center for Substance Abuse Treatment (CSAT): TI13190, TI13305, TI13313, TI13322, TI13323, TI13344, TI13345, TI13354, TI13356, TI13601, TI14090, TI14188, TI14189, TI14196, TI14252, TI14261, TI14267, TI14271, TI14272, TI14283, TI14311, TI14315, TI14376, TI15413, TI15415, TI15421, TI15433, TI15438, TI15446, TI15447, TI15458, TI15461, TI15466, TI15467, TI15469, TI15475, TI15478, TI15479, TI15481, TI15483, TI15485, TI15486, TI15489, TI15511, TI15514, TI15524, TI15527, TI15545, TI15562, TI15577, TI15584, TI15586, TI15670, TI15671, TI15672, TI15674, TI15677, TI15678, TI15682, TI15686, TI16386, TI16400, TI16414, TI16904, TI16928, TI16939, TI16961, TI16984, TI16992, TI17046, TI17070, TI17071, TI17433, TI17434, TI17446, TI17475, TI17476, TI17484, TI17486, TI17490, TI17517, TI17523, TI17534, TI17535, TI17547, TI17589, TI17604, TI17605, TI17638, TI17646, TI17648, TI17673, TI17702, TI17719, TI17728, TI17742, TI17744, TI17751, TI17755, TI17761, TI17763, TI17765, TI17769, TI17775, TI17779, TI17786, TI17788, TI17812, TI17817, TI17821, TI17825, TI17830, TI17831, TI17847, TI17864, TI18406, TI18671, TI18723, TI18735, TI18849, TI19313, TI19323, TI19942, TI20117, TI20759, TI20781, TI20798, TI20806, TI20827, TI20828, TI20847, TI20848, TI20849, TI20852, TI20865, TI20870, TI20910, TI20946, TI21551, TI21580, TI21595, TI21597, TI21632, TI21639, TI21682, TI21688, TI21705, TI21714, TI21774, TI21788, TI21815, TI21874, TI21883, TI21890, TI21892, TI22425, TI22513, TI22544, TI22622, TI22695, TI22838, TI22856, TI23037, TI23064, TI23174, TI23186, TI23188, TI23195, TI23196, TI23197, TI23200, TI23202, TI23204, TI23206, TI23224, TI23244, TI23247, TI23265, TI23270, TI23276, TI23278, TI23279, TI23296, TI23298, TI23304, TI23310, TI23311, TI23312, TI23316, TI23322, TI23323, TI23325, TI23336, TI23345, TI23346, TI23348, 655372, 655373, 655374, TI20084, TI20085, TI20086, TI20920, TI20921, TI20924, TI20925, TI20938, TI20941; Contract 207-98-7047, Contract 277-00-6500, Contract 270-2003-00006, Contract 270-07-0191, and Contract 270-12-0397. The opinions are those of the authors and do not reflect official positions of the contributing project directors or government.

References

American Psychiatric Association (APA). (2000). *Diagnostic and statistical manual of mental disorders version 4 text revised (DSM-IV-TR)*. Washington, DC: American Psychiatric Association.

American Psychiatric Association (APA). (2013). *Diagnostic and statistical manual of mental disorders* (5th ed.). Arlington, VA: American Psychiatric Publishing.

American Society of Addiction Medicine (ASAM). (1996). *Patient placement criteria for the treatment of psychoactive substance disorders* (2nd ed.). Chevy Chase, MD: American Society of Addiction Medicine.

American Society of Addiction Medicine (ASAM). (2001). *Patient placement criteria for the treatment for substance-related disorders* (2nd ed.). Chevy Chase, MD: American Society of Addiction Medicine.

Belenko, S., Knight, D., Wasserman, G. A., Dennis, M. L., Wiley, T., Taxman, F. S., … Sales, J. (2017). The juvenile justice behavioral health services cascade: A new framework for measuring unmet substance use treatment services needs among adolescent offenders. *Journal of Substance Abuse Treatment, 74*, 80–91.

Belur, V., Dennis, M. L., Ives, M. L., Vincent, R., & Muck, R. (2014). Feasibility and impact of implementing motivational enhancement therapy – Cognitive behavioral therapy as a substance use treatment intervention in school-based settings. *Advances in School Mental Health Promotion, 7*(2), 88–104.

Bickel, W. K., Johnson, M. W., Koffarnus, M. N., MacKillop, J., & Murphy, J. G. (2014). The behavioral economics of substance use disorders: Reinforcement pathologies and their repair. *Annual Review of Clinical Psychology, 10*(1), 641–677.

Bukstein, O. G. (2016). Understanding substance use problems in transitional age youth. *Child and Adolescent Psychiatric Clinics of North America, 26*(2), 253–269.

Carliner, H., Keyes, K. M., McLaughlin, K. A., Meyers, J. L., Dunn, E. C., & Martins, S. S. (2016). Childhood trauma and illicit drug use in adolescence: A population-based national comorbidity survey replication–adolescent supplement study. *Journal of the American Academy of Child & Adolescent Psychiatry, 55*(8), 701–708.

Chan, Y. F., Dennis, M. L., & Funk, R. R. (2008). Prevalence and comorbidity of major internalizing and externalizing problems among adolescents and adults presenting to substance abuse treatment. *Journal of Substance Abuse Treatment, 34*, 14–24.

Chestnut Global Partners (CGP). (2017). *Workplace outcome suite (WOS) annual report 2017*. Retrieved from http://chestnutglobalpartners.org/Portals/cgp/Publications/WOS-Annual-Report-2017-09-08.pdf

Coleman-Cowger, V. H., Baumer, P. C., Dennis, M. L., & Scott, C. K. (2015). L'impact de la concomitance de troubles liés à la consummation de substance et de troubles de santé mentale sur les comportements à risqué en function de l'âge. *Drogues, santé et société, 14*(1), 17–77.

Conrad, K. J., Bezruczko, N., Chan, Y. F., Riley, B., Diamond, G., & Dennis, M. L. (2010). Screening for atypical suicide risk with person fit statistics among people presenting to alcohol and other drug treatment. *Drug and Alcohol Dependence, 106*(2), 92–100.

Conrad, K. J., Conrad, K. M., Mazza, J., Riley, B. B., Funk, R., Stein, M. A., & Dennis, M. L. (2012). Dimensionality, hierarchical structure, age generalizability, and criterion validity of the GAIN's Behavioral Complexity Scale. *Psychological Assessment, 24*(4), 913–924.

Conrad, K. M., Conrad, K. J., Passetti, L. L., Funk, R. R., & Dennis, M. L. (2015). Validation of the full and short-form Self-Help Involvement Scale against the Rasch Measurement Model. *Evaluation Review, 39*(4), 395–427.

Conrad, K. M., Dennis, M. L., Bezruczko, N., Funk, R. R., & Riley, B. B. (2007). Substance use disorder symptoms: Evidence of differential item functioning by age. *Journal of Applied Measurement, 8*(4), 1–15.

Conrad, K. J., Riley, B. B., Conrad, K. M., Chan, Y. F., & Dennis, M. L. (2010). Validation of the Crime and Violence Scale (CVS) against the Rasch measurement model including differences by gender, race, and age. *Evaluation Review, 34*(2), 83–115.

Courtney, M. E., Barth, R. P., Berrick, J. D., Brooks, D., Needell, B., & Park, L. (1996). Race and child welfare service: Past research and future direction. *Child Welfare, 75*(2), 99–138.
Dakof, G. A., Henderson, C. E., Rowe, C. L., Bousanti, M., Greenbaum, P. E., Wang, W., … Liddle, H. A. (2015). A randomized clinical trial of family therapy in juvenile drug court. *Journal of Family Psychology, 29*(2), 232–241.
Dennis, M. L., Babor, T., Roebuck, M. C., & Donaldson, J. (2002). Changing the focus: The case for recognizing and treating marijuana use disorders. *Addiction, 97*(Suppl. 1), S4–S15.
Dennis, M. L., Baumer, P. C., & Stevens, S. (2016). The concurrent evolution and intertwined nature of juvenile drug courts and reclaiming futures approaches to juvenile justice reform. *Drug Court Review, X*(1), 6–30.
Dennis, M. L., Chan, Y. F., & Funk, R. (2006). Development and validation of the GAIN Short Screener (GSS) for internalizing, externalizing, and substance use disorders and crime/violence problems among adolescents and adults. *American Journal on Addictions, 15*(Suppl. 1), 80–91.
Dennis, M. L., Clark, H. W., & Huang, L. N. (2014). The need and opportunity to expand substance use disorder treatment in school-based settings. *Advances in School Mental Health Promotion, 7*(2), 75–87.
Dennis, M. L., Dawud-Noursi, S., Muck, R. D., & McDermeit (Ives), M. (2003). The need for developing and evaluating adolescent treatment models. In S. J. Stevens & A. R. Morral (Eds.), *Adolescent substance abuse treatment in the USA: Exemplary models from a National Evaluation Study* (pp. 3–34). Binghamton, NY: Haworth Press.
Dennis, M. L., Foss, M. A., & Scott, C. K. (2007). Correlates of long-term recovery after treatment. *Evaluation Review, 31*(6), 585–612.
Dennis, M. L., Godley, S. H., Diamond, G., Tims, F. M., Babor, T., Donaldson, J., … R, R. (2004). The Cannabis Youth Treatment (CYT) Study: Main findings from two randomized trials. *Journal of Substance Abuse Treatment, 27*(3), 197–213.
Dennis, M. L., Ives, M. L., White, M. K., & Muck, R. D. (2008). The Strengthening Communities for Youth (SCY) initiative: A cluster analysis of the services received, their correlates and how they are associated with outcomes. *Journal of Psychoactive Drugs, 40*(1), 3–16.
Dennis, M. L., Scott, C. K., & Funk, R. (2003). An experimental evaluation of recovery management checkups (RMC) for people with chronic substance use disorders. *Evaluation and Program Planning, 26*(3), 339–352.
Dennis, M. L., Scott, C. K., Funk, R., & Foss, M. A. (2005). The duration and correlates of addiction and treatment careers. *Journal of Substance Abuse Treatment, 28*(Suppl. 1), S51–S62.
Dennis, M. L., Titus, J. C., Diamond, G., Donaldson, J., Godley, S. H., Tims, F., … Steering Committee, C. Y. T. (2002). The Cannabis Youth Treatment (CYT) experiment: Rationale, study design, and analysis plans. *Addiction, 97*(Suppl. 1), S16–S34.
Dennis, M. L., Titus, J. C., White, M., Unsicker, J., & Hodgkins, D. (2003). *Global Appraisal of Individual Needs (GAIN): Administration guide for the GAIN and related measures* (5th ed.). Bloomington, IL: Chestnut Health Systems.
Dennis, M. L., White, M. K., & Ives, M. L. (2009). Individual characteristics and needs associated with substance misuse of adolescents and young adults in addiction treatment. In C. G. Leukefeld, T. P. Gullotta, & M. Stanton Tindall (Eds.), *Handbook on adolescent substance abuse prevention treatment: Evidence-based practice*. New York, NY: Springer.
French, M. T., Roebuck, M. C., Dennis, M. L., Diamond, G., Godley, S. H., Tims, F., … Herrell, J. M. (2002). The economic cost of outpatient marijuana treatment for adolescents: Findings from a multi-site field experiment. *Addiction, 97*(Suppl. 1), 84–97.
French, M. T., Zavala, S. K., McCollister, K. E., Waldron, H. B., Turner, C. W., & Ozechowski, T. J. (2008). Cost-effectiveness analysis of four interventions for adolescents with a substance use disorder. *Journal of Substance Abuse Treatment, 34*(3), 272–281.
Funk, R. R., McDermeit (Ives), M., Godley, S. H., & Adams, L. (2003). Maltreatment issues by level of adolescent substance abuse treatment: The extent of the problem at intake and relationship to early outcomes. *Child Maltreatment, 8*(1), 36–45.

Garner, B. R., Hunter, B. D., Smith, D. C., Smith, J. E., & Godley, M. D. (2014). The relationship between child maltreatment and substance abuse treatment outcomes among emerging adults and adolescents. *Child Maltreatment, 19*(3–4), 261–269.

Gerstein, D. R., & Johnson, R. A. (1999). *Adolescents and young adults in the National Treatment Improvement Evaluation Study (National Evaluation Data Services Report)*. Rockville, MD: Center for Substance Abuse Treatment.

Godette, D. C., Mulatu, M. S., Leonard, K. J., Randolph, S., & Williams, N. (2011). Racial/ethnic disparities in patterns and determinants of criminal justice involvement among youth in substance abuse treatment programs. *Journal of Correctional Health Care, 17*(4), 294–308.

Godley, M. D., Godley, S. H., Dennis, M. L., Funk, R., & Passetti, L. (2002). Preliminary outcomes from the assertive continuing care experiment for adolescents discharged from residential treatment. *Journal of Substance Abuse Treatment, 23*(1), 21–32.

Godley, M. D., Godley, S. H., Dennis, M. L., Funk, R. R., & Passetti, L. L. (2007). The effect of Assertive Continuing Care (ACC) on continuing care linkage, adherence and abstinence following residential treatment for adolescents. *Addiction, 102*(1), 81–93.

Government Accountability Office (GAO). (2007). *African American children in foster care*. Washington, DC: Author.

Grant, B. F., & Dawson, D. A. (1998). Age of onset of drug use and its association with DSM-IV drug abuse and dependence. *Journal of Substance Abuse, 10*(2), 163–173.

Green, B. L., Rockhill, A., & Furrer, C. (2007). Does substance abuse treatment make a difference for child welfare case outcomes? A statewide longitudinal study. *Children and Youth Services Review, 29*(4), 460–473.

Henggeler, S. W., Halliday-Boykins, C. A., Cunningham, P. B., Randall, J., Shapiro, S. B., & Chapman, J. E. (2006). Juvenile drug court: Enhancing outcomes by integrating evidence-based treatments. *Journal of Consulting and Clinical Psychology, 74*(1), 42–54.

Hser, Y. I., Grella, C. E., Hubbard, R. L., Hsieh, S. C., Fletcher, B. W., Brown, B. S., & Anglin, M. D. (2001). An evaluation of drug treatments for adolescents in four U.S. cities. *Archives of General Psychiatry, 58*(7), 689–695.

Hubbard, R. L., Cavanaugh, E. R., Craddock, S. G., & Rachal, J. V. (1985). Characteristics, behaviors, and outcomes for youth in the TOPS: Treatment services for adolescent substance abusers. In A. S. Friedman & G. M. Beschner (Eds.), *Treatment services for adolescent substance abusers* (pp. 49–65). Rockville, MD: National Institute on Drug Abuse.

Hunter, B. D., Godley, M. D., & Godley, S. H. (2014). Feasibility of implementing the Adolescent Community Reinforcement Approach in school settings for adolescents with substance use disorders. *Advances in School Mental Health Promotion, 7*(2), 105–122.

Ireland, T. O., Smith, C. A., & Walter, J. E. (2015). Maltreatment and damaging outcomes in adolescence. In M. D. Krohn & J. Lane (Eds.), *The handbook of juvenile delinquency and juvenile justice* (pp. 581–600). Chichester: John Wiley & Sons, Inc..

Ives, M. L., Chan, Y. F., Modisette, K. C., & Dennis, M. L. (2010). Characteristics, needs, services and outcomes of youths in juvenile treatment drug courts as compared to adolescent outpatient treatment. *Drug Court Review, 7*(1), 10–56.

Kelly, L. M., Becker, S. J., Wolff, J. C., Graves, H., & Spirito, A. (2017). Interactive effect of parent and adolescent psychiatric symptoms on substance use among adolescents in community treatment. *Community Mental Health Journal, 53*(4), 383–393.

Korchmaros, J. D., Baumer, P. C., & Valdez, E. S. (2016). Critical components of adolescent substance use treatment programs – The impact of juvenile drug court: Strategies in practice and elements of reclaiming futures. *Drug Court Review, X*(1), 60–79.

Lennox, R., Dennis, M. L., Ives, M., & White, M. K. (2006). The construct and predictive validity of different approaches to combining urine and self-reported drug use measures among older adolescents after substance abuse treatment. *American Journal on Addictions, 15*(Suppl. 1), 92–101.

Lennox, R. D., Dennis, M. L., Scott, C. K., & Funk, R. R. (2006). Combining psychometric and biometric measures of substance use. *Drug and Alcohol Dependence, 83*(2), 95–103.

Lu, Y. E., Landsverk, J., Ellis-Macleod, E., Newton, R., Ganger, W., & Johnson, I. (2004). Race, ethnicity, and case outcomes in child protective services. *Children and Youth Services Review, 26*(5), 447–461.

Luna, B., Padmanabhan, A., & O'Hearn, K. (2010). What has fMRI told us about the development of cognitive control through adolescence. *Brain and Cognition, 72*(1), 101–113.

Marlowe, D. B., Festinger, D. S., Dugosh, K. L., Lee, P. A., & Benasutti, K. M. (2007). Adapting judicial supervision to the risk level of drug offenders: Discharge and 6-month outcomes from a prospective matching study. *Drug and Alcohol Dependence, 88*(Suppl. 2), S4–S13.

Marsh, J. C., Ryan, J. P., Choi, S., & Testa, M. F. (2006). Integrated services for families with multiple problems: Obstacles to family reunification. *Children and Youth Services Review, 28*(9), 1074–1087.

McAlpine, C., Marshall, C. C., & Doran, N. H. (2001). Combining child welfare and substance abuse services: A blended model of intervention. *Child Welfare, 80*(2), 129–149.

McCollister, K., Yang, X., Sayed, B., French, M. T., Leff, J. A., & Schackman, B. R. (2017). Monetary conversion factors for economic evaluations of substance use disorders. *Journal of Substance Abuse Treatment, 81*, 25–34.

Mee-Lee, D., Shulman, G. D., Fishman, M. J., Gastfriend, D. R., & Miller, M. M. (Eds.). (2013). *The ASAM criteria: Treatment criteria for addictive, substance-related and co-occurring conditions* (3rd ed.). Carson City, NV: The Change Companies.

Merikangas, K. R., He, J. P., Swanson, S. A., Avenevoli, S., Cui, L., Benjet, C., … Swendsen, J. (2010). Lifetime prevalence of mental disorders in U.S. adolescents: Results from the National Comorbidity Replication-Adolescent supplement (NCS-A). *Journal of the American Academy of Child and Adolescent Psychiatry, 49*(10), 980–989.

Mulatu, M. S., Leonard, K. J., Godette, D. C., & Fulmore, D. (2008). Disparities in the patterns and determinants of HIV risk behaviors among adolescents entering substance abuse treatment programs. *Journal of the National Medical Association, 100*(12), 1405–1416.

Nagelhout, G. E., Hummel, K., de Goeij, C. M., de Vries, H., Kaner, E., & Lemmens, P. (2017). How economic recessions and unemployment affect illegal drug use: A systematic realist literature review. *International Journal of Drug Policy, 44*, 69–83.

National Research Council. (2012). *Reforming juvenile justice: A developmental approach*. Washington, DC: The National Academies Press.

Nissen, L. B., Hunt, S. R., Bullman, S., Marmo, J., & Smith, D. (2004). Systems of care for treatment of adolescent substance use disorders: Background, principles and opportunities. *Journal of Psychoactive Drugs, 36*(4), 429–438.

Office of Juvenile Justice and Delinquency Prevention (OJJDP). (2014). *Juvenile court statistics 2010*. Washington, DC: OJJDP Retrieved from http://www.ojjdp.gov/ojstatbb/nr2014/downloads/NR2014.pdf

Office of Juvenile Justice and Delinquency Prevention (OJJDP). (2016). Juvenile Drug Treatment Court guidelines. OJJDP Washington, DC. https://www.ojjdp.gov/pubs/250368.pdf

Piaget, J. (1972). Intellectual evolution from adolescence to adulthood. *Human Development, 15*(1), 1–12.

Ratterman, M. J. (2014). Measuring the impact of substance abuse on student academic achievement and academic growth. *Advances in School Mental Health Promotion, 7*(2), 123–135.

Riley, B. B., Conrad, K. J., Bezruczko, N., & Dennis, M. L. (2007). Relative precision, efficiency and construct validity of different starting and stopping rules for a computerized adaptive test: The GAIN Substance Problem Scale. *Journal of Applied Measurement, 8*(1), 48–64.

Riley, B. B., Dennis, M. L., & Conrad, K. J. (2010). A comparison of content-balancing procedures for estimating multiple clinical domains in computerized adaptive testing: Relative precision, validity, and detection of persons with misfitting responses. *Applied Psychological Measurement, 34*(6), 410–423.

Rounds-Bryant, J. L., Kristiansen, P. L., & Hubbard, R. L. (1999). Drug abuse treatment outcome study of adolescents: A comparison of client characteristics and pretreatment behaviors in three treatment modalities. *American Journal of Drug and Alcohol Abuse, 25*(4), 573–591.

Rounds-Bryant, J. L., & Staab, J. (2001). Patient characteristics and treatment outcomes for African American, Hispanic, and White adolescents in DATOS-A. *Journal of Adolescent Research, 16*(6), 624–641.

Sells, S. B., & Simpson, D. D. (1979). Evaluation of treatment outcome for youths in the Drug Abuse Reporting Program (DARP): A follow-up study. In G. M. Beschner & A. S. Friedman (Eds.), *Youth drug abuse: Problems, issues, and treatment* (pp. 571–628). Lexington, MA: DC Heath.

Shane, P., Diamond, G. S., Mensinger, J. L., Shera, D., & Wintersteen, M. B. (2006). Impact of victimization on substance abuse treatment outcomes for adolescents in outpatient and residential substance abuse treatment. *American Journal on Addictions, 15*(Suppl. 1), 34–42.

Shane, P., Jasiukaitis, P., & Green, R. S. (2003). Treatment outcomes among adolescents with substance abuse problems: The relationship between comorbidities and post-treatment substance involvement. *Evaluation and Program Planning, 26*(4), 393–402.

Simpson, D. D., Savage, L. J., & Sells, S. B. (1978). *Data book on drug treatment outcomes. Follow-up study of the 1969–1977 admissions to the Drug Abuse Reporting Program (IRB report no. 78-10).* Fort Worth, TX: Texas Christian University.

Smith, D. C., Bennett, K. M., Dennis, M. L., & Funk, R. R. (2017a). Sensitivity and specificity of the GAIN short-screener for predicting substance use disorders in a large national sample of emerging adults. *Addictive Behaviors, 68*, 14–17.

Smith, D. C., Bennett, K. M., Dennis, M. L., & Funk, R. R. (2017b). Screening, assessment and diagnosis of substance use disorders among emerging adults. In D. Smith (Ed.), *Emerging adults and substance use disorder treatment: Developmental considerations and innovative approaches* (pp. 38–70). New York, NY: Oxford University Press.

Spear, L. P. (2010). *The Behavioral Neuroscience of Adolescence*. New York, NY: W. W. Norton & Company, Inc.

Steinberg, L. (2005). Cognitive and affective development in adolescence. *Trends in Cognitive Sciences, 9*(2), 69–74.

Steinberg, L. (2010). A dual systems model of adolescent risk-taking. *Developmental Psychobiology, 52*(3), 216–224.

Substance Abuse and Mental Health Services Administration (SAMHSA). (2016a). *Key substance use and mental health indicators in the USA: Results from the 2015 National survey on drug use and health (NSDUH Series H-51, HHS Publication No. SMA 16–4984).* Author: Rockville, MD.

Substance Abuse and Mental Health Services Administration (SAMHSA). (2016b). *Treatment episode data set: Admissions 2014 data set (TEDS-A-2014-DS0001).* Rockville, MD: Author Retrieved from http://datafiles.samhsa.gov/study-dataset/treatment-episode-data-set-admissions-2014-teds-2014-ds0001-nid16950

Tanner-Smith, E. E., & Lipsey, M. W. (2015). Brief alcohol interventions for adolescents and young adults: A systematic review and meta-analysis. *Journal of Substance Abuse Treatment, 51*, 1–18.

Taxman, F. S., & Marlowe, D. B. (2006). Risk, needs, responsivity: In action or inaction? *Crime Delinquency, 52*(1), 3–6.

Titus, J. C., Dennis, M. L., White, W. L., Scott, C. K., & Funk, R. R. (2003). Gender differences in victimization severity and outcomes among adolescents treated for substance abuse. *Journal of Child Maltreatment, 8*(1), 19–35.

United States Bureau of Labor Statistics. (2017). *Current population survey (CPS)*. Washington, DC: USA Bureau of Labor Statistics Retrieved from https://www.bls.gov/cps/cpsaat03.htm

Van Etten, M. L., & Anthony, J. C. (1999). Comparative epidemiology of initial drug opportunities and transitions to first use: Marijuana, cocaine, hallucinogens and heroin. *Drug and Alcohol Dependence, 54*(2), 117–125.

Welty, L. J., Harrison, A. J., Abram, K. M., Olson, N. D., Aaby, D. A., McCoy, K. P., … Teplin, L. A. (2016). Health disparities in drug- and alcohol-use disorders: A 12-year longitudinal study of youths after detention. *American Journal of Public Health, 106*(5), 872–880.

White, M. (2005). Predicting violence in juvenile offenders: The interaction of individual, social, and environmental influences. *Offender Substance Abuse Report, 5*(6), 83–90.
White, M. K., Funk, R. R., White, W. L., & Dennis, M. L. (2004). Predicting violent behavior in adolescent cannabis users: The GAIN-CVI. In K. Knight & D. Farabee (Eds.), *Farabee treating addicted offenders: A continuum of effective practices* (pp. 3-1–3-7). Kingston, NJ: Civic Research Institute.
Winters, K. C., Tanner-Smith, E. E., Bresani, E., & Meyers, K. (2014). Current advances in the treatment of adolescent drug use. *Adolescent Health, Medicine and Therapeutics, 2014*(5), 199–210.

Adolescent Substance Abuse Treatment: A Review of Evidence-Based Research

Ken C. Winters, Andria M. Botzet, Randy Stinchfield, Rachel Gonzales-Castaneda, Andrew J. Finch, Timothy F. Piehler, Kadie Ausherbauer, Kristen Chalmers, and Anna Hemze

Introduction

Use of alcohol and other drugs (hereafter referred to as *drugs*) by American teenagers continues to present a significant public health concern. Whereas substance use among adolescents has leveled-off, and in some instances declined, in recent years (Miech, Johnston, O'Malley, Bachman, & Schulenberg, 2016)

K. C. Winters (✉)
Oregon Research Institute, Falcon Heights, MN, USA
e-mail: winte001@umn.edu

A. M. Botzet
Department of Psychiatry, University of Minnesota, Minneapolis, MN, USA
e-mail: botze003@umn.edu

R. Stinchfield
Saint Paul, MN, USA
e-mail: stinc001@umn.edu

R. Gonzales-Castaneda
Department of Psychology, Azusa Pacific University, Azusa, CA, USA
e-mail: rcastaneda@apu.edu

A. J. Finch
Peabody College, Vanderbilty University, Nashville, TN, USA
e-mail: andrew.j.finch@vanderbilt.edu

T. F. Piehler · K. Ausherbauer
Department of Family Social Science, University of Minnesota, Saint Paul, MN, USA
e-mail: tpiehler@umn.edu; aushe001@umn.edu

K. Chalmers · A. Hemze
Minneapolis, MN, USA
e-mail: chalm029@umn.edu; hemze004@umn.edu

C. G. Leukefeld, T. P. Gullotta (eds.), *Adolescent Substance Abuse*, Issues in Children's and Families' Lives, https://doi.org/10.1007/978-3-319-90611-9_5

the rates of use are still a public health concern (National Institute on Drug Abuse, 2014). Adolescence represents a critical period for the onset of drug use; onset of use during these years increases the likelihood of negative impacts on a range of developmental factors, including cognitive, physical, and psychosocial. Also, early onset use also increases the likelihood for developing a substance use disorder (SUD), and for some youth, it contributes to the progression of a long-term SUD (Volkow, Baler, Compton, & Weiss, 2014). There are concerns that recent trends in the USA to legalize marijuana for recreational or medical purposes may contribute to a rise in adolescent marijuana use. Marijuana is the most commonly used illicit drug among adolescents in the USA and is now used at higher rates than tobacco (Miech et al., 2016). Nearly one-quarter (23.4%) of high school students report use at least one or more times per month (Kann et al., 2014).

For youth who meet criteria for a SUD, treatment may be indicated. According to the National Survey on Drug Use and Health, approximately 1.3 million adolescents had a past year SUD (Center for Behavioral Health Statistics and Quality, 2015). Yet it is estimated that about 90% of youth with a SUD do not receive drug treatment (Substance Abuse and Mental Health Services Administration, 2013). There are several reasons for the large gap between SUDs and treatment utilization by youth: little if any local treatment options, poor health coverage, low motivation by the youth, and unsupportive parents.

Developmental Issues

The adolescent drug abuse treatment field continues to make significant strides in the expanding the field of evidence-based approaches. A common theme across contemporary approaches is their developmental relevance. Adolescents seeking treatment differ from their adult counterparts in many ways: the length and severity of substance use is usually less; typical patterns and context of use differ; the type of substance-related problems most often experienced also differ; and in most instances there is not a self-referral to treatment (National Institute on Drug Abuse, 2014). Moreover, developmental neuroscience research, which supports the view that brain develops during adolescence in a way that contributes to risky judgments, including the tendency to make choices based on heavily on emotion, (Spear, 2002; Volkow et al., 2014), have led to various speculations that youth may be less motivated to change drug use behaviors than adult clients, that advice alone may be ineffective for promoting change for a teenager, and that positive peer influences and interactions during treatment may be particularly important to treatment outcome (Riggs et al., 2007). Furthermore, because youth typically enter treatment because of a referral by a concerned parent, mental health clinician, or school staff) (Battjes, Gordon, O'Grady, & Kinlock, 2004), a negative attitude about drug treatment may be a prevalent among adolescents.

Intensity of Treatment

Based on several client characteristics (e.g., severity of drug involvement; mental health condition; current and past medical condition; environment support for recovery; readiness to change), it is advisable to initially place an adolescent into one of the following five treatment levels (American Society of Addiction Medicine, 2013): (1) brief intervention; (2) outpatient; (3) intensive outpatient; (4) residential/inpatient; or (5) medically managed inpatient treatment.

Treatment Approaches

Most adolescent drug treatment programs use an eclectic treatment approach, integrating multiple therapeutic strategies within their treatment service framework. Common themes among them are that they teach skills to resist the triggers associated with the individual's drug use pattern, address life functioning issues that likely contributed to the onset and maintenance of the drug use (e.g., mental health, family issues), and identify and build upon a youth's strengths.

Research has established that several types of therapeutic practices and approaches, regardless of intensity of treatment or therapeutic approach, are vital to providing effective treatment for adolescents with a drug problem. Recently the National Institute of Drug Abuse (2014) identified 13 practice principles that are elements of quality care spanning assessment, treatment and aftercare (see Table 1).

Treatment Outcome Research

Overview

Despite this issue of low treatment utilization, significant advances have been made since 1990 in the development and scientific evaluation of treatments for adolescent drug abuse (e.g., Winters, Tanner-Smith, Bresani, & Meyers, 2014). Perhaps the most significant sign of these advances is that the field is now characterized by rigorous controlled studies on the effectiveness of treatment approaches and strategies. Many treatments for adolescents with a SUD that are now considered evidenced based.

We focused our literature search on controlled evaluations of drug abuse treatment approaches for adolescent clients since 1990, owing to the principle that drug treatment for adolescents prior to that time may not be comparable to more contemporary and rigorous standards. The criteria for study inclusion were as follows: (1) adolescents had to be the primary target of the intervention or treatment; (2) drug use outcomes had to be measured; and (3) the study consisted of essential components of a controlled evaluation, including favorable sample sizes, com-

Table 1 Principles of adolescent substance use treatment

Principle	Description
1. Identify and address substance use as soon as possible	Identifying and addressing adolescent substance use as soon as possible is important due to the negative effects early use can have on the brain. Additionally, adults with substance use disorders often report using drugs as adolescents or young adults.
2. Adolescents do not have to be addicted to benefit from a substance use intervention	Interventions can successfully treat a range of substance use disorders from problematic use to severe addiction. Youth in particular can benefit from intervention at early stages. Even use that does not seem problematic can lead to heavier use and other risky behaviors.
3. Medical visits are an opportunity to ask about drug use	Medical doctors (e.g., pediatricians, emergency room doctors, dentists) can use standardized screenings to determine if an adolescent is using substances and if an intervention is warranted. In some instances, it is possible to provide a brief intervention in the physician's office and in other cases referral to treatment is more appropriate.
4. Legal or family pressure may be an important influence on adolescent's involvement in treatment	Most adolescents with a substance use disorder do not think they need treatment and rarely look for treatment. Treatment can be successful even if the adolescent is legally mandated to treatment or goes due to family pressures.
5. Treatment should be tailored to the adolescent's needs	Many factors need to be considered when developing a treatment plan for an adolescent including sex, family, and peer relationships, and community environment. Therefore, it is necessary to begin with a comprehensive assessment.
6. Treatment should not focus on just substance use	Treatment is most successful when it focuses on the whole person. Treatment should address housing, medical, social, and legal needs.
7. Behavioral therapies can effectively treat substance use disorders	Behavioral therapies have been shown to be an effective treatment. These therapies help build motivation to change by providing incentives for abstinence, teaching skills to deal with cravings, and finding positive and rewarding activities.
8. Family and community support are important features of treatment	There are several evidence-based interventions for adolescent substance use that involve family members and individuals in the community. These interventions try to improve family communication and provide the adolescent with support.
9. Mental health conditions need to be addressed in order to effectively treat substance use	Adolescents with a substance use disorder often have co-occurring mental health conditions. It is important that adolescents are screened and treated for these other conditions in order for substance abuse treatment to be successful.
10. Sensitive issues should be addressed and confidentiality maintained when possible	It is common for adolescents with substance use disorders to have a history of abuse or other trauma.69 whereas maintaining confidentiality with respect to sensitive issues is important in the therapeutic setting, appropriate authorities need to be informed if abuse is suspected.
11. Drug use should be monitored during treatment	It is important to monitor an adolescent's drug use while in treatment and identify a relapse early on. The relapse could indicate that treatment should be intensified or needs to be altered to better meet the adolescent's needs.

(continued)

Table 1 (continued)

Principle	Description
12. Completing treatment and having a continuing care plan are important	The length of treatment will vary based on the severity of the adolescent's substance use disorder; however, studies have shown outcomes are best when an individual is in treatment 3 months or longer. The adolescent can also benefit from continuing care.
13. Adolescents should be tested and treated for sexually transmitted diseases and hepatitis	Drug using adolescents are at an increased risk for sexually transmitted and blood borne diseases (e.g., human immunodeficiency virus, hepatitis B and C) due to the increase in high-risk behaviors that result from drug use. Addressing this in treatment can help decrease high-risk behaviors thereby reducing the likelihood of infection.

Note. From the National Institute on Drug Abuse. *Principles of Adolescent Substance Use Disorder Treatment: A Research-Based Guide*. Bethesda, MD: National institute on Drug Abuse, 2014. Available from http://www.drugabuse.gov/publications/principles-adolescent-substance-use-disorder-treatment-research-based-guide/principles-adolescent-substance-use-disorder-treatment

parison group (i.e., control group, waiting list control, or contrasting treatment group), use of standardized assessment instruments, treatment interventions that are well-described, and outcome evaluation ratings by individuals who did not conduct the therapy.

Treatment outcome studies were identified from a computerized literature search of standard journal databases (e.g., MEDLINE, PsychINFO, Social Sciences Abstracts), as well as from drug treatment websites and the sites of well-known treatment research organizations. Close reviews of the reference sections of relevant books, identified studies, and the handful of literature summaries and reviews were also conducted. We benefited from recent reviews of the literature (Deas & Thomas, 2001; Tanner-Smith, Wilson, & Lipsey, 2013; Vaughn & Howard, 2004).

The review is organized around these strategies or approaches: 12-step-based treatment, therapeutic community (TC), family-based interventions, behavioral therapy, cognitive behavioral therapy (CBT), motivational-based therapy (motivational enhancement and motivational interviewing), electronic and web-based therapy, and pharmacotherapy approaches (*see* Table 2 for an overview description of each). As noted above, multiple approaches are commonly integrated in clinical interventions, and thus, some overlap of approaches exists within the review presented here. Additionally we discuss these approaches aimed at maximizing outcome: recovery high schools, use of reinforcements, and adaptive strategies.

In addition to providing an overview of the prominent types of treatment approaches noted in Table 2, we also summarize a major multisite study (Cannabis Youth Treatment project) and highlight a recent meta-analysis on outpatient treatment (a meta-analysis refers to statistical techniques used to synthesize quantitative findings across multiple studies included in a review). Regardless of therapeutic modality, one underlying goal of adolescent treatment for drug abuse involves promoting recovery by preventing or minimizing relapse. The definition of relapse varies, but in most instances it refers to a return to drug use. Some definitions of relapse include categories for the level of problems resulting from the return to drug use or

Table 2 Descriptions of seven primary treatment approaches

Approach	Description
1. 12-step-based	The goal of 12-step therapy is to encourage the adolescent to become involved in a 12-step program. These programs incorporate a self-help approach centered within the context of reciprocal support. They are organized around the basic tenets of alcoholics anonymous (AA), and are a commonly applied strategy in inpatient and outpatient treatment programs, as well as a standalone approach (i.e., attending AA, narcotics anonymous, or cocaine anonymous meetings). Approximately 2.3% of AA members in the USA and Canada are under the age of 21.
2. Therapeutic community	The therapeutic community is typically rooted in self-help principles and experiential knowledge of the recovery community. This treatment option views the community as the key agent of change and emphasizes mutual self-help, behavioral consequences, and shared values for a healthy lifestyle. For adolescents, therapeutic communities use various therapeutic techniques which may include individual counseling sessions, family therapy, 12-step techniques, life skills techniques, and recreational techniques, and are usually long-term residential treatment programs.
3. Family-based	Family-based approaches seek to reduce an adolescent's use of drugs and correct the problem behaviors that often accompany drug use by addressing the mediating family risk factors, such as poor family communication, cohesiveness, and problem-solving. These approaches are based on the therapeutic premise that the family has the most profound and long-lasting influence on child and adolescent development. Family therapy typically includes the adolescent and at least one other parent or guardian, but can also include siblings, other family members, and friends. There are five evidence-based family-based treatments that are in use today: Brief strategic family therapy; family behavior therapy; functional family therapy; multidimensional family therapy; and multisystemic therapy.
4. Behavior therapy	Behavioral approaches generally focus on teaching and reinforcing new skills, behaviors, and new ways of thinking and coping so as to compete with or minimize drug-using behaviors. The ultimate goal is to reinforce desirable behaviors and eliminate unwanted or maladaptive ones.
5. Cognitive-behavior therapy	Cognitive-behavioral therapy (CBT) is centered on the notion that thoughts cause behaviors, and these thoughts determine the way in which people perceive, interpret, and assign meaning to the environment. Thus, maladaptive behaviors can be changed by modifying our thought processes, even if one's environment does not change. In the context of adolescent substance use, CBT encourages adolescents to develop self-regulation and coping skills by teaching youth to identify stimulus cues that precede drug use, to use various strategies to avoid situations that may trigger the desire to use, and to develop skills for communication and problem-solving.

(continued)

Table 2 (continued)

Approach	Description
6. Motivational enhancement therapy/brief intervention	Motivational enhancement therapy is based on motivational interviewing techniques that have come to the forefront of therapeutic approaches for addiction in the past decade, and even more so recently for adolescents. The goal of motivational enhancement therapy is to help encourage the adolescent to engage in treatment and stop using drugs. Motivational enhancement therapists use a person-centered, nonconfrontational style in assisting the youth to explore different facets of his or her use patterns. Adolescents are encouraged to examine the pros and cons of their use and to create goals to help them achieve a healthier lifestyle. The therapist provides personalized feedback and respects the youth's freedom of choice regarding his or her own behavior. Motivational enhancement therapy is typically delivered in conjunction with other treatment approaches, including brief interventions. Brief intervention often consists of educational or brief intervention services that aim to help the adolescent recognize the negative consequences of substance use and to understand and address the adolescent's problems that are likely related to their substance use.
7. Electronic and web-based therapy	Current use of electronic-assisted therapy includes internet "treatment programs" that employ various elements, such as psychoeducation, social support through chat rooms, monitoring of symptoms and progress, and feedback. Also included here are telephone-based treatment approaches.
8. Pharmacotherapy	This treatment approach uses medication to address various aspects of addiction, including craving reduction, aversive therapy, substitution therapy, and treatment of underlying psychiatric disorders. Specifically, medication can be used to treat addiction to opioids, alcohol, or nicotine in adults, but there are no medications approved by the US Food and Drug Administration to treat cannabis, cocaine, or methamphetamine abuse. Research is quite limited on this treatment strategy for adolescents, and there are no medications that are currently approved to treat adolescents. The applicability of adult findings to adolescents is unclear given that youth may react differently to the potential side effects of medications. However, doctors will sometimes prescribe medications to older adolescents.

Note. Adapted from "Adolescent Substance Abuse Treatment: A Review of Evidence-Based Research," by K. C. Winters, A. M. Botzet, T. Fahnhorst, R. Stinchfield, & R. Koskey, 2009, In C. G. Leukefeld, T. P. Gullotta & M. Staton-Tindall (Eds.), *Adolescent Substance Abuse: Evidence-Based Approaches to Prevention and Treatment*, pp. 73-96. New York, NY: Springer

for the levels of drug use frequency. Among youth receiving treatment for an SUD, it can be expected that from one-third to one-half are likely to return to some drug use at least once within 12 months following treatment (Grella, Joshi, & Hser, 2004; National Institute on Drug Abuse, 2014; Williams, Chang, & Addiction Centre Adolescent Research Group, 2000; Winters, 1999).

12-Step-Based Treatment

Organized around the basic tenets of Alcoholics Anonymous (AA), it is generally accepted in the field that this treatment approach is the most commonly applied strategy to youth with an SUD. It is estimated that about two-thirds of treatment programs utilize these basic principles as part of their approach, and some programs are primarily organized around the AA principles (Sussman, 2010). The first 5 steps of the 12 steps are typically addressed with adolescents during the primary treatment experience. These five steps are the following: (1) admitting that you are powerless over the addictive substance and that it has made life unmanageable, (2) believing that a power greater than yourself could restore you to health, (3) making a decision to turn your will over to a higher power as you interpret it to be, (4) taking moral inventory of yourself, and (5) admitting to yourself and to others the nature of your wrongs. One typically embarks upon the remaining seven steps during aftercare.

Applicability of the 12-step method for youth has been questioned due to limitations in developmentally appropriate content. Adolescence is a time of identifying a personal identity and independence from authority figures, developmental milestones that can be inconsistent with the main tenants of AA of acceptance and surrender. In addition, 12-step-based aftercare programs (e.g., AA, NA) are mainly composed of adults. It is estimated that only 2% of participants in self-help groups are under the age of 21 (Alcoholics Anonymous 2001 Membership Survey, 2001), which creates barriers for adolescents as they may struggle to relate to older group members (Kelly, Brown, Abrantes, Kahler, & Myers, 2008; Kelly & Urbanoski, 2012). Thus, efforts to adapt 12-step treatment for adolescents are important. Current adaptations of this approach include the Minnesota Model treatment approach for adolescents (Anderson, McGovern, & DuPont, 1999) and Jaffe's (1990) developmentally appropriate modifications of the first five steps of a 12-step program.

An approach that incorporates the 12-step method, the Minnesota Model, has been researched. The Minnesota Model includes a range of therapeutic elements (e.g., group and family therapy) in conjunction with the 12-step method (Winters, Stinchfield, Opland, Weller, & Latimer, 2000). Winters and colleagues followed a group of 179 adolescents who participated in either an outpatient or inpatient Minnesota Model treatment and a group of 66 adolescents who were on a treatment waiting-list (primarily due to insurance coverage limitations or no insurance). Results indicated that among the treated youth, those who finished the treatment program reported superior outcomes in contrast to those who left the program prior to completion and to a waiting-list group (Winters et al., 2000). At the 12-month follow-up, categorical data revealed that 53% of the treatment completers reported abstinence or minor relapse (used once or twice) compared to 15% for the treatment incompleters and to 27% for the waiting-list group. Continuous variable data revealed similar results. The comparison of setting (inpatient versus outpatient) did not yield any outcome differences. A longer-term follow-up study (approximately 5 years post-treatment) of the same youth (Winters, Stinchfield, Latimer, & Lee, 2007) showed a similar pattern of outcome, although the major predictor of favorable outcomes was involvement in aftercare. Whereas the studies above showed that favorable outcome is associated with treatment engagement, the study designs did not permit opportunity to evaluate the specific contribution of 12-step elements.

AA/NA attendance has been researched among teenagers who have received 12-step treatment. The prominent work by Kelly and colleagues suggests that despite spotty AA/NA attendance over time, adolescents with greater addiction severity and those who believed that they needed to maintain abstinence had higher attendance rates, and greater early participation was associated with more favorable long-term outcome (Kelly et al., 2008). As many have written (e.g., Kelly, Magill, & Stout, 2009), AA/NA's value to teenagers may be that it provides a free, semistructured therapeutic service with the flexibility allowing the youth to modulate level of involvement.

Therapeutic Community

Like the 12-step Minnesota Model, TC is typically classified as a community-based therapy based in self-help principles and experiential knowledge of the recovery community (Morral, McCaffrey, & Ridgeway, 2004). This treatment approach views the community as the key agent of change, and it emphasizes mutual self-help, behavioral consequences, and shared values for a healthy lifestyle (Jainchill, 1997). Adolescent TCs tend to be long-term residential treatment programs, and typically include a wide variety of therapeutic techniques, including (but not limited to) individual counseling sessions, family therapy, 12-step method, life-skills, and recreational techniques.

Morral et al. (2004) examined the TC approach using a rigorous evaluation design that compared nearly 450 adolescents in a 9- to 12-month residential TC program (Phoenix Academy) and a comparison group of treatment as usual (probation dispositions). The findings indicated that participation in Phoenix Academy was associated with significantly reduced drug use and improved psychological functioning outcomes compared to the comparison group at 12-month posttreatment.

Family-Based Therapy

The family therapy approach seeks to reduce an adolescent's use of drugs and correct the problem behaviors that often accompany drug use by addressing the mediating family risk factors such as poor family communication, cohesiveness, and problem solving. This approach is based on the therapeutic premise that the family carries the most profound and long-lasting influence on child and adolescent development (Szapocznik & Coatsworth, 1999). Family therapy typically includes the adolescent and at least one other parent or guardian. Ideally, siblings and other adult household members are included. Other approaches and theoretical positions are commonly integrated into family-based treatment, such as CBT (Latimer, Winters, D'Zurilla, & Nichols, 2003) and family empowerment theory (e.g., Dembo et al., 2000). In addition, social, neighborhood, community, and cultural factors are also considered within the treatment plan (Ozechowski & Liddle, 2002).

Austin and colleagues (Austin, Macgowan, & Wagner, 2005) identified and reviewed five family-based treatment approaches, all of which involved random assignment and other rigorous design features: (1) Brief strategic family therapy (BSFT; Santisteban et al., 2003); (2) Family behavior therapy (Azrin, Donohue, Besalel, Kogan, & Acierno, 1994); (3) Functional family therapy (FFT; Waldron, Slesnick, Brody, Turner, & Peterson, 2001); (4) Multidimensional family therapy (MDFT; also referenced in the Cannabis Youth Treatment, CYT, section of this chapter) (Liddle, Rowe, Dakof, Henderson, & Greenbaum, 2009); and (5) Multisystemic treatment (MST; Henggeler, Clingempeel, Brondino, & Pickrel, 2002; Henggeler, Pickrel, & Brondino, 1999). Of these five, MDFT demonstrated both clinically and statistically significant favorable drug use outcomes at the conclusion of treatment and at the 1-year post- treatment assessment. Whereas the other four approaches (BSFT, MST, FFT, and FBT) showed greater improvement compared to the control group at the completion of treatment, posttreatment follow-up assessments did not reveal group differences for MST and FFT, and there are no posttreatment outcomes reported for the BSFT and FBT studies (Austin et al., 2005).

Smith and colleagues (Smith, Hall, Williams, An, & Gotman, 2006) compared an outpatient family intervention (Strengths oriented family therapy, SOFT; Smith & Hall, 2008), with a group therapy approach (The Seven Challenges®; Schwebel, 2004) The SOFT intervention incorporated a pretreatment motivational family session, multifamily skills training, and case management. The comparison group (Seven Challenges) utilized interactive journaling, skills training, and motivational interviewing. Results at 6-month posttreatment revealed that the two interventions were comparable in terms of achieving abstinence (39% for SOFT and 31% for Seven Challenges), being symptom free (61% and 60%, respectively), and extent of reduction of drug use frequency and affiliated problems (Smith et al., 2006).

Some family therapy models being used to treat adolescent drug use were specifically designed to address the problem of drug use, such as Multidimensional Family Therapy (MDFT) and Brief Strategic Family Therapy (BSFT). Other family treatment models have been applied to adolescent drug use, but were initially designed to treat delinquency more generally. Functional Family Therapy (FFT) and Multisystemic Therapy (MST) are two such family treatment models that have been applied to adolescent drug use problems. Currently, these four family treatment models are the most prevalent in terms of clinical use and empirical research.

Multidimensional Family Therapy (MDFT) was designed to treat adolescent drug use as well as delinquency (Liddle, 2013). It employs a developmental model and considers risk and resilience factors in terms of their roles in developmental cascades. The treatment has elements that focus on the adolescent and the adolescent-parent relationship, while considering social and contextual factors (Liddle, 2013). MDFT has been tested in several randomized control trials. One review article compared results of randomized controlled trials (RCTs) testing MDFT to those testing

Cognitive Behavior Therapy (CBT) and Motivational Enhancement Therapy (MET), and found evidence in favor of MDFT on cannabis use outcomes for younger adolescents and those with more severe dependence (Walther, Gantner, Heinz, & Majic, 2016). The four RCTs evaluating MDFT reported on in the review were comprised of two studies comparing MDFT to a treatment-as-usual control and two studies comparing MDFT to a CBT control condition (Walther et al., 2016). Those adolescents in MDFT had greater reductions in cannabis use at the end of the treatment compared to treatment-as-usual, with comparable end-of-treatment cannabis outcomes when compared to CBT. However, in one study with a CBT control, there were reductions in dependence for youth in the MDFT treatment condition at a 12-month follow-up, with even greater gains among the higher severity of cannabis use sub-group. Multiple meta-analyses have evaluated the effect size of MDFT treatment from RCTs comparing MDFT to other treatment models (Liddle, 2016). The reductions of drug use outcomes of MDFT from RCTs, even when compared to other high-quality evidence-based treatments such as CBT, tend to be durable and often are preferable to other treatments at 1 year follow-ups (Liddle, 2016).

In a multisite, randomized control trial of outpatient drug treatment for adolescents between the ages of 13–18 in Western Europe, MDFT was compared to individual counseling for the treatment of cannabis use disorder (Rigter et al., 2013). Across five countries (Belgium, France, Germany, The Netherlands, and Switzerland) 450 youth were randomized to either individual psychotherapy (IP) (which referred to the current practice of the clinician or agency, including CBT and other models) or Multidimensional Family Therapy (MDFT). Clinicians administering the MDFT treatment condition reported higher rates of treatment retention to successful completion (90% of cases) than did the clinicians administering the IP treatment condition (48% of cases). For low-severity users (below the median of number of days used in past 90 days), MDFT and IP models were comparatively similar in reducing use at 3, 6, 9, and 12 months post-baseline (Rigter et al., 2013). However, for high-severity users, MDFT reduced the number of days of use notably more than did IP, with the high severity MDFT group nearly matching the 12 month outcome of the low-severity IP group. The effect size of this difference between IP and MDFT reduction in use for the high severity group across sites was medium to large ($d = 0.60$; Rigter et al., 2013).

Multisystemic Therapy (MST) was designed to treat antisocial behavior in youth who are at imminent risk of out-of-home placement and has been applied to drug-abuse populations (Sheidow & Houston, 2013). MST identifies antisocial behavior as resulting from multiple determinants; thus, treatment efforts are made to simultaneously generate change in family, school, community, and peer contexts (Sheidow & Houston, 2013). The modality of MST is intensive and generally involves approximately 60 h with the MST therapist over the course of three to five months. MST includes 24/7 on-call access to MST therapists (Sheidow & Houston, 2013). MST has been tested with many RCTs in terms of delinquency, with considerably fewer studies on MST measuring drug use outcomes. MST generally has greater impact on delinquency than on drug use (Henggeler & Schaeffer, 2016). However, in a meta-analysis of MST RCTs that considered included drug use among delinquency outcomes ($n = 5$), there was evidence of significant improvements in drug use compared to control groups with a mean of small to moderate effect size ($d = 0.291$) (van der Stouwe, Asscher, Stams, Deković, & van der Laan, 2014).

An adaptation of MST, coined as Multisystemic Therapy—Substance Abuse (MST-SA), was designed to treat adolescents with a substance use disorder (Swenson, Henggeler, Taylor, & Addison, 2005). Henggeler et al. (2006) conducted a randomized controlled trial in which MST-SA in a drug court was compared to three other conditions: family court with usual community services, drug court with usual community services, and drug court with MST. In general, findings supported the view that drug court was more effective than family court services in decreasing rates of adolescent substance use and criminal behavior. MST and MST-SA were equivalent on the drug use outcomes (Henggeler et al., 2006).

Brief Strategic Family Therapy (BSFT) was designed to treat conduct problems, delinquency, and drug use (Szapocznik, Muir, & Schwartz, 2013). BSFT incorporates traditional family therapy models of Structural Family Therapy and Strategic Family Therapy (Szapocznik et al., 2013). BSFT has been tested in fewer RCTs than MDFT and MST; however, there has been two RCTs with adolescents), including one efficacy trial and one effectiveness trial (Szapocznik et al., 2013). The efficacy trial measured marijuana use outcomes compared to group counseling control condition, and it was found that BSFT had preferable outcomes to group counseling. Notably, the group counseling consition demonstrated some potential iatrogenic effects with increased marijuana use among control participants. The effectiveness trial measured drug use through self-reported days of use per month in the past year, and compared BSFT) to a treatment-as-usual control condition (Szapocznik et al., 2013). Using a sample referred from juenvile justice or residential treatment settings with relatively limited drug use, the BSFT intervention group demonstrated fewer days of use per month when compared to the control condition.

Functional Family Therapy (FFT) was designed to treat adolescents with conduct disorder, delinquency, and disruptive behavior and their families, and has also been applied to youth with addictive behaviors (Waldron, Brody, Robbins, & Alexander, 2013). FFT considers alcohol and drug abuse as problems that develop in the context of maladaptive family relationships; thus, the mechanism of change is improving family interactions (Waldron et al., 2013). FFT targets the whole family and is designed for all family members who are living together. In three RCTs comparing FFT, CBT, and FFT plus CBT, the outcomes supported FFT as an equivalent or superior choice to CBT (Waldron et al., 2013). FFT had much higher rates of engagement than the comparison of a parenting intervention in one study (93% and 67%, respectively); however, both conditions resulted in equivalent significant reductions in drug use (Waldron et al., 2013). A RCT comparing FFT, FFT + CBT, and CBT found that the FFT conditions generated greater reductions in marijuana use in the first 4 months of treatment when compared to the CBT-only condition. However, by a follow-up assessment at 19 months, all conditions demonstrated comparable reductions in drug use, indicating that while both FFT and CBT are effective, FFT may produce an earlier reduction in drug use when compared to CBT (Waldron et al., 2013). In a second RCT, comparison groups were FFT, FFT + CBT, individual CBT, and group CBT to address adolescent alcohol-related problems. All four conditions were successful in reducing alcohol use from pretreatment to post-treatment, and additionally the FFT, individual CBT, and group CBT were effective in reducing marijuana use despite not being targeted in treatment (Waldron et al., 2013). In a third RCT comparing FFT + CBT to CBT, the researchers found that while the two conditions were comparably effective for reducing drug use in White, non-Hispanic youth, the FFT + CBT condition was more effective for Hispanic youth in reducing drug use (Waldron et al., 2013).

Whereas several of the family-based treatments show preferable outcomes for the targeted youth compared to traditional individual focused treatments (e.g., Latimer et al., 2003) a perhaps unique benefit of family based treatment is the implications for other members of the family. In MST and FFT, some RCTs have also measured the rates of drug use in siblings of the targeted adolescent. In both MST and FFT trials, the research teams found decreases in the drug use of siblings in the family, not just in the targeted youth (Henggeler & Schaeffer, 2016; Waldron et al., 2013). This has interesting implications for cost-effectiveness analysis from treatment and prevention perspectives if siblings are also reaping the benefits of family treatment modalities.

Behavioral Therapy

Therapeutic techniques based on behavioral psychology theories are another approach to treating adolescent substance abuse. Behavioral strategies, which target actions and behaviors presumed to be influenced by one's environment, include modeling, rehearsal, self-recording, stimulus control, urge control, and written assignments. In current practice, behaviorism is most often coupled with techniques that modify cognitions, referred to as CBT (which we review in the next section). We identified one behavioral study that met our review inclusion criteria. Azrin and colleagues randomly assigned drug-abusing youth to either a supportive counseling group (n = 11) or a behavioral treatment group (n = 15) for ~6 months of treatment (Azrin et al., 1994). The results indicated that drug use significantly decreased over the course of the treatment for the behavioral treatment group, with 73% reporting abstinence during the last month of treatment, compared to only 9% of the comparison group. Other drug use outcome measures were also significantly improved for the behavioral group.

A variant if behavioral treatment is the adolescent community reinforcement approach (A-CRA; Godley et al., 2014, 2017). This intervention targets areas of the adolescent's life and surrounding community that reinforce reducing or eliminating substance use and helps the adolescent to replace these negative influences with healthier prosocial behaviors. A-CRA can address problem-solving, communication skills, relapse prevention, and encourage participation in positive social and community activities.

Cognitive Behavioral Therapy

CBT is based in the belief that thoughts cause behaviors, and these thoughts determine the way in which people perceive, interpret, and assign meaning to the environment (Beck & Weishaar, 2005). Thus, by changing our thought processes, maladaptive behaviors can be changed even if our environment does not change. When used within the context of adolescent substance use, CBT encourages adolescents to develop self-regulation and coping skills. Techniques commonly used include the identification of stimulus cues preceding drug use, the use of strategies to avoid situations that may trigger the urge to use, and skill development for refusal techniques, communication, and problem solving (Waldron et al., 2001). CBT is a frequently used therapeutic approach, but it is commonly integrated into other approaches (Beck & Weishaar, 2005), especially family systems therapy and motivational enhancement/brief interventions (BIs). For this reason, some CBT methods are also mentioned in other sections of this chapter as an integral part of another therapeutic approach.

Barrett and colleagues (Barrett, Slesnick, Brody, Turner, & Peterson, 2001) conducted a randomized clinical trial that compared CBT, family therapy, combined individual and family therapy, and a group intervention for 114 substance-abusing adolescents. Drug use outcomes were the percentage of days that marijuana was used and the percentage of youths achieving minimal use. Each intervention demonstrated some efficacy. From pretreatment to 4 months, significantly fewer days of use were found for the family therapy alone and the combined interventions. Significantly more youths achieved minimal use levels in the CBT, family, and combined conditions. From pretreatment to 7 months, reductions in percentage of days of use were significant for the combined and group interventions, and changes in minimal use levels were significant for the family, combined, and group interventions.

Kaminer, Burleson, and Goldberger (2002) examined a sample of 51 adolescents who were randomly assigned to a CBT intervention in comparison to 37 adolescents who received psychoeducational treatment. A greater reduction in substance use was found for older adolescents and for males in the CBT group at a 3-month follow-up, as compared to the psychoeducational group, but at 9-month follow-up the two groups did not differ on drug use outcome.

Motivational Enhancement Therapy (MET)/Brief Intervention

MET techniques have recently come to the forefront of therapeutic approaches for addiction, and even more so recently for adolescents. MET (also referred to as motivational interviewing) utilizes a person-centered, nonconfrontational approach to assist the youth to explore the different facets of their use patterns. Clients are encouraged to examine the pros and cons of their use and to create goals to help them achieve a healthier lifestyle. The therapist provides personalized feedback and respects the youth's freedom of choice regarding his/her own behavior. Although the relationship between the therapist and client is more of a partnership than an expert/recipient role, the therapist is directive in assisting the individual to examine and resolve ambivalence and to encourage the client's responsibility for selecting and working on healthy changes in behavior (Rollnick & Miller, 1995).

MET is frequently incorporated into a brief intervention format, in which a therapist meets with the client for only a brief period, anywhere from a single 10-min session to multiple 1-h sessions (Winters, 2016). BIs are becoming an attractive therapeutic approach due to cost-containment policies of managed care, and many BIs are included in a more comprehensive model, Screening, Brief Intervention and Referral to Treatment (SBIRT; Vendetti et al., 2017). They may be particularly attractive to youth because of the brief number of therapeutic contacts, and the approach is developmentally fitting given that many drug-abusing youth are not "career" drug abusers and young people are likely to be more receptive to self-guided behavior change strategies, a cornerstone of MET (Miller & Sanchez, 1994; Winters, Leitten, Wagner, & O'Leary Tevyaw, 2007).

There is growing support for the efficacy of MET/BI. We located eight published meta-analyses or literature reviews of this model for adolescents (Carney & Myers, 2012; Erickson, Gerstle, & Feldstein, 2005; Grenard, Ames, Pentz, & Sussman, 2006; Jensen et al., 2011; Macgowan & Engle, 2010; Tait & Hulse, 2003; Tanner-Smith & Lipsey, 2015; Wachtel & Staniford, 2010). These meta-analyses concur that, despite some exceptions (see Haller et al., 2014; McCambridge & Strang, 2004; Walker et al., 2011; Walker, Roffman, Stephens, Berghuis, & Kim, 2006), the efficacy of MET/BI is generally encouraging. These findings have occurred in multiple settings, including schools (e.g., Winters, Lee, Botzet, Fahnhorst, & Nicholson, 2014), juvenile offender (e.g., Dembo et al., 2014; Stein et al., 2006), primary care (e.g., Levy & Knight, 2008), and emergency departments (e.g., Monti et al., 1999; Walton et al., 2010). Of note is that this approach significantly outperformed control or comparison conditions, which include education (e.g., Ögel & Coskun, 2011) and assessment-only conditions (e.g., Conrod, Castellanos-Ryan, & Mackie, 2011; Goti et al., 2010; Winters, Lee, et al., 2014; Winters, Tanner-Smith, et al., 2014).

Electronic-Based Therapy

The use of technology for behavioral interventions and therapies has become an emerging approach for supporting the delivery of treatment and aftercare for youth populations challenged with substance use disorders. With increasing advances in technology, the types of technology-based applications have grown in diversity over the years, ranging from computers/Internet, tablets, iPads, mobile apps, and text messaging. Access to, and usage of such devices among youth populations is common. According to the International Telecommunications Union (2012), ownership of mobile phones is particularly pervasive within youth culture, with roughly 90% of this segment of the population having access to mobile devices and texting being "the preferred form of communication" (Campbell & Park, 2014; ITU, 2012;

Madden, Lenhart, Duggan, Cortesi, & Gasser, 2013). Such high access increases the possibility of reaching youth who are unlikely to return to the traditional system for aftercare services, for example (Moore, Dickson-Deane, & Galyen, 2011).

Computer-based interventions and text-messaging resources have become embraced and accepted as a promising and effective technology-based health tools within behavioral health systems for preventing, treating, and supporting therapeutic regimens (i.e., medication compliance) for a wide array of health issues, including but not limited to diabetes, mental health (schizophrenia, depression, anxiety), smoking cessation, sexual and reproductive health, asthma, alcohol drinking and substance use (e.g., Bickel, Christensen, & Marsch, 2011; Kaltenthaler, Parry, Beverley, & Ferriter, 2008; Rooke, Thorsteinsson, Karpin, Copeland, & Allsop, 2010). Online consultation is also available in which individuals can chat online with therapists who have verified credentials (e.g., the International Society for Mental Health Online, www.ismpo.org). Feasibility studies have demonstrated high acceptance and satisfaction for using cell phones as a means of communicating about health and service delivery (e.g., Gonzales, Ang, Murphy, Glik, & Anglin, 2014).

Based on a systematic review of the literature, there have been growing outcome-based studies conducted on the efficacy and effectiveness of technology-based approaches. Collective results show high promise: lowering rates of impairment, improving functioning, decreasing risk behaviors, and increasing adherence or compliance with therapeutic/recovery regimens. Unfortunately, to date, few studies are available that examine the cost efficiency of technology-based approaches.

There are several benefits to integrating technology based approaches for supporting the delivery of treatment and aftercare for youth populations challenged with substance use disorders. One major advantage is maintaining therapeutic fidelity, i.e., ensuring the delivery of evidence based content effectively, reliably, and flexibly. Workforce costs are also minimized with such methods (Newman, Szkodny, Llera, & Przeworski, 2011), as the majority of costs are directed to development rather than delivery; however there is monitoring and follow-up that needs to be built in. Also, technology-based approaches increase the degree of therapeutic flexibility a program or provider has to address treatment and aftercare participation barriers linked to youth concerns about physically attending programs to receive services. Studies support that youth in particular are a group that tends to prefer such interactions more favorably than face-to-face meetings with providers (Pilowsky & Wu, 2013). Technology is also a way to address access and service obstacles specific to youth with unstable housing as they are not required to have a physical residence address to receive services as is required of most treatment programs. Technology devices also enhance the system's ability to readily monitor and assess for youth progress and outcomes via the collection of real time data (in the moment during lived recovery experiences), as well as, increase the likelihood of honest reporting linked to privacy and confidentiality provided by such devices (Turner et al., 1998; Weisband & Kiesler, 1996). Lastly, such technologies allow for potential tailoring and personalization of services (Ondersma, Chase, Svikis, & Schuster, 2005), which is important for youth with substance use issues who tend to have divergent experiences, risk and protective factors, and pathways to recovery.

Pharmacotherapy

Various medications with different approaches have been used to address addiction. These approaches include craving reduction, aversion aversive therapy, substitution therapy, and treatment of underlying psychiatric disorders. Medications approved by the US Food and Drug Administration can be used to treat addiction to opioids, alcohol, or nicotine in adults, but there are no approved medications to treat cannabis, cocaine, or methamphetamine addiction, and no medications are currently approved to treat adolescents. Anecdotal reports indicate that doctors will sometimes prescribe addiction-treatment medications to older adolescents, but the applicability of adult findings to adolescents is unclear given that youth may react differently to the potential side effects of medications (Deas & Thomas, 2001). The approved medications that target alcohol dependence are disulfiram (Fuller et al., 1986), a type of aversive therapy that causes severe nausea, vomiting, and flushing (via the blockage of an enzyme involved in the metabolism of alcohol), and two that seek to reduce cravings—Naltrexone (ReVia) (Morris, Hopwood, Whelan, Gardiner, & Drummond, 2001) and Acamprosate (Campral) (Mann, Lehert, & Morgan, 2004).

Cannabis Youth Treatment Study

One of the largest and most comprehensive research studies to examine the effectiveness of adolescent drug treatment. The Cannabis Youth Treatment Study (CYT), initiated by the Center for Substance Abuse Treatment, was designed to compare the clinical efficacy and cost-effectiveness of multiple short-term (less than 3 months) interventions for adolescents who have a cannabis use problem (Dennis et al., 2004). Researchers from four sites [University of Connecticut Health Center (UCHC), Operation PAR, Inc. (PAR), Chestnut Health Systems (CHS), and Children's Hospital of Philadelphia (CHOP)], along with other community stakeholders, formed a 35-member steering committee and selected five short-term, manual-driven interventions to investigate. Feasibility limitations guided the study to be divided into two trials. Trial 1, implemented at UCHC and PAR, compared three interventions (1) MET and five sessions of CBT; (2) MET and 12 sessions of CBT; and (3) Family Support Network (FSN). Trial 2, conducted at CHS and CHOP, also compared three interventions: (1) MET and five sessions of CBT; (2) Adolescent community reinforcement approach (A-CRA); and (3) MDFT. Participants were randomly assigned to the various interventions per site and qualified for this study if they were 12–18 years old, reported one or more cannabis abuse or dependence symptom(s) (*DSM-IV*; American Psychiatric Association, 1994), and qualified for outpatient treatment (American Society of Addiction Medicine, 2013). Additional information about participant qualifications and other methodological specifications of this study are reported elsewhere (Dennis et al., 2004; Diamond et al., 2002).

Favorable treatment effects, as defined by increased days of abstinence during the 12 months following treatment and percentage of adolescents in recovery at the end of the study were found to be stable across sites and conditions (Dennis et al., 2004). Highly similar clinical outcomes were also observed across sites and conditions. Additional findings were that increased dosage was not necessarily associated with improved outcomes and a cost-effectiveness analysis indicated that FSN in Trial 1 and MDFT in Trial 2 were the least cost-effective.

Meta-Analysis of Outpatient Treatment

Given that outpatient treatment is the predominant setting in which adolescents receive drug treatment, it is pertinent to highlight the recent analyses performed by Tanner-Smith and colleagues (Tanner-Smith et al., 2013). They conducted a meta-analysis on the effects of outpatient treatment on substance use outcomes for adolescents with substance use disorders. Whereas a systematic literature review identifies and summarizes the empirical evidence from the studies that fits prespecified eligibility criteria, a meta-analysis is the use of statistical methods to summarize the results of these studies.

The authors located 45 eligible experimental or quasi-experimental studies reporting 73 treatment–comparison group pairs, with many of the comparison groups also receiving some treatment. The most prevalent treatment types were family therapy, MET/motivational interviewing, psychoeducational therapy (PET), adolescent community reinforcement approach (ACRA), and CBT. In order to assess the comparative effectiveness, the authors examined the effect sizes for pre–post changes in substance use of each treatment type compared to whatever diverse treatment or control conditions was used in the respective studies.

Results from the pre–post analysis indicated an almost universal reduction in substance use between treatment entry and termination regardless of treatment type. A closer look at the results indicated that family therapy, behavioral therapy, CBT and MET were among the treatment types showing the largest substance use reductions. The most convincing and consistent comparative effectiveness finding was for family therapy, which showed relatively large positive effects relative to other treatments in both analyses. Not surprisingly, placebo and no treatment controls were among those showing the smallest reductions.

The authors reported an additional exploratory analysis of pooled data from Chestnut Health System's GAIN database pertaining to outpatient treatment (Dennis, White, Titus, & Unsicker, 2008). They conducted a meta-analysis analogous to that reported above. Analyses were based on data from 102 outpatient treatment programs serving over 9000 adolescents across the United States. Those results provided convergent results - there was almost universal reduction in substance use between treatment entry and termination regardless of treatment type.

Thus, one major take-away from the Tanner-Smith et al. (2013) work is that most types of treatment appear to be beneficial in helping adolescents reduce their substance use. As the authors note, "given the indications that at least some treatments are effective in reducing substance use, it is encouraging to see widespread reductions among the adolescents in the research studies" (p. 154–155).

A final topic addressed in this study was the issue of outcome and adolescent characteristics. The authors coded all the baseline information reported in the studies about those characteristics and included them in the analysis to identify subgroups more or less responsive to treatment. The analysis of pre–post reductions in substance use showed that, save for one variable, there were no differences related to gender, race/ethnicity, age, baseline substance use severity, comorbidity, or delinquency level. Also, the authors examined the interactions of these variables with the different distinct treatment types and found only a handful of chance levels of statistical significance. The one participant variable related to outcome was type of substance. The pre–post comparison showed that reductions in substance use were smaller for alcohol and other substances (e.g., heroin and cocaine) than for marijuana. But in the main, these analyses, albeit far short of definitive, suggest that treatments are relatively effective across a wide range of youth that differ in terms of demographics and problem severity.

Approaches Aimed at Maximizing Outcome

Recovery Schools

School is a critically important social environment for adolescents with SUDs. Developing new, sober peer groups is an important yet challenging aspect of recovery for youth completing SUD treatment. Given the documented environmental substance-exposure risk in high schools, and the vulnerability to early relapse following SUD treatment, school environments play a vital role in maintaining or undermining treatment gains.

On the one hand, school sits at the heart of the threat of relapse and other unhealthy and maladaptive behaviors. For youth in recovery from SUDs, traditional high school is a context likely to involve interactions with peer groups who are actively using alcohol and other drugs. The National Survey of American Attitudes on Substance Abuse annual survey of students ages 12–17 found that about two-thirds of high school students say drugs are used, kept, or sold on the grounds of their schools (Johnson, Shapiro, & Zill, 2009). Association with drug-using peers, alcohol or drug availability, and academic challenges are significant relapse-risk factors for youth after drug treatment (Clark & Winters, 2002; Svensson, 2000). For the student who attempts to resist peer pressure, difficulty coping with negative feelings and interpersonal conflict may endanger a teen's newly established sobriety.

Conversely, schools can be opportunities for promoting recovery and protecting students. Treatment for substance use disorders in any age group does not produce certain remission. The course of substance use disorders is characterized by cycles of recovery and relapse (Dennis & Scott, 2007), which may endanger academic achievement and social functioning. Abstaining represents a challenge for students, who are especially vulnerable to relapse during the 6- to 12-month post-treatment period (Winters, Stinchfield, et al., 2007).

Any approach addressing recovery from substance use disorders among youth therefore must involve school settings. School bonding, school interest, and academic achievement are negatively associated with substance use, particularly among low-achieving students (Bryant, Schulenberg, O'Malley, Bachman, & Johnston, 2003). Succeeding academically can help students stay sober and ultimately graduate, given that "connectedness with school" is a protective factor for adolescents (Resnick et al., 1997). Continuing care and peer networks are integral to sustaining long-term sobriety (Brown, 2004; Karakos, 2014; McKay et al., 2009; Stout, Kelly, Magill, & Pagano, 2012). For high school students, knowing how to relate and respond to peers given newfound sobriety is a difficult challenge (Finch & Wegman, 2012) and increasing social interaction with non-substance-using peers is associated with greater odds of remission and recovery. Youth who abstain from substance use posttreatment report a higher number of non-using social supports (including peers) than youth who return to heavy drug use (Anderson, Ramo, Schulte, Cummins, & Brown, 2007; Richter, Brown, & Mott, 1991).

Recovery high schools are an alternative high school option that provides recovery support and a protective environment for students with SUDs and related behavioral, emotional, or mental health needs. Having been diagnosed with a substance use disorder is not a requirement of most recovery high schools, but SUDs and prior treatment are the norm for recovery high school students (Moberg & Finch, 2008; Moberg, Finch, & Lindsley, 2014).

The first recovery high school opened in Maryland in 1979 as a public alternative school called "Phoenix". The Association of Recovery Schools (ARS) was formed in 2002 to advocate for "the promotion, strengthening, and expansion of secondary and postsecondary programs designed for students and families committed to achieving success in both education and recovery" (Association of Recovery Schools, 2016). There are currently 40 recovery high schools in 16 states, with at least five additional schools under development. Over 85 recovery high schools have operated since 1979 (Association of Recovery Schools; https://recoveryschools.org/).

Recovery support programs such as recovery high schools enhance "recovery capital," which encompasses all resources related to the recovery process, including financial, human, social, and community factors (Granfield & Cloud, 1999; Hennessy & Finch, 2015; Kelly & Hoeppner, 2015). Recovery high schools provide services supporting both the academic and therapeutic needs of students. The schools attempt to support recovery and academic achievement by creating connectedness and building social and recovery capital in a context with clear pathways to success.

Recovery high schools are typically small, with an average enrollment of about 30 students. The programs are schools of choice for which the willingness of a student to attend is an enrollment criterion. Students ultimately may either graduate from the recovery high school or transition to a more traditional school. While there is no one recovery high school model, certain elements are common (Finch, Moberg, & Krupp, 2014; Hennessy & Finch, 2015; Moberg & Finch, 2008):

1. Building a base of peer/family connection, social structures, accountability, psychoeducational information, and recovery resources;
2. Repairing/replacing disconnected or unhealthy peer, family, and authority relationships and minimizing contact with high-risk peers during school hours;
3. Providing students the opportunity to meet other students with similar histories and goals and to practice skills, including how to have sober fun;
4. Identifying and responding to behaviors indicating potential substance use or the symptoms of a co-occurring disorder by taking advantage of smaller school environments and specialized staff;
5. Requiring participation in support and mutual aid groups outside school to promote contact with additional positive peers and mentors; and
6. Providing an individualized, accredited curriculum taught by licensed teachers to give students a chance to stay on-course for earning a high school diploma.

Recovery high school-specific research has expanded in recent years (Botzet, McIlvaine, Winters, Fahnhorst, & Dittel, 2014; Finch et al., 2014; Finch, Tanner-Smith, Hennessy, & Moberg, 2017; Karakos, 2014; Moberg et al., 2014; Moberg & Finch, 2008). Finch et al. (2017) provides the strongest evidence yet of a positive effect of RHSs for adolescents who have received treatment for SUDs. This article emerges from the first NIH-funded comparative outcomes study of recovery high schools (RHS). The study used a longitudinal quasi-experimental design to examine the effects of RHS attendance on adolescents' outcomes, specifically examining whether students *who have received treatment for SUDs* and who subsequently attend RHSs, experience significantly better behavioral outcomes (less alcohol and other drug use) and educational outcomes (higher GPA, better attendance) compared to recovering students who attend school in other settings. The study was unique in the inclusion of propensity score modeling of a wide range of important correlates of outcomes selected based on prior meta-analytic research on adolescent treatment outcomes.

Results at 6 months compared adolescents attending RHSs following treatment for SUDs to non-RHS students who had received similar SUD treatment:

- RHS students were twice (59% versus 30%) as likely to report complete abstinence from alcohol, marijuana, and other drugs at the 6-month follow-up.
- RHS students reported significantly fewer days of marijuana use (9 days compared to 26 days in the past 3 months), and
- RHS students reported significantly less absenteeism from school.

While studies suggest recovery high schools offer a promising approach to improve both academic and behavioral outcomes, more research is needed (US Office of the Surgeon General, 2016), especially with regard to diverse populations and long-term (i.e., post-high school) trajectories.

Overall, reports indicate that recovery high schools are feasible to implement and sustain, and participating students and staff believe they have positive educational and behavioral outcomes (Moberg & Finch, 2008). Assuming overall effectiveness continues to be demonstrated, additional analyses to characterize the most effective program elements will be needed to guide policy and service development.

Employing Reinforcements to Promote Recovery

Incentive-based approaches, which include contingency management, encourages healthy changes in behavior by providing adolescents with immediate rewards contingent on positive changes in behavior, such as negative urine tests or meeting treatment goals. This approach is based on the operant conditioning principle that the use of consequences can modify behavior. Rewards are often in the form of award prizes (e.g., dollar prizes) (Sindelar, Elbel, & Petry, 2007). Community reinforcement plus vouchers approach (CRA) is an example. Key features of this strategy are vouchers to reward treatment compliance and abstinence, frequent and random urine screens to detect drug use, and several tools to support successful recovery (e.g., functional analyses to identify triggers for drug use; self-management plans to address identified triggers; and the development of drug avoidance skills). Incentive-based strategies merit greater research attention and utilization in the treatment field; they can be readily integrated into the variety of treatment approaches that are becoming the mainstay in adolescent treatment, including behavior therapy, cognitive behavior therapy, family therapy, and motivational enhancement.

Adapting Treatment

A promising model to optimize treatment effectiveness is personalizing the content and or delivery to address those who do not respond readily to the first-line treatment offered. This model, referred to as a "SMART" (Sequential Multiple Assignment Randomized Trials) approach (Murphy, Lynch, Oslin, McKay, & TenHave, 2007) applies an algorithm of enhanced treatment for poor responders. Given that many youth do not initially respond to treatment, the field may benefit from use of this strategy. The adaptive approach has the potential to increase rates of participation; the burden on the patient is lower at the outset, and the tailoring that occurs for nonresponders may be perceived favorably by these clients. Adaptive care may also increase cost-effectiveness and cost benefit, because lower intensity treatments are also often less costly.

A challenge of adaptive treatment models is how to define poor treatment response and when to apply the next step of treatment. Should the client be switched from initial treatment and switched to a different strategy? If so, what type of second-line treatment? Perhaps the client should receive a more intensive version of the first-line treatment, or have a supplemental treatment to augment what the client is already receiving (McKay, 2009).

Adaptive or stepped care treatment algorithms have been developed and evaluated for adults. McKay (2009) summarized 15 adult drug treatment studies; most of these studies concluded that the adaptive approach was associated with either better drug use outcomes or equivalent outcomes compared to treatments with other advantages (e.g., lower cost and lower patient burden). The senior author knows of several SMART studies in progress for youth but no published results yet.

Summary

Overall, great advances have been made since 1990 in the development and evaluation of treatments for adolescent drug abuse. This body of research reflects a greater focus on varying interventions using different theory-based psychotherapies, as well as a recognition of the unique developmental milestones specific to adolescents. The field is revealing its maturity in several ways: the use of assessment tools developed and validated on adolescent populations is the norm; many treatment approaches target multiple drugs, reflecting the fact that most clinical populations of teenagers abuse multiple substances; treatment manuals and specific protocols that permit treatment replication are available; and an increased rigor in evaluating the effectiveness of these approaches. We can now say with relative certainty that several modalities and approaches meet standards of evidence-based treatments, and that, in general, they are comparable in terms of outcomes.

It is our assessment of the treatment outcome studies that family systems-based treatments and MET/BI approaches have received the most empirical support compared to other modalities. Two approaches that have been applied to drug-abusing youth over time and still retain a core position among treatment options—the 12-step approach and TCs—have received very little investigation with clinical trials. Also, few pharmacological treatments of adolescents with an SUD have been published; their role as an effective adjunct to psychosocial-based approaches merits more research.

Moreover, very little is still known as to what extent community programs provide essential clinical elements or characteristics of effective treatment (e.g., use of standardized adolescent assessment measures and developmentally adjusted strategies for treatment engagement). Also, the use by community programs of treatment reinforcements, adaptive treatment strategies, and electronic resources to supplement treatment and promote recovery is an open question.

Despite a maturing treatment outcome research field, important knowledge gaps exist. Because most treatment research in this field examines stand-alone approaches, it is not clear to what extent this body of work generalizes to the wider treatment community field where electric approaches are commonly utilized. Addressing this issue, along with cost-efficient and sustainable ways to translate research findings into day-to-day practice with fidelity, is needed. One effort along these lines is the use of the Screening, Brief Intervention and Referral to Treatment (SBIRT) approach as means to expand the identification of and treatment for youth with a substance use problem (Vendetti et al., 2017; Winters, 2016). Other research needs include the following: which pharmacological treatments for substance use disorders are effective for adolescents; what factors mediate and moderate engagement in the behavior change process; what variables may be related to treatment effectiveness for specific substances (e.g., marijuana; opioids); how to maximize the role of parents in treatment engagement and support of recovery; the role of technology to promote treatment effectiveness; and understanding how to make quality treatment across the entire continuum of care accessible to adolescents with varying degrees of substance use.

In summary, the adolescent substance abuse treatment field has benefitted by targeted research resulting in evidence-based treatments and practices that are associated with reductions in substance use and the associated short-term individual and societal costs that result from this disorder. Quality treatment approaches are now available for a wide range of youth suspected of a substance use problem.

Acknowledgement This work was supported in part by grants DA015347 (Winters) and DA029785 (Finch) from the National Institute on Drug Abuse.

We gratefully acknowledge the contribution of Tamara Fahnhorst and Rachel Koskey to the prior version of this chapter.

References

Alcoholics Anonymous 2001 Membership Survey. (2001). *Alcoholics anonymous 2001 membership survey*. New York, NY: AA Grapevine Inc.

American Psychiatric Association. (1994). *Diagnostic and statistical manual of mental disorders* (4th ed.). Washington, DC: American Psychiatric Association Author.

American Society of Addiction Medicine. (2013). *Patient placement criteria for the treatment of psychoactive substance disorders* (3rd ed.). Chevy Chase, MD: American Society of Addiction Medicine Author.

Anderson, D. J., McGovern, J. P., & DuPont, R. L. (1999). The origins of the Minnesota model of addiction treatment: A first person account. *Journal of Addictive Diseases, 18*(1), 107–114.

Anderson, K. G., Ramo, D. E., Schulte, M. T., Cummins, K., & Brown, S. A. (2007). Substance use treatment outcomes for youth: Integrating personal and environmental predictors. *Drug and Alcohol Dependence, 88*(1), 42–28.

Association of Recovery High Schools. (2016). *State of recovery high schools, 2016 biennial report*. Denton, TX: Association of Recovery High Schools.

Austin, A. M., Macgowan, M. J., & Wagner, E. F. (2005). Effective family-based interventions for adolescents with substance use problems: A systemic review. *Research on Social Work Practice, 15*(2), 67–83.

Azrin, N. H., Donohue, B., Besalel, V. A., Kogan, E. S., & Acierno, R. (1994). Youth drug abuse treatment: A controlled outcome study. *Journal of Child & Adolescent Substance Abuse, 3*(3), 1–16.

Barrett, H., Slesnick, N., Brody, J. L., Turner, C. W., & Peterson, T. R. (2001). Treatment outcomes for adolescent substance abuse at 4-and 7-month assessments. *Journal of Consulting and Clinical Psychology, 69*(5), 802–813.

Battjes, R. J., Gordon, M. S., O'Grady, K. E., & Kinlock, T. W. (2004). Predicting retention of adolescents in substance abuse treatment. *Addictive Behaviors, 29*(2), 1021–1027.

Beck, A., & Weishaar, M. (2005). Cognitive therapy. In R. J. Corsini & D. Wedding (Eds.), *Current psychotherapies* (7th ed., pp. 238–268). Belmont, CA: Thomson Brooks/Cole Publishing.

Bickel, W. K., Christensen, D. R., & Marsch, L. A. (2011). A review of computer-based interventions used in the assessment, treatment, and research of drug addiction. *Substance Use & Misuse, 46*(1), 4–9.

Botzet, A., McIlvaine, P. W., Winters, K. C., Fahnhorst, T., & Dittel, C. (2014). Data collection strategies and measurement tools for assessing academic and therapeutic outcomes in recovery schools. *Peabody Journal of Education, 89*(2), 197–213.

Brown, S. A. (2004). Measuring youth outcomes from alcohol and drug treatment. *Addiction, 99*(s2), 38–46.

Bryant, A. L., Schulenberg, J. E., O'Malley, P. M., Bachman, J. G., & Johnston, L. D. (2003). Substance use during adolescence: A 6-year, multiwave national longitudinal study. *Journal of Research on Adolescence, 13*(3), 361–397.

Campbell, S. W., & Park, Y. J. (2014). Predictors of mobile sexting among teens: Toward a new explanatory framework. *Mobile Media & Communication, 2*(1), 20–39.

Carney, T., & Myers, B. (2012). Effectiveness of early interventions for substance-using adolescents: Findings from a systematic review and meta-analysis. *Substance Abuse Treatment, Prevention, and Policy, 7*(1), 1–15.

Center for Behavioral Health Statistics and Quality. (2015). *Behavioral health trends in the United States: Results from the 2014 National Survey on drug use and health (HHS publication no. SMA 15-4927, NSDUH series H-50)*. Rockville, MD: Substance Abuse and Mental Health Services Administration.

Clark, D., & Winters, K. C. (2002). Measuring risks and outcomes in substance use disorders prevention research. *Journal of Consulting and Clinical Psychology, 70*(6), 1207–1223.

Conrod, P. J., Castellanos-Ryan, N., & Mackie, C. (2011). Long-term effects of a personality-targeted intervention to reduce alcohol use in adolescents. *Journal of Consulting and Clinical Psychology, 79*(3), 296–306.

Deas, D., & Thomas, S. E. (2001). An overview of controlled studies of adolescent substance abuse treatment. *The American Journal on Addictions, 10*(2), 178–189.

Dembo, R., Briones-Robinson, R., Ungaro, R., Barrett, K., Gulledge, L., Winters, K. C., … Karas, L. (2014). Brief intervention for truant youth sexual risk behavior and marijuana use. *Journal of Child & Adolescent Substance Abuse, 23*(6), 218–333.

Dembo, R., Shemwell, M., Pacheco, K., Seeberger, W., Rollie, M., Schmeidler, J., … Wothke, W. (2000). A longitudinal study of the impact of a family empowerment intervention on juvenile offender psychosocial functioning: An expanded assessment. *Journal of Child & Adolescent Substance Abuse, 10*(1), 1–7.

Dennis, M. L., Godley, S. H., Diamond, G., Tims, F. M., Babor, T., Donaldson, J., … Funk, R. (2004). The cannabis youth treatment (CYT) study: Main findings from two randomized trials. *Journal of Substance Abuse Treatment, 27*(3), 197–213.

Dennis, M. L., & Scott, C. K. (2007). Managing addiction as a chronic condition. *Addiction Science & Clinical Practice, 4*(1), 45–55.

Dennis, M. L., White, M., Titus, J. C., & Unsicker, J. (2008). *GAIN: Global appraisal of individual needs: Administration guide for the GAIN and related measures (version 5)*. Bloomington, IL: Chestnut Health Systems.

Diamond, G. S., Godley, S. H., Liddle, H. A., Sampl, S., Webb, C., Tims, F. M., … Meyers, R. (2002). Five outpatient treatment models for adolescent marijuana use: A description of the cannabis youth treatment interventions. *Addiction, 97*(s1), S70–S83.

Erickson, S. J., Gerstle, M., & Feldstein, S. W. (2005). Brief interventions and motivational interviewing with children, adolescents, and their parents in pediatric health care settings: A review. *Archives of Pediatric Adolescent Medicine, 159*(12), 1173–1180.

Finch, A., & Wegman, H. (2012). Recovery high schools: Opportunities for support and personal growth for students in recovery. *Prevention Researcher, 19*(5), 12–16.

Finch, A. J., Moberg, D. P., & Krupp, A. L. (2014). Continuing care in high schools: A descriptive study of recovery high school programs. *Journal of Child & Adolescent Substance Abuse, 23*(2), 116–129.

Finch, A. J., Tanner-Smith, E., Hennessy, E., & Moberg, D. P. (2017). Recovery high schools: Effect of schools supporting recovery from substance use disorders. *The American Journal of Drug and Alcohol Abuse, 44*(2), 175–184 1-10. Advance online publication. Retrieved from. https://doi.org/10.1080/00952990.2017.1354378

Fuller, R. K., Branchey, L., Brightwell, D. R., Derman, R. M., Emrick, C. D., Iber, F. L., … Maany, I. (1986). Disulfiram treatment of alcoholism. *Journal of the American Medical Association, 256*(11), 1449–1455.

Godley, M. D., Godley, S. H., Dennis, M. L., Funk, R. R., Passetti, L. L., & Petry, N. M. (2014). A randomized trial of assertive continuing care and contingency management for adolescents with substance use disorders. *Journal of Consulting and Clinical Psychology, 82*(1), 40–51.

Godley, M. D., Passetti, L. L., Subramaniam, G. A., Funk, R. R., Smith, J. E., & Meyers, R. J. (2017). Adolescent community reinforcement approach implementation and treatment outcomes for youth with opioid problem use. *Drug and Alcohol Dependence, 174*, 9–16.

Gonzales, R., Ang, A., Murphy, D. A., Glik, D. C., & Anglin, M. D. (2014). Substance use recovery outcomes among a cohort of youth participating in a mobile-based texting aftercare pilot program. *Journal of Substance Abuse Treatment, 47*(1), 20–26.

Goti, J., Diaz, R., Serrano, L., Gonzalez, L., Calvo, R., Gual, A., … Castro, J. (2010). Brief intervention in substance-use among adolescent psychiatric patients: A randomized controlled trial. *European Child & Adolescent Psychiatry, 19*(6), 503–511.

Granfield, R., & Cloud, W. (1999). *Coming clean: Overcoming addiction without treatment*. New York, NY: New York University Press.

Grella, C. E., Joshi, V., & Hser, Y. I. (2004). Effects of comorbidity on treatment processes and outcomes among adolescents in drug treatment programs. *Journal of Child & Adolescent Substance Abuse, 13*(4), 13–31.

Grenard, J. L., Ames, S. L., Pentz, M. A., & Sussman, S. (2006). Motivational interviewing with adolescents and young adults for drug-related problems. *International Journal of Adolescent Medicine and Health, 18*(1), 53–67.

Haller, D. M., Meynard, A., Lefebvre, D., Ukoumunne, O. C., Narring, F., & Broers, B. (2014). Effectiveness of training family physicians to deliver a brief intervention to address excessive substance use among young patients: A cluster randomized controlled trial. *Canadian Medical Association Journal, 186*(8), E263–E272.

Henggeler, S. W., Clingempeel, W. G., Brondino, M. J., & Pickrel, S. G. (2002). Four year follow-up of multisystemic therapy with substance-abusing and substance-dependent juvenile offenders. *Journal of the American Academy of Child & Adolescent Psychiatry, 41*(7), 868–874.

Henggeler, S. W., Halliday-Boykins, C. A., Cunningham, P. B., Randall, J., Shapiro, S. B., & Chapman, J. E. (2006). Juvenile drug court: Enhancing outcomes by integrating evidence-based treatments. *Journal of Consulting and Clinical Psychology, 74*(1), 42–54.

Henggeler, S. W., Pickrel, S. G., & Brondino, M. J. (1999). Multisystemic treatment of substance abusing and dependent delinquents: Outcomes, treatment fidelity, and transportability. *Mental Health Services Research, 1*(3), 171–184.

Henggeler, S. W., & Schaeffer, C. M. (2016). Multisystemic therapy®: Clinical overview, outcomes, and implementation research. *Family Process, 55*(3), 514–528.

Hennessy, E. A., & Finch, A. J. (2015). Recovery capital: A systematic review and application to adolescent recovery. Poster presented at the Society for Community Research and Action, Lowell, MA.

International Telecommunications Union. (2012). *Measuring the information society*. Geneva, Switzerland: International Telecommunications Union [ITU] Author.

Jaffe, S. (1990). *Step workbook for adolescent chemical dependence recovery*. Washington, DC: American Academy of Child and Adolescent Psychiatry.

Jainchill, N. (1997). Therapeutic communities for adolescents: The same and not the same. In G. DeLeon (Ed.), *Community as method: Therapeutic communities for special populations and special settings* (pp. 161–178). Westport, CT: Praeger.

Jensen, C. D., Cushing, C. C., Aylward, B. S., Craig, J. T., Sorell, D. M., & Steele, R. G. (2011). Effectiveness of motivational interviewing interventions for adolescent substance use behavior change: A meta-analytic review. *Journal of Consulting and Clinical Psychology, 79*(4), 433–440.

Johnson, T., Shapiro, R., & Zill, N. (2009). *National survey of American attitudes on substance abuse XIV: Teens and parents* (pp. 3–4). New York, NY: The National Center on Addiction and Substance Abuse.

Kaltenthaler, E., Parry, G., Beverley, C., & Ferriter, M. (2008). Computerised cognitive–behavioural therapy for depression: Systematic review. *The British Journal of Psychiatry, 193*(3), 181–184.

Kaminer, Y., Burleson, J. A., & Goldberger, R. (2002). Cognitive-behavioral coping skills and psychoeducation therapies for adolescent substance abuse. *The Journal of Nervous and Mental Disease, 190*(11), 737–745.

Kann, L. K., Shanklin, S. L., Flint, K. H., Hawkins, J., Harris, W. A., Lowry, R., … Zaza, S. (2014). *Youth risk behavior surveillance–United States, 2013*. Rockville, MD: ICF International, Westat.

Karakos, H. L. (2014). Positive peer support or negative peer influence? The role of peers among adolescents in recovery high schools. *Peabody Journal of Education, 89*(2), 214–228. https://doi.org/10.1080/0161956X.2014.897094

Kelly, J. F., Brown, S. A., Abrantes, A., Kahler, C. W., & Myers, M. (2008). Social recovery model: An 8-year investigation of adolescent 12-step group involvement following inpatient treatment. *Alcoholism: Clinical and Experimental Research, 32*(8), 1468–1478.

Kelly, J. F., & Hoeppner, B. (2015). A biaxial formulation of the recovery construct. *Addiction Research and Theory, 23*(1), 5–9.

Kelly, J. F., Magill, M., & Stout, R. L. (2009). How do people recover from alcohol dependence? A systematic review of the research on mechanisms of behavior change in alcoholics anonymous. *Addiction Research and Theory, 17*(3), 236–259.

Kelly, J. F., & Urbanoski, K. (2012). Youth recovery contexts: The incremental effects of 12 – Step attendance and involvement on adolescent outpatient outcomes. *Alcoholism: Clinical and Experimental Research, 36*(7), 1219–1229.

Latimer, W. W., Winters, K. C., D'Zurilla, T., & Nichols, M. (2003). Integrated family and cognitive-behavior therapy for adolescent substance abusers: A stage I efficacy study. *Drug and Alcohol Dependence, 71*(3), 303–317.

Levy, S., & Knight, J. R. (2008). Screening, brief intervention, and referral to treatment for adolescents. *Journal of Addiction Medicine, 2*(4), 215–221.

Liddle, H. A. (2013). Multidimensional family therapy for adolescent substance abuse: A developmental approach. In P. Miller (Ed.), *Interventions for addiction: Comprehensive addictive behaviors and disorders* (pp. 87–96). San Diego, CA: Academic Press.

Liddle, H. A. (2016). Multidimensional family therapy: Evidence base for trans-diagnostic treatment outcomes, change mechanisms, and implementation in community settings. *Family Process, 55*(3), 558–576.

Liddle, H. A., Rowe, C. L., Dakof, G. A., Henderson, C. E., & Greenbaum, P. E. (2009). Multidimensional family therapy for young adolescent substance abuse: Twelve-month outcomes of a randomized controlled trial. *Journal of Consulting and Clinical Psychology, 77*(1), 12–25.

Macgowan, M. J., & Engle, B. (2010). Evidence for optimism: Behavior therapies and motivational interviewing in adolescent substance abuse treatment. *Child and Adolescent Psychiatric Clinics of North America, 19*(3), 527–545.

Madden, M., Lenhart, A., Duggan, M., Cortesi, S., & Gasser, U. (2013). *Teens and technology 2013* (pp. 1–19). Washington, DC: Pew Internet & American Life Project.

Mann, K., Lehert, P., & Morgan, M. Y. (2004). The efficacy of acomprosate in the maintenance of abstinence on alcohol-dependent individuals: Results of a meta-analysis. *Alcohol Clinical and Experimental Research, 28*(1), 51–63.

McCambridge, J., & Strang, J. (2004). The efficacy of a single-session motivational interviewing in reducing drug consumption and perceptions of drug-related risk and harm among young people: Results from a muli-site cluster randomized trial. *Addiction, 99*(1), 39–52.

McKay, J. R. (2009). *Treating substance use disorders with adaptive continuing care*. Washington, DC: American Psychological Association Press.

McKay, J. R., Carise, D., Dennis, M. L., Dupont, R., Humphreys, K., Kemp, J., … Schwartzlose, J. (2009). Extending the benefits of addiction treatment: Practical strategies for continuing care and recovery. *Journal of Substance Abuse Treatment, 36*(2), 127–130.

Miech, R. A., Johnston, L. D., O'Malley, P. M., Bachman, J. G., & Schulenberg, J. E. (2016). *Monitoring the future national survey results on drug use, 1975–2015: Volume I, secondary school students*. Ann Arbor, MI: Institute for Research for Social Research, The University of Michigan.

Miller, W. R., & Sanchez, V. C. (1994). Motivating young adults for treatment and lifestyle change. In G. S. Howard & P. E. Nathan (Eds.), *Alcohol use and misuse by young adults* (pp. 55–81). Notre Dame, IN: University of Notre Dame Press.

Moberg, D. P., & Finch, A. J. (2008). Recovery high schools: A descriptive study of school programs and students. *Journal of Groups in Addiction & Recovery, 2*(2-4), 128–161.

Moberg, D. P., Finch, A. J., & Lindsley, S. M. (2014). Recovery high schools: Students and responsive academic and therapeutic services. *Peabody Journal of Education, 89*(2), 165–182.

Monti, P. M., Colby, S. M., Barnett, N. P., Spirito, A., Rohsenow, D. J., Myers, M., … Lewander, W. (1999). Brief intervention for harm reduction with alcohol-positive older adolescents in a hospital emergency department. *Journal of Consulting and Clinical Psychology, 67*(6), 989–994.

Moore, J. L., Dickson-Deane, C., & Galyen, K. (2011). E-learning, online learning, and distance learning environments: Are they the same? *The Internet and Higher Education, 14*(2), 129–135.

Morral, A. R., McCaffrey, D. F., & Ridgeway, G. (2004). Effectiveness of community-based treatment for substance-abusing adolescents: 12-month outcomes of youth entering phoenix academy or alternative probation dispositions. *Psychology of Addictive Behaviors, 18*(3), 257–268.

Morris, P. L., Hopwood, M., Whelan, G., Gardiner, J., & Drummond, E. (2001). Naltrexone for alcohol dependence: A randomized controlled trial. *Addiction, 96*(11), 1565–1573.

Murphy, S. A., Lynch, K. G., Oslin, D., McKay, J. R., & TenHave, T. (2007). Developing adaptive treatment strategies in substance abuse research. *Drug and Alcohol Dependence, 88*(2), S24–S30.

National Institute on Drug Abuse. (2014). *Principles of adolescent substance use disorder treatment: A research-based guide*. Bethesda, MD: National Institute on Drug Abuse.

Newman, M. G., Szkodny, L. E., Llera, S. J., & Przeworski, A. (2011). A review of technology-assisted self-help and minimal contact therapies for anxiety and depression: Is human contact necessary for therapeutic efficacy? *Clinical Psychology Review, 31*(1), 89–103.

Ögel, K., & Coskun, S. (2011). Cognitive behavioral therapy-based brief intervention for volatile substance misusers during adolescence: A follow-up study. *Substance Use & Misuse, 46*(Suppl. 1), 128–133.

Ondersma, S. J., Chase, S. K., Svikis, D. S., & Schuster, C. R. (2005). Computer-based brief motivational intervention for perinatal drug use. *Journal of Substance Abuse Treatment, 28*(4), 305–312.

Ozechowski, T. J., & Liddle, H. A. (2002). Family-based therapy. In C. A. Essau (Ed.), *Substance abuse and dependence in adolescence: Epidemiology, risk factors, and treatment* (pp. 203–226). East Sussex, UK: Brunner-Routledge.

Pilowsky, D. J., & Wu, L. T. (2013). Screening instruments for substance use and brief interventions targeting adolescents in primary care: A literature review. *Addictive Behaviors, 38*(5), 2146–2153.

Resnick, M., Bearman, P., Blum, R., Bauman, K., Harris, K., Jones, J., … Udry, J. (1997). Protecting adolescents from harm: Findings from the national longitudinal study on adolescent health. *Journal of the American Medical Association, 278*(10), 823–832.

Richter, S. S., Brown, S. A., & Mott, M. A. (1991). The impact of social support and self-esteem on adolescent substance abuse treatment outcome. *Journal of Substance Abuse, 3*(4), 371–385.

Riggs, P. D., Thompson, L. L., Tapert, S. F., Frascella, J., Mikulich-Gilbertson, S., Dalwani, M., … Lohman, M. (2007). Advances in neurobiological research related to interventions in adolescents with substance use disorders: Research to practice. *Drug and Alcohol Dependence, 91*(2-3), 306–311.

Rigter, H., Henderson, C. E., Pelc, I., Tossmann, P., Phan, O., Hendriks, V., … Rowe, C. L. (2013). Multidimensional family therapy lowers the rate of cannabis dependence in adolescents: A randomised controlled trial in western European outpatient settings. *Drug and Alcohol Dependence, 130*(1), 85–93.

Rollnick, S., & Miller, W. R. (1995). What is motivational interviewing? *Behavioural and Cognitive Psychotherapy, 23*(4), 325–334.

Rooke, S., Thorsteinsson, E., Karpin, A., Copeland, J., & Allsop, D. (2010). Computer-delivered interventions for alcohol and tobacco use: A meta-analysis. *Addiction, 105*(8), 1381–1390.

Santisteban, D. A., Coatsworth, J. D., Perez-Vidal, A., Kurtines, W. M., Schwartz, S. J., LaPerriere, A., … Szapocznik, J. (2003). Efficacy of brief strategic family therapy in modifying Hispanic adolescent behavior problems and substance use. *Journal of Family Psychology, 17*(1), 121–133.

Schwebel, R. (2004). *The seven challenges manual*. Tucson, AZ: Viva Press.

Sheidow, A. J., & Houston, J. L. (2013). Multisystemic therapy for adolescent substance use. In P. Miller (Ed.), *Interventions for addiction: Comprehensive addictive behaviors and disorders* (pp. 77–86). San Diego, CA: Academic Press.

Sindelar, J., Elbel, B., & Petry, N. M. (2007). What do we get for our money? Cost-effectiveness of adding contingency management. *Addiction, 102*(2), 309–316.

Smith, D. C., & Hall, J. A. (2008). Strengths oriented family therapy for adolescents with substance abuse problems. *Social Work, 53*(2), 185–188.

Smith, D. C., Hall, J. A., Williams, J. K., An, H., & Gotman, N. (2006). Comparative efficacy of family and group treatment for adolescent substance abuse. *The American Journal on Addictions, 15*(Suppl. 1), 131–136.

Spear, L. P. (2002). Alcohol's effects on adolescents. *Alcohol Health and Research World, 26*(4), 287–291.

Stein, L. A., Colby, S. M., Barnett, N. P., Monti, P. M., Golembeske, C., & Lebeau-Craven, R. (2006). Effects of motivational interviewing for incarcerated adolescents on driving under the influence after release. *The American Journal on Addictions, 15*(s1), 50–57.

Stout, R. L., Kelly, J. F., Magill, M., & Pagano, M. E. (2012). Association between social influences and drinking outcomes across three years. *Journal of Studies on Alcohol and Drugs, 73*(3), 489–497.

Substance Abuse and Mental Health Services Administration. (2013). *Results from the 2012 national survey on drug use and health: Summary of national findings*. Rockville, MD: Substance Abuse and Mental Health Services Administration.

Sussman, S. (2010). A review of alcoholics anonymous/narcotics anonymous programs for teens. *Evaluation & the Health Professions, 33*(1), 26–55.

Svensson, R. (2000). Risk factors for different dimensions of adolescent drug use. *Journal of Child & Adolescent Substance Abuse, 9*(3), 67–90.

Swenson, C. C., Henggeler, S. W., Taylor, I. S., & Addison, O. W. (2005). *Multisystemic therapy and neighborhood partnerships: Reducing adolescent violence and substance abuse*. New York, NY: Guilford Press.

Szapocznik, J., & Coatsworth, D. (1999). An ecodevelopmental framework for organizing the influences on drug abuse: A developmental model of risk and protection. In M. D. Glantz

(Ed.), *Drug abuse: Origins and interventions* (pp. 331–366). Washington, DC: American Psychological Association.
Szapocznik, J., Muir, J. A., & Schwartz, S. J. (2013). Brief strategic family therapy for adolescent drug abuse: Treatment and implementation. In P. Miller (Ed.), *Interventions for addiction: Comprehensive addictive behaviors and disorders* (pp. 97–108). San Diego, CA: Academic Press.
Tait, R. J., & Hulse, G. K. (2003). A systematic review of the effectiveness of brief interventions with substance using adolescents by type of drug. *Drug and Alcohol Review, 22*(3), 337–346.
Tanner-Smith, E. E., & Lipsey, M. W. (2015). Brief alcohol interventions for adolescents and young adults: A systematic review and meta-analysis. *Journal of Substance Abuse Treatment, 51*, 1–18.
Tanner-Smith, E. E., Wilson, S. J., & Lipsey, M. W. (2013). The comparative effectiveness of outpatient treatment for adolescent substance abuse: A meta-analysis. *Journal of Substance Abuse Treatment, 44*(2), 145–158.
Turner, C. F., Ku, L., Rogers, S. M., Lindberg, L. D., Pleck, J. H., & Sonenstein, F. L. (1998). Adolescent sexual behavior, drug use, and violence: Increased reporting with computer survey technology. *Science, 280*(5365), 867–873.
U.S. Office of the Surgeon General. (2016). *Reports of the surgeon general: Facing addiction in America: The surgeon general's report on alcohol, drugs, and health*. Washington, DC: U.S. Department of Health and Human Services.
van der Stouwe, T., Asscher, J. J., Stams, G. J. J., Deković, M., & van der Laan, P. H. (2014). The effectiveness of multisystemic therapy (MST): A meta-analysis. *Clinical Psychology Review, 34*(6), 468–481.
Vaughn, M. G., & Howard, M. O. (2004). Adolescent substance abuse treatment: A synthesis of controlled evaluations. *Research on Social Work Practice, 14*(5), 325–335.
Vendetti, J., Gmyrek, A., Damon, D., Singh, M., McRee, B., & Del Boca, F. (2017). Screening, brief intervention and referral to treatment (SBIRT): Implementation barriers, facilitators and model migration. *Addiction, 112*(S2), 23–33.
Volkow, N. D., Baler, R. D., Compton, W. M., & Weiss, S. R. (2014). Adverse health effects of marijuana use. *New England Journal of Medicine, 370*(23), 2219–2227.
Wachtel, T., & Staniford, M. (2010). The effectiveness of brief interventions in the clinical setting in reducing alcohol misuse and binge drinking in adolescents: A critical review of the literature. *Journal of Clinical Nursing, 19*(5-6), 605–620.
Waldron, H. B., Brody, J. L., Robbins, M. S., & Alexander, J. F. (2013). Functional family therapy for adolescent substance use disorders. In P. Miller (Ed.), *Interventions for addiction: Comprehensive addictive behaviors and disorders* (pp. 109–116). San Diego, CA: Academic Press.
Waldron, H. B., Slesnick, N., Brody, J. L., Turner, C. W., & Peterson, T. R. (2001). Treatment outcomes for adolescent substance abuse at 4- and 7-month assessments. *Journal of Consulting and Clinical Psychology, 69*(5), 802–813.
Walker, D. D., Roffman, R. A., Stephens, R. S., Berghuis, J., & Kim, W. (2006). Motivational enhancement therapy for adolescent marijuana users: A preliminary randomized controlled trial. *Journal of Consulting and Clinical Psychology, 74*(3), 628–632.
Walker, D. D., Stephens, R., Roffman, R., Demarce, J., Lozano, B., Towe, S., & Berg, B. (2011). Randomized controlled trial of motivational enhancement therapy with nontreatment-seeking adolescent cannabis users: A further test of the teen marijuana check-up. *Psychology of Addictive Behaviors, 25*(3), 474–484.
Walther, L., Gantner, A., Heinz, A., & Majic, T. (2016). Evidence-based treatment options in cannabis dependency. *Deutsches Ärzteblatt International, 113*(39), 653–659.
Walton, M. A., Chermack, S. T., Shope, J. T., Bingham, C. R., Zimmerman, M. A., Blow, F. C., … Cunningham, R. M. (2010). Effects of a brief intervention for reducing violence and alcohol misuse among adolescents: A randomized controlled trial. *Journal of the American Medical Association, 304*(5), 527–535.

Weisband, S., & Kiesler, S. (1996). Self disclosure on computer forms: Meta-analysis and implications. In M. J. Tauber (Ed.), *CHI '96 Proceedings of the SIGCHI conference on human factors in computing systems* (pp. 3–10). New York: NY: ACM Digital Library. https://doi.org/10.1145/238386.238387

Williams, R. J., Chang, S. Y., & Addiction Centre Adolescent Research Group. (2000). A comprehensive and comparative review of adolescent substance abuse treatment outcome. *Clinical Psychology: Science and Practice, 7*(2), 138–166.

Winters, K. C. (1999). Treating adolescents with substance use disorders: An overview of practice issues and treatment outcomes. *Substance Abuse, 20*(4), 203–225.

Winters, K. C. (2016). Adolescent brief interventions. *Journal of Drug Abuse, 2*(1), 1–3.

Winters, K. C., Lee, S., Botzet, A., Fahnhorst, T., & Nicholson, A. (2014). One-year outcomes of a brief intervention for drug abusing adolescents. *Psychology of Addictive Behaviors, 28*(2), 464–474.

Winters, K. C., Leitten, W., Wagner, E., & O'Leary Tevyaw, T. (2007). Use of brief interventions in a middle and high school setting. *Journal of School Health, 77*(4), 196–206.

Winters, K. C., Stinchfield, R. D., Latimer, W. W., & Lee, S. (2007). Long-term outcome of substance dependent youth following 12-step treatment. *Journal of Substance Abuse Treatment, 33*(1), 61–69.

Winters, K. C., Stinchfield, R. D., Opland, E., Weller, C., & Latimer, W. W. (2000). The effectiveness of the Minnesota model approach in the treatment of adolescent drug abusers. *Addiction, 95*(4), 601–612.

Winters, K. C., Tanner-Smith, E., Bresani, E., & Meyers, K. (2014). Current advances in the treatment of adolescent substance use. *Adolescent Health, Medicine and Therapeutics, 5*, 199–210.

Evidence-Based Family Treatment of Adolescent Substance-Related Disorders

Shaun I. Calix, Kevin C. Garrett, and Mark A. Fine

Introduction

Adolescence is an important period of individual development. It is a time wherein youth develop the ability to reason in more sophisticated ways than done previously. During this crucial period, youth often explore and shift their identity, behavior, and relationships (Arnett, 2013). Some degree of risk-taking and other externalizing problem behaviors are normal during this period of exploration and change. Although potentially dangerous, these behaviors help adolescents learn the importance of boundaries regarding their physical and emotional safety, as well as appropriate ways to assert their independence. Many adolescents discover these limits by experiencing punishments imposed by caregivers and authority figures, along with natural consequences when their behaviors are inappropriate. These repercussions often help to decrease problem behaviors by the time youth reach adulthood. However, the cessation of problem behaviors often is frustrated by adolescent substance abuse and addiction. Additionally, family, peer, and other contexts in which teens live have the potential to contribute to the development and continuation of their problem behaviors and substance abuse.

S. I. Calix (✉)
Department of Psychology, School of Graduate and Professional Studies, Cameron University, Lawton, OK, USA
e-mail: scalix@cameron.edu

K. C. Garrett
Oregon Institute of Technology, Klamath Falls, OR, USA
e-mail: kevin.garrett@oit.edu

M. A. Fine
Human Development and Family Studies, School of Health and Human Sciences, The University of North Carolina at Greensboro, Greensboro, NC, USA
e-mail: mafine@uncg.edu

C. G. Leukefeld, T. P. Gullotta (eds.), *Adolescent Substance Abuse*, Issues in Children's and Families' Lives, https://doi.org/10.1007/978-3-319-90611-9_6

Repetti, Taylor, and Seeman (2002) outlined the characteristics of both healthy and unhealthy family systems. These authors point to the increased risk of youth raised in unhealthy families to develop mental and physical problems in adolescence and later in life, including smoking, alcohol abuse, and drug abuse. To help youth exhibiting substance-related disorders, clinical interventions are crucial. Due to the interconnectedness of youth and their families, only treating the youth involved will be likely to result in failure because the family systems will not have adapted to support the individual's changes. Weidman (1987) recognized that the families of adolescent drug abusers can either help or hinder treatment, and proposed that families should be at least minimally involved in the treatment of adolescents and preferably engaged in family therapy.

Family systems researchers also assert that not only do individuals and families mutually influence one another, but individuals and families experience mutual influences with their surrounding systems as well (Bronfenbrenner, 1988). For instance, teens who engage in problem behavior, including substance use, often develop adversarial relationships with school officials, law enforcement, and others. When such teens begin to make changes aimed at eliminating problem behaviors, if their schools and law enforcement do not change the way they interact with the teens (i.e., continue to treat them as adversaries), the changes the teens are making will not be supported and may be jeopardized.

On the basis of a review of the clinical literature, Liddle (2004) concluded that family-based treatments of adolescent substance abuse have been shown to be more effective than alternative treatments in producing short-term and long-term change. To bring about lasting change, clinicians have proposed that treatments must not only intervene with the family system in which the adolescent develops, but also address extrafamilial systems. Sexton and Alexander (2005) identified several approaches that fulfill those criteria: multisystemic therapy (MST), multidimensional family therapy (MDFT), functional family therapy (FFT), and brief strategic family therapy (BSFT). After reviewing the recent clinical literature (i.e., the last 10 years) on family treatments of adolescent substance abuse, including two meta-analyses (Baldwin, Christian, Berkeljon, Shadish, & Bean, 2012; Tanner-Smith, Wilson, & Lipsey, 2013) published in the last 5 years, the authors of this chapter decided to include these four models in this chapter under the heading of "evidence-based family treatments." Other promising models will be discussed briefly, but MST, MDFT, FFT, and BSFT will receive the most attention.

Prevalence of Substance Use

Illicit Drugs

It is important to note two factors when considering rates of illicit drug use among adolescents: grade level of the child and type of drug use being reported (Johnston, O'Malley, Miech, Bachman, & Schulenberg, 2017). Grade level of the child often is used instead of the child's age in reports of substance use rates because it better captures developmental context, particularly the peer context. Adolescents tend to share the peer context most often with peers in the same grade level, and drug use among adolescents is most likely to occur in peer contexts.

Children at higher grade levels are more likely than those in lower grade levels to use illicit drugs as they spend less time in the family context and more in the peer context (Johnston et al., 2017). The type of drug used also tends to vary by grade level of child. Children at lower grade levels are more likely than children at higher grade levels to use easily accessed substances (e.g., inhalants), while children in higher grade levels are more likely to use "harder" drugs (e.g., marijuana, cocaine, heroin). Finally, rates of illicit drug use are often impacted by the fact that marijuana, especially among older children, is the most frequently used illicit drug and tends to drive indices of illicit drug use; therefore, it is useful to consider rates of illicit drug use, excluding marijuana, to better detect trends in overall illicit drug use rates. This also should be in considered in the context of changing laws on recreational marijuana use; although it is still illegal for those under 21 to possess marijuana in states where recreational marijuana use has been legalized, the punishments may be less severe.

Although researchers have observed declines in adolescent drug abuse with regard to specific classes of drugs since 2014 (Johnston et al., 2017), the rate of drug use still is high. According to Johnston et al., (2017), the average lifetime rate of any illicit drug use 8th, 10th, and 12th graders combined was 32.6% in 2016. The average lifetime rate of illicit drug use for drugs other than marijuana was 14.3% in 2016. By grade level, the rates of lifetime use of any illicit drug are as follows: 17.2% for 8th graders, 33.7% for 10th graders, and 48.3% for 12th graders. A notable difference exists between these rates and those that exclude use of marijuana, which are significantly lower: 8.9% for 8th graders, 14% for 10th graders, and 20.7% for 12th graders.

Alcohol Abuse

The Monitoring the Future survey (Johnston et al., 2017) also revealed that statistics varied widely by grade level for alcohol use. Among 8th graders, 22.8% had ever used alcohol, followed by 43.4% of 10th graders, and 61.2% of 12th graders. In terms of those who had been drunk, 8.6% of 8th graders, 26% of 10th graders, and 46.3% of 12th graders reported ever being intoxicated.

Long-Term Impacts of Adolescent Substance Use

Substance abuse that begins in adolescence can have long-term consequences. The National Survey on Drug Use and Health (Substance Abuse and Mental Health Services Administration, 2013) found that adults who first used marijuana at age 14 or younger were over four times more likely to be classified with substance use or dependence as those who first used marijuana at or after age 18 (11.5% vs. 2.6% respectively). Adults who first consumed alcohol at age 14 or younger also were over four times more likely to be classified at any point in their lives with alcohol abuse or dependence compared with those who first consumed alcohol at or after age 18 (15.4% vs. 3.8% respectively).

Treatment Gaps

The Substance Abuse and Mental Health Services Administration (2013) estimates that 1.5% of teens in the US population at or above age 12 received treatment for either illicit drug use or alcohol use in 2013. This remained stable from the previous year and is comparable to 2002. According to the Substance Abuse and Mental Health Services Administration (2013) the percentage of adolescents currently dependent on or abusing illicit drugs in 2013 was 5.2% (2.8% for alcohol); comparison of these statistics indicates that there may be a significant gap between the number of adolescents who need treatment and those who actually receive it.

Evidence-Based Family Treatments

Family-based treatments are clinical approaches wherein the adolescent battling with a substance-related disorder is treated with members of his or her family system. Considerable research supports the importance of including more than just the adolescent in treatment, as the adolescents' families are often affected by the adolescents' substance abuse and the adolescents' substance abuse is also influenced by family interactions in a bidirectional manner (Alexander, Waldron, Robbins, & Neeb, 2013).

Several family-based treatments have displayed varying, yet promising, levels of success in treating adolescent substance abuse. Some of the treatments considered in this chapter (e.g., MST, MDFT, FFT, and a combination of FFT and cognitive-behavioral therapy) are integrative therapy models because they employ the use of multiple therapeutic models. Other family treatments (e.g., BSFT) are more narrowly focused family interventions, and adhere more closely to traditional family therapy models. In addition to providing treatment to the family system, MDFT, MST, and FFT also qualify as ecological models in that they include other external systems in treatment (e.g., law enforcement, schools, religious groups) to encourage change in those systems that would support changes in the family and individual who are the focus of treatment.

MST (Henggeler, Schoenwald, Borduin, Rowland, & Cunningham, 2009), MDFT (Liddle, 2002), FFT (Alexander & Parsons, 1982), and BSFT (Szapocznik, Hervis, & Schwartz, 2003) are four family treatments that have shown, through multiple and rigorous studies, effectiveness in treating adolescent substance abuse

(Baldwin et al., 2012; Tanner-Smith et al., 2013). Descriptions of each family-based treatment model and its respective empirical evidence will be elucidated hereafter.

Multisystemic Therapy

MST (Henggeler et al., 2009) is based on the ecological theory of human development (Bronfenbrenner, 1979) and early family therapy approaches including structural (Minuchin, 1974) and strategic family therapy (Haley, 1976). Bronfenbrenner's ecological theory posits that human beings develop in the context of multiple nested systems. Beyond the developing individual, the most basic and important of these systems is the family. Other systems include the community, school, work, and larger society in general. These systems shape the individual both directly (through interaction with the individual) and indirectly (through interaction with other systems). In addition, the individual and the systems interact with each other in a reciprocal manner; individuals shape the systems just as the systems shape individuals. Bronfenbrenner's theory is central to the practice of MST because the MST therapist acts as an advocate for and intervention specialist within the adolescent, family, and the extrafamilial systems (Schoenwald & Henggeler, 2005).

Bronfenbrenner's ecological theory is central to the MST theory of change (Henggeler et al., 2009), which posits that adolescent antisocial behavior, which includes substance abuse, develops in the context of intersecting risk factors whose origins are in the multiple systems with which the adolescents interact, either directly or indirectly. For therapy to be effective, MST interventions must address these risk factors and develop protective factors in their place. These protective factors are important because they support the changes made by the individuals and families through the course of treatment; without such supports, changes made are likely to break down. In addition, MST assumes that caregivers play a central role in change, and need the resources and skills to make changes to become more effective caregivers (Henggeler et al., 2009). The development of protective factors in systems external to the family is accomplished in partnership with caregivers.

MST is a home-based therapy. A primary therapist, who is part of a larger treatment team, implements MST by providing therapy to the adolescent, family, and other systems in their environments (Henggeler et al., 2009; Schoenwald & Henggeler, 2005). The prescribed use of a treatment team is the most unique aspect of MST, and one that is necessary due to the intensive nature of MST. The treatment team consists of the primary therapist, a supervisor, and one to three other MST therapists. Although the primary therapist is ultimately responsible for carrying out the treatment interventions, the treatment team helps in assessment and provides feedback on the therapist's conceptualization of the case. Assessment is constantly occurring in MST, so the treatment team monitors and makes changes to the treatment plan based on whether targeted changes are taking place. In addition, the treatment team makes it possible for an MST therapist to be available to clients 24 h a day, 7 days a week by making a treatment team member available as a therapist in the absence of the primary therapist. The supervisor's role is to ensure treatment fidelity. The treatment team is essential to the successful implementation of MST.

MST has a well-defined analytical process known as the "Do Loop" (Henggeler et al., 2009; Swenson, Henggeler, Taylor, & Addison, 2005). The "Do Loop" is a series of steps that guide the MST treatment team in assessment and intervention. First, the therapist assesses what problems brought about the family's referral to MST. Next, the therapist assesses the goals of the key players involved in the process (e.g., adolescent, parents, school officials, coworkers, or work supervisors). Once those goals are decided upon, the treatment team formulates overarching goals for the family. The therapist then begins to determine the fit between the referral problems and the ecology of the youth (Henggeler et al., 2009; Swenson et al., 2005). To do so, the therapist observes the strengths of the family and the surrounding systems, and refines the assessment as information is discovered. Next, the therapist formulates short-term treatment goals that are linked to the overarching goals.

When all the goals are formulated, the therapist begins to implement interventions meant to help the family and extrafamilial systems accomplish those goals (Henggeler et al., 2009; Schoenwald & Henggeler, 2005). During this period, the therapist monitors the success of the interventions. When a barrier to success appears (whether at the family, extrafamilial, or therapeutic level), the treatment team formulates strategies to overcome those barriers. The therapist implements those strategies and reevaluates. Another unique aspect of MST is that, at any point in the therapeutic process, MST prescribes a self-reflexive process for the therapists and treatment teams. Success and failure of treatment are evaluated by both the therapist and the treatment team. The therapist, treatment team, and supervisor monitor their own behavior in relation to the therapeutic process. The self-reflexive process is unique because many other therapies do not prescribe it as a crucial part of therapy, and because a treatment team plays an integral role in the process. Although other therapies, in theory, can function without such a process, MST requires it as a part of a faithful adherence to the treatment model.

MST has been evaluated as an effective treatment for youth violence, delinquency, and substance use (Curtis, Ronan, & Borduin, 2004; Henggeler, Clingempeel, Brondino, & Pickrel, 2002; Henggeler, Melton, Brondino, Scherer, & Hanley, 1997; Henggeler, Melton, & Smith, 1992; Henggeler, Pickrel, & Brondino, 1999; Liddle, 2004; Liddle & Dakof, 1995). Henggeler et al. (1991) reported that 4% of all juvenile offenders in the MST condition had a substance-related arrest in a 4-year follow-up, compared to 15% of those in individual therapy. In a 14 year follow-up to this study, Schaeffer and Borduin (2005) found that juvenile offenders who received MST were less than half as likely as those who received individual therapy (13% vs. 33.3% respectively) to be arrested for a later substance-related offense. In another 4-year follow-up study, Henggeler et al. (2002) found that adolescents in the MST condition abstained from marijuana significantly more frequently than did adolescents in the treatment-as-usual condition (55% vs. 28%, respectively). Finally, in a study of substance abusing juvenile offenders (Henggeler et al., 2006), researchers found that MST was more effective than other treatments at decreasing substance use over a one year period.

Multidimensional Family Therapy

MDFT (Liddle, 2002) is based on several frameworks: risk and protective factors, developmental perspectives, and ecological theory (Liddle, 2016). The risk and protective factors framework provides information to clinicians about various factors that facilitate or hinder healthy development (e.g., peer networks, early physical maturation, community resources, neighborhood violence). Developmental perspectives provide information to clinicians about normative developmental transitions and youths' ability to cope with the developmental tasks associated with such transitions (Rohde et al., 2007). Ecological perspectives provide a framework for understanding not only the individual and family, but interacting social influences (e.g., mesosystems; Bronfenbrenner, 1979) that form unique and whole systems of influence on individual development (e.g., peer and school, school and home). Such systems need to be a focus of intervention (Liddle, 2016) because it helps to reinforce longer lasting systemic change for individuals and families if the systems surrounding them are supportive of changes made at the individual and family level.

One of the primary guiding principles of how change occurs in MDFT is that "adolescent problems are multidimensional phenomena" (Liddle, 2016, p. 233). In other words, substance abuse problems in adolescents are associated with a myriad of interconnected factors that are biological, psychological, and social in nature. Therefore, the MDFT therapist must intervene with not only the individual, but also family, peers, school, and other social systems, to name a few. In addition, MDFT assumes that "family functioning is instrumental in creating developmentally healthy lifestyle alternatives for adolescents" (Liddle, 2016, p. 233). In MDFT, the family is a target in assessment and intervention because of its direct influence on adolescents. It is the therapist's role to create individual therapeutic alliances with the family and other multiple systems in which the adolescent is embedded.

MDFT is a manualized treatment system, which is published online (Liddle, 2002; Liddle, Rodriguez, Dakof, Kanzki, & Marvel, 2005). MDFT is designed to tailor the treatment to the characteristics of the adolescent, family, and their involvement with extrafamilial systems. For that reason, MDFT has been modified into several formats to account for varying individual and family circumstances (Liddle, 2004). MDFT is similar to MST in its goals and some of its concepts, but MDFT takes a different approach to the process of therapy, mainly in its prescription for individual sessions and meetings with the adolescent and with the family, and the lack of a dedicated treatment team that is available 24/7 as in MST.

MDFT is implemented in stages with modules within each stage (Liddle, 2002, 2016). Initially, the therapist meets with the entire family to begin assessing family interactions, and then the therapist moves on to the first stage. The first stage is *engagement*. Within this stage, the MDFT therapist usually meets with the adolescent (module 1) and parents (module 2) separately for a few sessions to allow for engagement and to gain information about the unique perspectives of each individual. In individual sessions with the adolescent, therapists focus on current pressures the adolescent is experiencing, motivation for substance use, identity, and future dreams and goals (Liddle, 2016). In individual sessions with parents, therapists focus on environmental challenges parents experience in their parenting, along with gaining information about parenting practices and their relationship with their child (Liddle, 2016). Some interventions take place in the engagement stage as well. After the individual sessions are complete, the therapist brings the family together (module 3) to further assess family interactions and history, as well as to begin to define the therapeutic process. The therapist also begins to shape family interactions on a smaller scale (e.g., the therapist may ask family members to use I-statements or may have family members explore one another's perspectives or emotions). Larger scale, and more stress-inducing, changes and interventions (e.g., enactments, prescribed changes to interactions outside of therapy) are accomplished in later stages. In module 4, the therapist makes contact with representatives from the extrafamilial systems that have an interest in the adolescent's well-being. The therapist assesses the needs of the extrafamilial systems in relation to the adolescent and establishes a working relationship with them. Of course, as with MST, the therapist receives the parents' permission to contact those systems.

The second stage is the *primary intervention* stage (Liddle et al., 2005). Module 1 is insight-oriented, skill-oriented, and solution-focused. The therapist encourages self-examination in the adolescent, helps to improve functioning in critical areas (e.g., anger management), and focuses on solutions and alternatives for living. The therapist also collaborates with other treatment systems (e.g., psychiatrists) with which the adolescent is involved. In module 2, the therapist helps the parents to learn how to engage in self-care activities (e.g., stress-reduction, and assessing needs and desires), employs parenting training, and helps solve interparental conflict (i.e., help them work as a team). In module 3, the therapist facilitates discussion among family members to bring conflict into the open and to deal with it directly. The therapist also encourages the discussion of past hurts and emotions surrounding the problem and parental attempts to solve the problem.

In the third stage, the therapist acknowledges changes that have been made by the family, making them overt and visible to the family (Liddle et al., 2005). MDFT emphasizes that treatment is not perfect, and that all changes, whether desirable or imperfect, are part of the family's narrative about a future that includes those changes. In this stage, the therapist also explores termination of therapy with the family.

MDFT has been effective in reducing substance abuse in adolescent client populations (Liddle et al., 2001; Liddle, Rowe, Dakof, Ungaro, & Henderson, 2004). In a randomized clinical trial, MDFT, compared to adolescent group therapy and a multifamily educational intervention, yielded clinically significant and greater reductions in substance abuse and improved family functioning between pretreatment and posttreatment, and at 6- and 12-month follow-ups (Liddle et al., 2001). Clinically significant reductions were judged to be a reduction in substance abuse below the threshold set for entry into the study (i.e., marijuana use at least three times per week over a period of a month, or an instance of using "hard drugs"). Liddle et al. (2004) found that MDFT led to greater maintenance of treatment gains when compared to peer group treatment.

Comparison of MDFT and MST

On the surface, MDFT and MST are very similar therapeutic models. Although the overarching goals and targets of treatment are quite similar, there are noticeable treatment process differences. Similarly to MST, in the treatment of adolescent substance abuse, MDFT targets the adolescent, family, and extrafamilial systems. MDFT emphasizes that adolescent substance abuse develops along various contextual pathways that sometimes intersect (Liddle et al., 2005). In other words, the MDFT therapist assumes that adolescent substance abuse develops along pathways involving peer relationships, family relationships, individual psychological issues, and interactions between those systems and educational and justice systems (i.e., mesosystemic interactions; Bronfenbrenner, 1988). For example, MDFT may target an adolescent's peer relationships in the context of the school setting or examine how relationships with peers are affecting interactions with parents.

Despite their similarities, MST and MDFT take different approaches to the therapeutic process. While MST permits individual sessions, it is preferred that the therapist intervene with the entire family; MDFT prescribes individual sessions. In addition, unlike MST, there is no prescription for a treatment team to be involved in each case for MDFT. The therapists in MST and MDFT are self-reflexive, but MST therapists have the added advantage of a treatment team that is available to be actively involved in the therapeutic process as both observers and actors (i.e., meeting with extrafmailial systems, providing back-up to the lead therapist in case of absence). Finally, MDFT seems to emphasize the role of the therapist in creating therapeutic alliances between and among involved systems, where MST emphasizes the family as the active agent in setting up therapeutic alliances with the coaching of the therapist.

Functional Family Therapy

FFT (Alexander et al., 2013; Alexander & Parsons, 1982) follows many of the same theoretical principles and therapy models as Multisystemic Therapy and Brief Strategic Family Therapy (e.g., family systems theory, structural family therapy, and strategic family therapy). In addition, as is often the case with other therapeutic approaches, FFT explicitly emphasizes that the therapist is an integral part of the therapeutic system. Because of FFT's assumption that every family is different, the therapist must be creative in the treatment of the family (Sexton & Alexander, 2005).

However, the need for creativity does not preclude the need for structure in the therapeutic process. The FFT therapist must be attuned to the dialectic tension between creativity and structure, and be able to balance the two (Sexton & Alexander, 2005).

FFT developed out of the earlier family therapy models of structural and strategic family therapy (Sexton & Alexander, 2005). Those two models, as with other therapies discussed in this chapter, emphasize assessing repeated patterns of interactions in families and intervening in an active and purposeful manner by targeting the problems that are most amenable to change. FFT has more recently included social constructionist and ecological theories to provide (1) an approach that is open to therapist creativity and (2) a comprehensive approach that considers the multiple systemic interactions that difficult client populations (such as substance abusing adolescents) experience (Sexton & Alexander, 2005). Additionally, FFT is a short-term, intensive, strength-based model, which is usually completed over an average of 12 sessions spanning 3–4 months (Alexander et al., 2013).

To provide the structure needed for sound therapy, the creators of FFT developed a clinical model that consists of five treatment phases: Engagement, Motivation, Relational Assessment, Behavior Change, and Generalization (Alexander et al., 2013). The goal of the Engagement Phase is "to enhance family members' perceptions of responsiveness and credibility" (Alexander et al., 2013, p. 8). This phase is completed in a culturally sensitive manner, wherein the therapist attends to the myriad needs of the family and meets them where they are. Families may have transportation issues or speak a different language. Therefore, therapy may need to be performed in the families' homes and the therapist may need to arrange for a translator or for another therapist who is fluent in the families' native tongue (Alexander et al., 2013).

FFT involves as many family members in treatment as possible and, whereas other treatment models focus much more on individual behavior change in the adolescent (and sometimes the parents), FFT emphasizes that the family's interactions are central to problem development (Alexander et al., 2013). Therefore, the overarching goal of the Motivation Phase is to help engage all family members, thus helping to increase their motivation for change as a result of treatment. Specifically, "The goals of this phase include creating a positive motivational context, minimizing hopelessness and low self-efficacy, and changing the meaning of family relationships to emphasize possible hopeful experiences" (Alexander et al., 2013, p. 12).

In the Relational Assessment phase, the therapist attends to whether each family member's statements or behaviors seek to build connection or to distance within the family system, as well as to establish hierarchy (Alexander et al., 2013). In the Behavior Change phase, change occurs through family-based interventions such as skill building, changing habitual problematic interactions, and other coping skills being taught at both the individual and relational levels. Other creative interventions and skills aimed at changing negative behavioral and cognitive patterns are utilized during this phase (Alexander et al., 2013; Sexton & Alexander, 2005). FFT therapists work with family risk and protective factors to activate change. For example, the FFT therapist may target a particular family strength (e.g., positive regard for one another) to reduce negative affect or poor communication in interactions.

Lastly, the Generalization Phase is used to help individuals and families maintain the changes they have made or are in the process of making on multiple systemic levels (Alexander et al., 2013). This involves the therapist linking changes in the family to other areas of family functioning peripheral to the original presenting problem, with the goal of transferring treatment gains into multiple areas of family functioning. The FFT therapist also makes connections between the family and other community resources. For example, the FFT therapist may link the family with support groups or community recreation centers (Alexander et al., 2013).

Although all the therapies mentioned in this chapter are attuned to the same guiding principles of family therapy as FFT, there are notable differences among them. For example, FFT does not prescribe individual sessions with the adolescent or other family members as in MDFT. According to FFT, individual behavior change is best accomplished in the context of the family; therefore, the preferred tool is relational interventions.

Another difference among FFT, MST, and MDFT is in the level of focus on extrafamilial systems. While FFT considers extrafamilial systems (e.g., relationships with peers, the family's support network) in the generalization phase, there is no direct consultation or intervention with those systems during the first two stages of therapy. Both MST and MDFT therapists interact directly with extrafamilial systems during the entire course of therapy.

According to several clinical trials, FFT has demonstrated effectiveness in reducing delinquency and substance abuse (Liddle, 2004; Waldron, 1997; Waldron, Slesnick, Brody, Turner, & Peterson, 2001). Liddle cited FFT as one of the more effective models of family therapy for adolescent drug abuse. Friedman (1989) found that FFT significantly reduced substance use and improved psychiatric and family functioning, but the effects were not significantly greater than those in the other treatment condition (i.e., parent training group). However, in a randomized clinical trial, FFT demonstrated significantly greater effectiveness in reducing heavy to minimal adolescent marijuana use at 7 months posttreatment than did cognitive-behavioral therapy (CBT) alone and group interventions (Waldron et al., 2001). Another study demonstrated that FFT (office based) was more effective than treatment as usual in reducing alcohol and other drug use among runaway youth (Slesnick & Prestopnik, 2009). However, the same authors found that families took part in and completed more treatment sessions when they received a home-based ecologically based family therapy approach versus FFT. The authors point to the likelihood that the setting (i.e., office-based versus home-based) in which the therapy is provided influences the number of sessions families complete (Slesnick & Prestopnik, 2009).

Brief Strategic Family Therapy

Another family-based treatment that has demonstrated effectiveness is BSFT (Szapocznik et al., 2003). Like the other approaches reviewed in this chapter, BSFT adheres to family systems theory, as well as structural and strategic family therapy models (Horigian et al., 2005). BSFT is different than the others in that it is a short-term therapy alternative. BSFT is intended to be completed within 12–16 sessions, with booster sessions after termination as needed (Horigian et al., 2005). BSFT subscribes to the same theories as FFT, but it has different emphases within its process. BSFT has three main stages: joining, diagnosing, and restructuring (Horigian et al., 2005). During the joining phase, the therapist focuses on engaging the adolescent and family in therapy. The therapist attempts to form a new system with the family—the therapeutic system. The therapeutic system includes all members of the family and the therapist, with the therapist acting as both an observer and a change agent. As both an observer and a change agent, the BSFT therapist is very active. Joining is crucial to the therapist becoming a change agent because the therapist must gain the family's trust in order to direct change in an active way. Joining involves simultaneously attending to the individuals within the family and patterns of family interaction. Because the therapist must assess family functioning as it typically and naturally occurs during the joining phase, substantive interventions are not implemented during this stage.

At the diagnosing stage, the therapist begins to more actively assess the family. Part of the diagnosing stage involves creating enactments (Horigian et al., 2005). Enactments should fulfill two purposes: (1) create an atmosphere in which family members can interact as they normally do and (2) provide the therapist with an assessment opportunity to passively observe the family. The therapist should intervene in early enactments to redirect the family members to interact with each other during the enactment rather than to talk to the therapist.

The therapist attends to several factors during assessment (Horigian et al., 2005). Paying attention to family hierarchy, subsystem organization, and the communication flow enable the therapist to understand how the family organizes itself around interactions. The therapist also focuses on the connections and responsiveness among family members. It is important for the therapist to assess the family's developmental stage, especially when children are in adolescence. One of the family interactional patterns most closely associated with adolescent behavior problems occurs when one or both parents do not allow for developmentally appropriate autonomy (Micucci, 1998). Finally, the therapist attends to family interactions organized around maintaining the adolescent as the identified patient. In doing so, the therapist identifies who blames the adolescent for family problems, and who contributes to the adolescent maintaining that role (Horigian et al., 2005).

The final stage before termination of treatment is restructuring (Szapocznik et al., 2003). Once the therapist has assessed the family, clinical goals are formulated and interventions are assigned to each goal. Interventions focus on reshaping present interactions. That is, therapists work to pinpoint what is happening in the therapy room and use those interactions as the basis for change (Horigian et al., 2005). Families in therapy often want to focus on the content of their past interactions ("he said/she said"), but it is the therapist's responsibility to redirect the family to process-oriented interactions in the here-and-now.

The therapist uses reframing to motivate change. When reframing, the therapist helps the family create alternative meanings behind interactions. Reframing is not meant to change individual cognitions, but to create an alternate frame of reality in which the family can successfully operate (Worden, 2003). For instance, in the context of exploring what parents term as an adolescent's "rebellion," the therapist may reframe the rebellion as an attempt by the adolescent to become more independent from the parents so that he or she can one day live without the parents' assistance. If the parents buy into the reframe, then they can set up a system in which they feel less need to control the adolescent and will be able to help develop that autonomy in more adaptive ways.

The BSFT therapist also works to change the family's boundaries to de-emphasize alliances that are maintaining maladaptive behavior in the adolescent (Horigian et al., 2005). For instance, if the adolescent has an overinvolved relationship with one parent, the therapist might assign tasks designed to increase the frequency of positive interactions with the other parent. The BSFT therapist also assigns tasks to the family to be completed outside of sessions (Horigian et al., 2005). Assigning tasks accomplishes two goals: (1) it maintains the family's effort outside of therapy sessions, and (2) it helps the family continue its success following treatment. The belief is that if the family members can successfully complete tasks while outside of the therapy room, then they will continue to carry their success and new tools after treatment.

BSFT differs from the other therapies mentioned in this chapter in several ways. First, it is a brief therapy option, and is less intensive than MST and MDFT. It is a viable alternative when a therapist does not have the resources to be available to clients 24 h a day, 7 days a week (as MST requires), or to engage in prolonged treatment. It is meant to be completed within a relatively brief time period; MST, MDFT, and FFT do not have a set number of sessions. BSFT also differs in that there is no prescription for intervention with extrafamilial systems.

BSFT has been shown to be effective in treating adolescent drug abuse (Santisteban et al., 2003; Szapocznik et al., 1988; Szapocznik, Kurtines, Foote, Perez-Vidal, & Hervis, 1986). Santisteban et al. (2003) found that 60% of BSFT participants reliably decreased marijuana usage, compared to 17% in the group therapy condition. In a recent clinical trial comparing BSFT to treatment-as-usual conditions (e.g., group therapy, parent education, case management), Robbins et al. (2011) found that BSFT resulted in a significant reduction in number of days of self-reported drug use among adolescents compared to the treatment-as-usual, as well as higher success in engaging adolescents and their families in treatment, and improvements in family functioning.

Promising Family Treatments

Certainly, treatments with strong empirical support are the best options for clinicians who wish to ensure they are utilizing the best available treatments. However, there are alternative approaches that show promise. Some treatments have not been developed fully into a treatment model or have not yet been shown to be effective, yet they show promise as viable treatment alternatives. The most promising of these is described below.

Cognitive-Behavioral Therapy and FFT (Integrative Treatment)

Integrative treatment has shown promise in recent research, but has not been institutionalized in the form of a manual or developed beyond being a treatment condition in clinical trials. Waldron et al. (2001) combined CBT and FFT to serve as a treatment condition in testing the effectiveness of FFT as a treatment for adolescent substance abuse. Waldron et al. (2001) also tested CBT by itself in the study. The CBT model used in the study focused on developing self-control and coping skills to help the adolescents avoid substance abuse. When combined with a family therapy model such as FFT, this rendition of CBT adds an additional skill-based component that is not always present in traditional family therapy.

When combined, FFT and CBT offered an integrative treatment that (1) identifies and intervenes in family interactions that maintain adolescent substance abuse and (2) initiates behavioral change in the adolescent and helps the adolescent gain skills to avoid the use of substances. Waldron et al. (2001) found that the condition that combined FFT and CBT outperformed both component treatments. The FFT/CBT combination resulted in a greater reduction in heavy to minimal marijuana usage from pretreatment to 7 months posttreatment (89.7% vs. 55.6%) than did the FFT condition (86.6% vs. 62.1%).

Family Treatments for Specific Abused Substances

There are no family treatment approaches to our knowledge that are *designed* to target a specific drug. However, some treatment models have shown effectiveness in decreasing use of specific substances. For instance, Santisteban et al. (2003) found that BSFT was more effective than adolescent group therapy in the treatment of adolescents who abused marijuana. At posttreatment, 60% of the adolescents in the BSFT condition improved (i.e., decreased use) and 15% deteriorated (i.e., increased use), while 17% of those in the group therapy condition improved and 50% deteriorated.

Parental substance abuse can also be a target of family therapy interventions with adolescent substance users. Parental substance abuse is a systemic issue that needs to be addressed when it occurs in the home of an adolescent. It is not uncommon for adolescents to abuse drugs or alcohol that they witness their parents using. It is somewhat less common, but possibly more therapeutically significant, that some parents abuse drugs *with* their children. It may be helpful for the therapist to target those specific drugs that the parents abuse, whether alone or with their children, when facilitating family therapy.

Conclusion: Treatment Recommendations

Our overarching treatment recommendation is that clinicians treating substance abusing adolescents or their families should strive to use those treatment strategies that have been shown to be empirically effective. Researchers testing the effectiveness of MST, MDFT, FFT, and BSFT have demonstrated their ability to produce both short-term and long-term reductions in substance misuse of adolescents, above and beyond the effects of other treatments popular in treatment communities (Curtis et al., 2004; Henggeler et al., 1991, 2002; Liddle et al., 2001, 2004). Many available treatment options have shown some effectiveness in treating other disorders and family problems. It is a natural tendency of treatment professionals to gravitate toward the treatment models under which they trained, and with which they have experienced some success in other contexts. However, it should be the goal of every clinician to utilize treatment approaches that are effective for the specific populations and problems with which the clinician works (e.g., adolescent substance abuse).

There are specific aspects of evidence-based family treatments that have been connected with treatment success with substance abusing adolescent populations. The following aspects of evidence-based treatments could be used as criteria for discerning effective treatment protocols from ineffective ones.

- *Engagement.* Researchers examining evidence-based treatments have demonstrated the effectiveness of family-based treatments in engaging adolescents and their families in treatment (Curtis et al., 2004; Liddle, 2016; Liddle et al., 2001, 2005; Schoenwald & Henggeler, 2005). The engagement process is also referred to as joining (Horigian et al., 2005). Engaging adolescents and their families in treatment is important to keeping them in treatment long enough for treatment to have a significant effect on the identified problems. Family-based treatments emphasize engaging the entire family, not just the adolescent with the identified problem.
- *A present- and problem-focused approach.* Evidence-based treatments emphasize the use of both present- and problem-focused approaches to therapy (Horigian et al., 2005; Schoenwald & Henggeler, 2005; Sexton & Alexander, 2005). Present-focused approaches rely on family interaction patterns that take place during and between therapy sessions for both assessment and intervention.

MDFT therapists encourage clients to talk about past hurts, but they make sure that clients talk to each other about such things rather than to the therapist in order to maintain a process focus (Liddle et al., 2005).

- *A multisystemic (ecological systems) orientation.* Most evidence-based treatments for adolescent substance abuse incorporate multisystemic interactions and how they are related in a reciprocal manner to the identified problem (Liddle et al., 2005; Schoenwald & Henggeler, 2005; Sexton & Alexander, 2005). Interventions with the systems surrounding the adolescent and family (e.g., work, school, legal system, and peers) produce changes in the systems, beyond the family, that maintain the adolescent's substance misuse.

Our recommendation for the treatment of adolescents battling with substance-related disorders is a family-based approach that encompasses all of the above criteria. MST, MDFT, and FFT all meet these criteria. BSFT includes the first two criteria listed above, but does not explicitly focus on multisystemic processes early in therapy. However, BSFT is a brief therapy option; a multisystemic orientation requires more long-term and intensive therapy. However, even with a short intervention, it might be advisable for BSFT therapists to consider multisystemic influences on the family in assessment and intervention.

A final recommendation is that clinicians should choose a therapy approach geared toward the context within which each client/family operates. MST, MDFT, and FFT have been validated with juvenile-justice populations, and are more appropriate for them. BSFT, as a brief therapy option, may be more appropriate for adolescents and families who are not or are minimally involved with the legal system due to its less intense focus on extrafamilial systems.

References

Alexander, J. F., & Parsons, B. V. (1982). *Functional family therapy: Principles and procedures.* Carmel, CA: Brooks & Cole.

Alexander, J. F., Waldron, H. B., Robbins, M. S., & Neeb, A. A. (2013). *Functional family therapy for adolescent behavior problems.* Washington, DC: American Psychological Association.

Arnett, J. (2013). *Adolescence and emerging adulthood: A cultural approach* (5th ed.). Boston, MA: Pearson.

Baldwin, S. A., Christian, S., Berkeljon, A., Shadish, W. R., & Bean, R. (2012). The effects of family therapies for adolescent delinquency and substance abuse: A meta-analysis. *Journal of Marital and Family Therapy, 38*(1), 281–304.

Bronfenbrenner, U. (1979). *The ecology of human development: Experiments by nature and design.* Cambridge, MA: Harvard University Press.

Bronfenbrenner, U. (1988). Strengthening family systems. In E. F. Zigler & M. Frank (Eds.), *The parental leave crisis: Toward a national policy* (pp. 143–160). New Haven, CT: Yale University Press.

Curtis, N. M., Ronan, K. R., & Borduin, C. M. (2004). Multisystemic treatment: A meta-analysis of outcome studies. *Journal of Family Psychology, 18*, 411–419.

Friedman, A. S. (1989). Family therapy vs. parent groups: Effects on adolescent drug abusers. *American Journal of Family Therapy, 17*(4), 335–347.

Haley, J. (1976). *Problem solving therapy*. San Francisco, CA: Jossey-Bass.
Henggeler, S. W., Borduin, C. M., Melton, G. B., Mann, B. J., Smith, L., Hall, J. A., ... Fucci, B. R. (1991). Effects of multisystemic therapy on drug use and abuse in serious juvenile offenders: A progress report from two outcome studies. *Family Dynamics of Addiction Quarterly, 1*(3), 40–51.
Henggeler, S. W., Clingempeel, W. G., Brondino, M. J., & Pickrel, S. G. (2002). Four-year follow-up of multisystemic therapy with substance-abusing and substance-dependent juvenile offenders. *Journal of the American Academy of Child and Adolescent Psychiatry, 41*(7), 868–874.
Henggeler, S. W., Halliday-Boykins, C. A., Cunningham, P. B., Randall, J., Shapiro, S. B., & Chapman, J. E. (2006). Juvenile drug court: Enhancing outcomes by integrating evidence-based treatments. *Journal of Consulting and Clinical Psychology, 74*(1), 42–54.
Henggeler, S. W., Melton, G. B., Brondino, M. J., Scherer, D. G., & Hanley, J. H. (1997). Multisystemic therapy with violent and chronic juvenile offenders and their families: The role of treatment fidelity in successful dissemination. *Journal of Consulting and Clinical Psychology, 65*(5), 821–833.
Henggeler, S. W., Melton, G. B., & Smith, L. A. (1992). Family preservation using multisystemic therapy: An effective alternative to incarcerating serious juvenile offenders. *Journal of Consulting and Clinical Psychology, 60*(6), 953–961.
Henggeler, S. W., Pickrel, S. G., & Brondino, M. J. (1999). Multisystemic treatment of substance-abusing and dependent delinquents: Outcomes, treatment fidelity, and transportability. *Mental Health Services Research, 1*(3), 171–184.
Henggeler, S. W., Schoenwald, S. K., Borduin, C. M., Rowland, M. D., & Cunningham, P. B. (2009). *Multisystemic treatment of antisocial behavior in children and adolescents* (2nd ed.). New York, NY: Guilford Press.
Horigian, V. E., Suarez-Morales, L., Robbins, M. S., Zarate, M., Mayorga, C. C., Mitrani, V. B., & Szapocznik, J. (2005). Brief strategic family therapy for adolescents with behavior problems. In J. L. Lebow (Ed.), *Handbook of clinical family therapy* (pp. 73–102). Hoboken, NJ: Wiley.
Johnston, L. D., O'Malley, P. M., Miech, R. A., Bachman, J. G., & Schulenberg, J. E. (2017). *Monitoring the future national survey results on drug use, 1975–2016: Overview, key findings on adolescent drug use*. Ann Arbor, MI: Institute for Social Research, The University of Michigan.
Liddle, H. A. (2002). *Multidimensional family therapy for adolescent cannabis users, Cannibis Youth Treatment (CYT) Series, Volume 5*. Rockville, MD: Center for Substance Abuse Treatment, Substance Abuse and Mental Health Services Administration.
Liddle, H. A. (2004). Family-based therapies for adolescent alcohol and drug use: Research contributions and future research needs. *Addiction, 99*(2), 76–92.
Liddle, H. A. (2016). Multidimensional family therapy. In T. Sexton & J. Lebow (Eds.), *Handbook of family therapy* (pp. 231–249). New York, NY: Routledge.
Liddle, H. A., & Dakof, G. A. (1995). Efficacy of family therapy for drug abuse: Promising but not definitive. *Journal of Marital and Family Therapy, 21*(4), 511–543.
Liddle, H. A., Dakof, G. A., Parker, K., Diamond, G. S., Barrett, K., & Tejeda, M. (2001). Multidimensional family therapy for adolescent drug abuse: Results of a randomized clinical trial. *The American Journal of Drug and Alcohol Abuse, 27*(4), 651–688.
Liddle, H. A., Rodriguez, R. A., Dakof, G. A., Kanzki, E., & Marvel, F. A. (2005). Multidimensional family therapy: A science-based treatment for adolescent drug abuse. In J. L. Lebow (Ed.), *Handbook of clinical family therapy* (pp. 128–163). Hoboken, NJ: Wiley.
Liddle, H. A., Rowe, C. L., Dakof, G. A., Ungaro, R. A., & Henderson, C. (2004). Early intervention for adolescent substance abuse: Pretreatment to posttreatment outcomes of a randomized controlled trial comparing multidimensional family therapy and peer group treatment. *Journal of Psychoactive Drugs, 36*(1), 2–37.
Micucci, J. A. (1998). *The adolescent in family therapy: Breaking the cycle of conflict and control*. New York, NY: Guilford Press.
Minuchin, S. (1974). *Families and family therapy*. Cambridge, MA: Harvard University Press.

Repetti, R. L., Taylor, S. E., & Seeman, T. E. (2002). Risky families: Family social environments and the mental and physical health of offspring. *Psychological Bulletin, 128*(2), 330–366.
Robbins, M. S., Feaster, D. J., Horigian, V. E., Rohrbaugh, M., Shoham, V., Bachrach, K., … Vandermark, N. (2011). Brief strategic family therapy versus treatment as usual: Results of a multisite randomized trial for substance using adolescents. *Journal of Consulting and Clinical Psychology, 79*(6), 713–727.
Rohde, P., Lewinsohn, P. M., Seeley, J. R., Klein, D. N., Andrews, J. A., & Small, J. W. (2007). Psychosocial functioning of adults who experienced substance use disorders as adolescents. *Psychology of Addictive Behaviors, 21*(2), 155–164.
Santisteban, D. A., Coatsworth, J. D., Perez-Vidal, A., Kurtines, W. M., Schwartz, S. J., LaPerriere, A., & Szapocznik, J. (2003). Efficacy of brief strategic family therapy in modifying Hispanic adolescent behavior problems and substance use. *Journal of Family Psychology, 17*(1), 121–133.
Schaeffer, C. M., & Borduin, C. M. (2005). Long-term follow-up to a randomized clinical trial of multisystemic therapy with serious and violent juvenile offenders. *Journal of Consulting and Clinical Psychology, 73*(3), 445–453.
Schoenwald, S. K., & Henggeler, S. W. (2005). Multisystemic therapy for adolescents with serious externalizing problems. In J. L. Lebow (Ed.), *Handbook of clinical family therapy* (pp. 103–127). Hoboken, NJ: Wiley.
Sexton, T. L., & Alexander, J. F. (2005). Functional family therapy for externalizing disorders in adolescents. In J. L. Lebow (Ed.), *Handbook of clinical family therapy* (pp. 164–191). Hoboken, NJ: Wiley.
Slesnick, N., & Prestopnik, J. L. (2009). Comparison of family therapy outcome with alcohol-abusing, runaway adolescents. *Journal of Marital and Family Therapy, 35*(3), 255–277.
Substance Abuse and Mental Health Services Administration. (2013). *National survey on drug use and health: Summary of national findings*. Retrieved from www.drugabusestatistics.samhsa.gov.
Swenson, C. C., Henggeler, S. W., Taylor, I. S., & Addison, O. W. (2005). *Multisystemic therapy and neighborhood partnerships: Reducing adolescent violence and substance abuse*. New York, NY: Guilford.
Szapocznik, J., Hervis, O. E., & Schwartz, S. (2003). *Brief strategic family therapy for adolescent drug abuse (NIDA Therapy Manuals for Drug Addiction Series)*. Rockville, MD: NIDA.
Szapocznik, J., Kurtines, W. M., Foote, F., Perez-Vidal, A., & Hervis, O. (1986). Conjoint versus one-person family therapy: Further evidence for the effectiveness of conducting family therapy through one person. *Journal of Consulting and Clinical Psychology, 54*(3), 395–397.
Szapocznik, J., Perez-Vidal, A., Brickman, A. L., Foote, F. H., Santisteban, D., Hervis, O., & Kurtines, W. M. (1988). Engaging adolescent drug abusers and their families in treatment: A strategic structural systems approach. *Journal of Consulting and Clinical Psychology, 56*(4), 552–557.
Tanner-Smith, E. E., Wilson, S. J., & Lipsey, M. W. (2013). The comparative effectiveness of outpatient treatment for adolescent substance abuse: A meta-analysis. *Journal of Substance Abuse Treatment, 44*(2), 145–158.
Waldron, H. (1997). Adolescent substance abuse and family therapy outcome: A review of randomized trials. In T. H. Ollendick & R. J. Prinz (Eds.), *Advances in clinical child psychology* (Vol. 19, pp. 199–234). New York, NY: Plenum Press.
Waldron, H. B., Slesnick, N., Brody, J. L., Turner, C. W., & Peterson, T. R. (2001). Treatment outcomes for adolescent substance abuse at 4- and 7-month assessments. *Journal of Consulting and Clinical Psychology, 69*(5), 802–813.
Weidman, A. A. (1987). Substance-abusing adolescents in family therapy. *International Journal of Family Psychiatry, 8*(3), 211–219.
Worden, M. (2003). *Family therapy basics* (3rd ed.). Toronto, ON: Brooks-Cole.

Residential Treatment of Adolescents with Substance Use Disorders: Evidence-Based Approaches and Best Practice Recommendations

Emily K. Lichvar, Sally Stilwell, Tanvi Ajmera, Andrea L. Alexander, Robert W. Plant, Peter Panzarella, and Gary M. Blau

Introduction

The rate of alcohol and drug abuse among adolescents and the number of youth at risk for the development of substance use disorders later in life remain a serious, national health concern. Intervention and prevention in adolescence is particularly, indicated considering that most long-term patterns of abuse and dependence originate in youth or young adulthood. Although most of the early efforts to address adolescent substance abuse utilized adult treatment models, more recent efforts have been based on research with adolescent populations and are informed by theories and knowledge of adolescent development. Recently, the National Institute of Drug Abuse (2014) put forth recommendations for adolescent substance abuse

---

The content of this publication does not necessarily reflect the views, opinions, or policies of the Center for Mental Health Services (CMHS), the Substance Abuse and Mental Health Services Administration (SAMHSA), or the Department of Health and Human Services (DHHS).

E. K. Lichvar (✉) · T. Ajmera · A. L. Alexander
Child, Adolescent & Family Branch, Center for Mental Health Services,
Substance Abuse and Mental Health Services Administration, Rockville, MD, USA
e-mail: emily.lichvar@samhsa.hhs.gov; Tanvi.Ajmera@samhsa.hhs.gov; Andrea.Alexander@samhsa.hhs.gov

S. Stilwell
Jacksonville, FL, USA

R. W. Plant
Middlefield, CT, USA

P. Panzarella
North Franklin, CT, USA

G. M. Blau
SAMHSA, MD, USA
e-mail: gary.blau@samhsa.hhs.gov

C. G. Leukefeld, T. P. Gullotta (eds.), *Adolescent Substance Abuse*, Issues in Children's and Families' Lives, https://doi.org/10.1007/978-3-319-90611-9_7

treatment in a research-based guide that highlighted best practice principles. Residential care of adolescents with substance abuse disorders represents one level of care in the continuum of treatment approaches. A residential treatment center has been defined as a 24-h facility designed for the treatment of mental health disorders (including substance abuse) that is not licensed or designated as a hospital (Connor, Miller, Cunningham, & Melloni, 2002). Leichtman (2006) and, others note that there is no consensus on the defining characteristics of residential treatment and that there is tremendous heterogeneity among programs. This makes the measurement of effectiveness extremely difficult. Although many programs have incorporated group, family and individual therapies, the essence of residential treatment has often resided in the concept of the "milieu," an elusive concept that is not well articulated. One often cited core aspect of the therapeutic milieu is that the most powerful therapeutic intervention is the moment-to-moment, and day-to-day interactions between direct care staff and program participants. The purpose and intent of those interactions and the methods used to structure them are at the core of residential care.

Residential substance abuse treatment for adolescents has continued to lack adequate research regarding its practices and outcomes. However, it should be noted that separately there are best practices, principles and strategies in both residential treatment and in adolescent substance abuse treatment. In this chapter both are summarized for the best possible care.

Residential Treatment

It should be understood that residential treatment is a highly complex treatment intervention that encompasses all of the rules, therapies, staff interactions, structures, philosophies, etc. involved in 24-h care, 7 days a week, typically lasting 6 months or longer. Beyond this general and overarching definition of residential, there are no specific models of adolescent substance abuse residential treatment have been sufficiently articulated and/or investigated. Programs are characterized by a high degree of variability and heterogeneity. There has been controversy regarding whether or not residential treatment is effective, in general, or in the treatment of adolescent substance abuse, in particular.

The use of residential treatment for adolescents with behavioral, psychiatric, and substance use disorders had been growing steadily since the early 1900s, and according to Leichtman had "assumed a prominent place among mental health services for children" (Leichtman, 2006, p. 285). Connor et al. (2002) reported that the number of youth receiving this form of treatment grew steadily between 1982 (29,000 youth) and 1997 (117,720 youth). However, "by the 1990s, residential treatment had lost much of its luster" (Leichtman, 2006, p. 286).

In response to system of care and other community mental health movements, residential care underwent significant scrutiny and was found lacking due to the practice of separating children from their parents, little to no involvement of family in treatment, poor aftercare planning, and a general failure to maintain treatment gains in the community post discharge. In a special issue of the *American Journal of Orthopsychiatry*, Pumariega (2006a) concluded that there is limited evidence for the effectiveness of residential treatment.

A major review of evidence-based treatments (Hoagwood, Burns, Kiser, Ringeisen, & Schoenwald, 2001) concluded that residential treatment for children and adolescents is a widely used but empirically unjustified service, and that any gains made during treatment are seldom maintained once the adolescent returns to the community. A further concern regarding residential treatment is the potential iatrogenic effects of placing youth with substance abuse problems in settings that may be dominated by a deviant peer culture where drug use is glorified and antisocial behavior encouraged. This issue is a particular concern in the case of placing "light" users in the same program with "heavier" users. In light of these challenges, the clinical management and composition of the group experiences that form the core of the milieu take on added importance (Kaminer, Blitz, Burleson, Kadden, & Rounsaville, 1998).

On the other side of the debate regarding the effectiveness of residential care, Lyons and McCulloch (2006, p. 251) warn that "it is important that residential treatment not be dismissed as an ineffective intervention because of the barriers that its complexity poses for conducting randomized clinical trials." In a position statement on residential care, the Child Welfare League of America (Child Welfare League of America (CWLA), 2005) maintains that residential treatment is an important component in the continuum of care and cites several studies of effectiveness while acknowledging the limitation of much of the research in the field.

In response to the issues identified in research specific to outcomes for youth in residential treatment centers there are now best practice solutions that engage youth, families, providers, and communities in a collaborative process that improves treatment outcomes for youth. One of these best practice solutions is the Building Bridges Initiative (BBI). BBI was created as a way to better engage residential interventions and their community counterparts, along with youth and families, and has created tip sheets, monographs, and other materials and resources to help improve practices. More information about BBI can be found at: www.buildingbridges4youth.org.

BBI's strategies incorporate and address (a) the negative concerns found in the research, such as high recidivism, use of seclusion and restraint, and long lengths of stay; (b) the positive practices known to improve outcomes for youth in residential treatment which include shorter lengths of stay, increased family and community involvement, and stability and support in the post residential environment, and (c) the administrative, fiscal, treatment, and policy realities of residential treatment providers who implement BBI in the community (Walter & Petr, 2008).

The key BBI strategies are as follows:

1. Establish relationships and dialogue across all constituent groups, including families, youth, community-based and residentially based treatment and service providers, advocates, and policy makers.
2. Identify and promote best practices and innovative solutions.
3. Identify and propose recommendations to overcome fiscal, licensing, regulatory, and practice barriers.
4. Identify needed technical assistance, training, and support for providers, policy makers, families, and youth.

5. Identify or develop measures that provide information and feedback about system efforts to coordinate and integrate services and supports, and to implement the values and principles described in the Building Bridges Joint Resolution.
6. Develop and implement dissemination and marketing strategies to communicate the critical importance of creating a coordinated and comprehensive array of community-based and residential treatment services and supports that are family-driven, youth-guided, strength-based, culturally and linguistically competent, and focused on sustained positive outcomes.

Another best practice solution is the Six Core Strategies for Reducing Seclusion and Restraint Use. Disseminated by the National Association of State Mental Health Program Directors (NASMHPD), these strategies were developed through extensive literature reviews and input from experts who have successfully reduced the use of S/R in a variety of mental health settings for children and adults across the USA and internationally (NASMHPD, 2008). In addition to developing strategies, NASMHPD also provides a planning guide and tool, and examples of policies to support the cultural change necessary throughout the facility. The strategies are:

1. Consistent, Continuous and Engaged Leadership to Guide Organizational Change
2. Use Data to Inform Practice Throughout the Facility
3. Create a Treatment Environment through Workforce Development
4. Reducing the Use of Seclusion and Restraint Prevention Tools
5. Inclusion of Consumer Roles in Inpatient Settings
6. Debriefing Techniques for every Seclusion Restraint Event

Recently, there has been pressure on the residential field to provide data on outcomes associated care. Assembled in 2014, the BBI Outcomes Workgroup, was brought together to develop and implement guidelines and practices to promote self-assessment among residential treatment and service providers. In 2015, the Outcomes Workgroup, together with Chapin Hall and other national partners, articulated that long-term outcomes for young people should be researched across four functional domains: Home, Purpose, Community, and Health. These domains provide a framework for measuring long-term well-being, and a benchmark to achieve comprehensive, coordinated care for youth and families. Further, the Outcomes Workgroup, conducted a feasibility pilot aimed to test methods for collecting functional outcomes data among youth 6 months post discharge from residential care; to identify barriers to data collection; and to test the feasibility of provider-based data management, case identification, and data collection. The results are in press but the major take away is that collecting outcome data is feasible post discharge. This data is needed to understand the long term impact of residential care (Blau, Caldwell, & Lieberman, 2014).

Finally, the accreditation processes for residential facilities for youth provide standards of care with which a facility must be compliant in order to attain and sustain accreditation. The Joint Commission on Accreditation of Hospital Facilities (JCAHO: https://www.jointcommission.org/) and the Commission on Accreditation of Rehabilitation Facilities (CARF: https://www.carf.org) both have standards for residential facilities that serve the adolescent population, as well as other healthcare facilities. As the funders and payors of adolescent and substance abuse services require accreditation for licensing, those standards support and even require the utilization of BBI and 6-core strategies or other improvement processes for care and treatment outcomes for our youth and their families.

Substance Abuse

In general, most adolescents receiving residential substance abuse treatment (RSAT) show reduction in use and associated problems in the year following treatment (Williams & Chang, 2000). According to Sealock, Gottfredson, and Gallagher (1997), substance abusing youthful offenders randomly assigned to residential vs outpatient treatment reported decreased drug use and delinquent behavior and exhibited a longer time till rearrest. Leichtman, Leichtman, Barber, and Neese (2001), reported that intensive, short-term residential treatment can be an effective treatment intervention with adolescents when it includes family therapy, connection to community activities, and effective discharge planning. A meta-analysis of adjudicated, adolescents in residential treatment reviewed 111 studies (Garrett, 1985) and reported that recidivism was modestly improved as were adjustments in the institution, academic performance, and psychological adjustment. The authors concluded that residential treatment does "work." Frensch and Cameron (2002) conducted a review of studies of adolescent residential treatment centers. They determined that despite the lack of a uniform treatment approach and numerous methodological limitations, some youth appear to show improvement in functioning, although that improvement tends to dissipate post discharge. Hooper and colleagues (Hooper, Murphy, Devaney, & Hultman, 2000) reported that 60% of youth receiving residential care demonstrated successful outcomes and that long-term treatments that incorporated home and school components were most successful. In a review of 18 outcomes studies conducted, between 1993 and 2000, Hair (2005) concluded that residential treatment is beneficial in both the short-term and the long-term. Finally, researchers in Washington State evaluated the economic costs and benefits of adolescent RSAT (French, Salome, & Carney, 2002) and found that the benefits outweighed the costs by a factor of 4.34 to 1 for a net cost-savings of $16,418 per treatment episode.

Taking into account the preceding review, a reasonable adolescent, parent, provider, or policy maker might conclude that some but not all adolescents are likely to show, some level of improvement following a period of residential treatment. However, to justify the costs, removal from the community, and disruption of family life associated with residential care, the need for evidence that residential care is superior to other forms of less intrusive treatment, even if only for a specific subpopulation of adolescents that use drugs and alcohol. The American Academy of Child and Adolescent Psychiatry (2005) practice parameter on adolescent substance abuse treatment recommends that treatment should always occur in the least restrictive environment and residential treatment should be recommended only when previous treatment efforts have failed, when there is a need for additional structure and supervision that cannot be provided in a less restrictive setting, or when there are specific goals of treatment that cannot be accomplished in community-based settings.

Given the paucity of randomized clinical trials of well-defined and adequately articulated residential models for the treatment of adolescents with drug and alcohol problems, this chapter focuses on the features of successful residential programs and the integration of evidence-based treatment approaches into the residential milieu.

Prevalence, Need for Treatment, and Population Parameters

The Prevalence of Alcohol Use

Alcohol use among adolescents has declined. According to the Monitoring the Future national survey results, 1975–2016, all alcohol measures, including lifetime, annual, and binge drinking prevalence, were at a historic low for 8th, 10th, and 12th graders. Lifetime alcohol prevalence in teenagers has declined, with the rate of teens reporting they have "been drunk" in the past year at the survey's lowest rates ever. 37.3% of 12th graders reported they have been drunk at least once, down from a peak of 53.2% in 2001. In 2016, the proportions of 8th, 10th, and 12th graders who reported drinking an alcoholic beverage in the 30-day period prior to the survey were 7%, 20%, and 33%, respectively (Johnston, O'Malley, Miech, Bachman, & Schulenberg, 2017).

Alcohol use steadily rises until age 30, with use higher in young adults compared to high school age, and age 30 being the peak at 76%, compared to 33% among 18 year olds. These increases are interpreted to be due to age-related life events such as leaving the parental home and attending college. Binge drinking follows a similar trend, with an occurrence in the past two weeks of 16% at age 18, 23% between ages 19 and 20, and reaching a peak at ages 21–22 at 38%, then slowly decreasing with age (Schulenberg et al., 2017).

The Prevalence of Marijuana Use

Like alcohol, there has also been no increase in marijuana use among adolescents. In fact, marijuana use has remained stable since 2011. Among 12th graders, use increased from 2006 to 2011 and then has held level through 2016. Daily use has increased in 8th, 10th, and 12th grades after 2007, reaching peaks in 2011. Daily prevalence rates in 2016 were 0.7% for 8th graders, 2.5% for 10th graders, and 6.0% for 12th graders, respectively, with one in seventeen 12th graders smoking daily.

Recent research indicates that marijuana use among adolescents may be related to the laws permitting use by state. According to Monitoring the Future national survey results, 1975–2016, there is a higher rate of marijuana use among 12th graders in states with medical marijuana laws, compared to states without them. For example, in 2016, 38.3% of high school seniors in states with medical marijuana laws reported past year marijuana use, compared to 33.3% in nonmedical marijuana states (Johnston et al., 2017).

Over the past 5 years, states have legalized marijuana for medicinal use, recreational use, or decriminalized possession of the drug. States with recreational legalization of marijuana include—Nevada, Colorado, Washington, Oregon, Alaska, California, Maine and Massachusetts. States with medicinal legalization of marijuana include—Arkansas, Florida, North Dakota, Minnesota, Montana, Michigan, Ohio, Pennsylvania, New York, Illinois, Arizona, New Mexico, Hawaii, New Jersey, Delaware, Maryland, District of Columbia, Vermont, Connecticut, and New Hampshire (Governing the States and Localities, 2017). At the federal level marijuana is still considered an illicit substance and is classified as *Schedule I* under the Controlled Substance Act.

Perceived risk associated with use has continued a steep decline since the mid-2000s without a concomitant further rise in overall use. Disapproval and availability may be constraining factors offsetting the effects of risk. Recent, sharp declines in the use of "gateway drugs"—in particular cigarette smoking, with which marijuana use has been highly correlated— may also be playing a role. In terms of access to marijuana, 81% of 12th graders state they can get marijuana easily if they wanted to (Johnston et al., 2017).

Although marijuana laws pertaining to this drug are changing, as with any mind altering substance, marijuana use should be taken into account and targeted adolescents entering treatment.

In general, adolescent use of illicit drugs has gradually declined over the past 20 years. There have been some slight increases in use of substances in different adolescent age groups at random between 2007 and 2011, including use of amphetamines, MDMA, and narcotics other than heroin. However, rates of use have continued to slowly decline in a broad spectrum of substances in general since the 1990s (Miech et al., 2017).

Need for Treatment

According to the 2015 Behavioral Health Barometer, 5.1% of adolescents needed substance use treatment in 2014, yet only 6.3% received treatment; or 80,000 out of 1.3 million adolescents. Between 2005 and 2015, marijuana and alcohol represented the most common drugs targeted for treatment in adolescent substance abuse programs accounting for 83% and 87% of all adolescent substance abuse treatment episodes, including outpatient, partial hospitalization, and residential treatment types (SAMHSA, 2015a).

An increase in treatment admissions for opioids was recorded over this time span as well, with opioid use representing 2% of admissions between 2005 and 2008 but increasing to 3–4% of admissions between 2009 and 2015. For those adolescents reporting treatment in the past year, 10–12% reported that they received treatment in a residential facility, 1–2% received treatment in an inpatient hospital facility, and 87–89% received treatment in an outpatient setting. The 2015 National Survey of Substance Abuse Treatment Facilities found that in 2015, there were 729,771 clients under the age of 18 in substance abuse treatment, making up 6–8% of the substance abuse treatment population. 75% of those under 18 were in specialty programs designed just for adolescents, a 26% decrease from 2005 (SAMHSA, 2015b). The age of first use is an important factor in adolescent admissions. The average age of first use of lower level substances, such as alcohol, is 13.2 years, and 15.2 years for higher level substances, such as cocaine (Bracken, Rodolico, & Hill, 2013).

Another cause for concern is the heroin specific deaths which have tripled between 2010 and 2015 (12,989 heroin related deaths in 2015) (Rudd, Seth, David, & Scholl, 2016). The largest increase in overdose deaths in that same year was for those involving synthetic opioids (other than methadone)—5544 deaths in 2014 to 9580 deaths in 2015. Fentanyl (an illegal synthetic opioid) drove this increase. According to findings by CDC, from 2002–2013, use of heroin (both in terms of the past month and past year), as well as dependence defined by the DSM-IV criteria, all increased among young adults ages 18–25.

In light of this, the US Department of Health and Human Services is spearheading an interagency collaboration to maximize the effect of programs related to the Comprehensive Addiction and Recovery Act (CARA) and twenty-first Century Cures Act (Cures Act). Additionally, the President's Commission on Combating Drug Addiction and the Opioid Crisis was created to provide guidance to the nation for an emergency response plan starting in December of 2016.

Population Parameters

Co-occurrence of substance use problems and psychiatric disorders occurs in adolescents more often than not. Common co-occurring disorders in adolescents with a substance use disorder include conduct disorder, ADHD, trauma-related disorders, and mood disorders. Recent findings show that 29% of adolescent males and 49% of adolescent females had both a mood disorder and substance use disorder. Co-occurring disorders are also associated with more severe substance use disorder symptoms and less treatment success (Hulvershorn, Quinn, & Scott, 2015). Subramanian, Stitzer, Clemmey, Kolodner, and Fishman (2007) found that over 50% of adolescents in RSAT had clinically elevated scores on the Beck Depression Inventory and the presence of depression at intake was associated with increased post discharge substance use. The data also shows that depression, victimization, and other mental health conditions are related to an earlier age of initiation and increased consequences of use at an early age. Adolescents with a major depressive episode in the past year were twice as likely to use alcohol and other drugs. Early intervention with depressed adolescents may reduce the onset of substance abuse.

Another study by Chan, Dennis, and Funk (2008) showed that two thirds of adolescents and young adults had a co-occurring mental health problem in the year prior to treatment admission for substance use. Further, adolescents' and young adults' self-reporting criteria for past-year substance use disorder were more likely than those who did not report to have other co-occurring mental health problems. Young adults (ages 18–25) were found to be most vulnerable to co-occurring problems. Considering the high prevalence and cost (e.g., increased risk of serious medical and legal problems, incarceration, suicide, school difficulties and dropout, unemployment, and poor interpersonal relationships) of untreated co-occurring disorders, RSAT must consider targeting both issues for intervention (Hawkins, 2009), especially as problems may worsen into young adulthood.

Youth with lower SES were also more likely to have a comorbid disorder. Although high rates of dual diagnosis among adolescents with substance abuse problems are well documented, most children are placed in residential settings without consideration given to matching the adolescent's individual treatment needs with the particular expertise and service package of the treatment program (Weiner, Abraham, & Lyons, 2001). Boys and girls with dual diagnoses were more likely to have problems with suicidality, development, and delinquency. Those who have co-occurring mental health and psychiatric disturbance, early onset delinquency and conduct disorder or a history of abuse have poorer outcomes. It has been noted that the most vulnerable children who are most often referred to residential care may be the least suited to benefit from it (Connor et al., 2002).

Commenting on the rate and variability of relapse, Tomlinson, Brown, and Abrantes (Tomlinson, Brown, & Abrantes, 2004, p. 168) noted that "heterogeneity within substance abusing samples including co-morbid psychopathology may account for a portion of the variability in relapse rates." Those adolescents with comorbid psychiatric conditions returned to substance use more quickly and at a higher rate following discharge from short-term RSAT. In addition to comorbid psychiatric conditions, youth receiving treatment in residential substance abuse programs are very likely to have experienced trauma in their lives and to demonstrate symptomatic responses to traumatic exposure. In one study, 71% of residential program participants reported lifetime exposure to trauma, and 29% met criteria for PTSD. Trauma-exposed adolescents reported more behavioral problems and were more likely to leave treatment sooner (Jaycox, Ebener, Damesek, & Becker, 2004).

Gender differences in overall substance use are present within the adolescent population, with males having somewhat higher rates in overall illicit drug use. However, specific drugs of choice show varying differences, with females having higher misuse rates of prescription drugs such as amphetamines, tranquilizers, and sedatives. Race and ethnicity differences are also present within this population. Hispanic adolescents currently have the highest rates of substance use in the past few years, mainly due to their increase in use of marijuana. Yet, they also have higher reported use rates in almost every class of drug, except for prescription drugs, in which White adolescents have the highest rates of misuse. African-American adolescents have usually had lower rates of overall illicit drug use than Hispanic and

White adolescents, but the gap is narrowing more with recent increases in marijuana over the past couple of years (Johnston et al., 2017).

While ethnic disparities in healthcare methods and outcomes are common in general medical practice as well as specialty treatments, the findings here are similarly troubling and suggest that criteria regarding what constitutes "least restrictive care" may be unevenly applied. In an investigation of the role of client factors in treatment retention, Edelen et al. (2007) reported that positive self-attitude, problem recognition, and having a strong social network predicted retention in care for 90 days or more. Remaining in care for 90 days or more is a known predictor of better outcome post discharge.

Youth who do better in residential care also include those with better overall functioning and academic ability, lower rates of conduct problems, and the involvement of a child's family in treatment (Connor et al., 2002). Other client factors often related to successful outcome include completing treatment, low pretreatment use of substances, peer and parent social support, and nonuse of substances by the youth's familial and social network (Williams & Chang, 2000). Researchers have found that laboratory measures of distress tolerance (e.g., cold pressor tests and stressful cognitive challenges as measures of an individual's general ability to tolerate distress) can predict early dropout from adolescent residential treatment (Daughters et al., 2005). The study authors suggest that efforts be taken to improve distress tolerance of children and youth in residential care given the significance of dropout in this level of care.

Theoretical Background and Principal Interventions

Recent research has highlighted trends and successes in adolescent substance abuse treatment across settings. Trends in clinical approaches include identifying the youth's strengths and building upon them, teaching skills to resist triggers specific to the individual and their drug use pattern, and address contributing factors to the onset or continuation of drug use, such as mental illness, trauma, and negative family or peer relationships. Treatment centers also are usually using an eclectic intervention model, using traditionally single approaches in a combined manner. Treatment centers are treating adolescents in mostly outpatient settings, with the most progress using family-based approaches and motivational enhancement techniques. Overall, the results are positive with decreases being seen in adolescent substance use following treatment.

Despite these findings, studies have also highlighted areas of need and found that there is a multitude of short-comings in current interventions. This includes the lack of specialized, developmentally focused treatment options as well as inconsistency in the overall quality of treatment and too short of durations of treatment. These findings also come from the acknowledgement of the difference in needs of adults and adolescents in treatment. One of these areas of difference is in treatment need motivation; motivational enhancement techniques should be utilized on the front end of all treatment to increase treatment motivation and the belief that drug use is not a problem.

The majority of adolescent substance abuse treatment should and does occur in outpatient settings, but severe dependence should be addressed in longer, more intensive treatment settings such as residential. During or after treatment in these settings, lapses and relapses should be considered the norm and continuity of care should be utilized. Because of these factors, including things such as self-help programs, recovery high schools, alternative peer groups, and the adolescent community reinforcement approach (A-CRA) have proven beneficial (Winters, Tanner-Smith, Bresani, & Meyers, 2014).

In the minimal research that has been conducted in residential settings, there are a few primary approaches to residential treatment for adolescent substance use. They include the Minnesota Model (12, steps), Multidisciplinary Team Model, The Seven Challenges, and the Therapeutic Community (TC).

The Minnesota Model, also known as 12 Steps, is based on Alcoholics Anonymous (AA) and Narcotics Anonymous (NA). This model is widely used in adolescent substance use treatment and views addiction as a disease that is consistently treated throughout one's life with abstinence as the goal (Muck et al., 2001). The Minnesota Model includes elements of social support, relationship to a "higher power," motivation for change, and the importance of lifestyle. 12-Step approaches have been adapted for adolescents and have been shown to have some, effectiveness (Winters, Stinchfield, Opland, Weller, & Latimer, 2000). The limited availability of adolescent 12-step groups in community settings has been identified as a limitation of this approach, but adolescents participation in adult 12-step groups have been shown to lead to positive outcomes (Brown, Myers, Abrantes, & Kahler, 2008). The social networking opportunities afforded by, the Internet could be helpful in connecting youth with 12-step groups and like-minded peers interested in recovery. Application of the 12 steps is a common element of most adolescent residential treatment programs.

The Minnesota Model is an effective model of treatment resulting in decreased use of substances post treatment, particularly for those who completed treatment (Winters et al., 2000). Fishman, Clemmey, and Hoover (2003) describe the treatment approach of the Mountain Manor Treatment Center, an exemplary model of adolescent substance abuse treatment. They report positive results with an eclectic milieu therapy approach that incorporates elements of the 12 steps, as well as TC, motivational enhancement therapy (MET), and multisystemic approaches.

The Multidisciplinary Team Model includes a variety of professionals, often led by a physician, who provide a range of treatment modalities across several primary domains: substance use/abuse, education/vocation, social/leisure, medical, family, and legal. While this approach has been widely utilized in residential treatment programs and in many evidence-based treatments for substance abuse, the approach itself has not been well defined, is often combined with other approaches, and there is scant quality treatment outcome research supporting its effectiveness.

The Seven Challenges is a relatively new approach to treatment of adolescent, substance abuse that originated in the field and has received recent research, attention. The Seven Challenges incorporates knowledge of adolescent development (Schwebel, 2004). The program has been found to be effective in multiple, treatment settings (e.g., outpatient and residential or milieu-based settings) and, is considered a promising practice (Dennis & Kaminer, 2006). The model is a relationship-based approach that incorporates aspects of motivational enhancement therapy, cognitive behavioral approaches, and health decision making focusing on the adolescent's particular need for autonomy, self-determination, and choice. Seven Challenges meets adolescents at the stage of treatment they are at, even if it is a stage of complete denial. The model then goes through seven steps, or as noted "challenges" which address the client's use in a multitude of manners; including the manner of their use, the issues it caused, the reasons behind the use, the future with being sober, and how to address any relapses (The Seven Challenges, 2017).

The TC is a well-established model of residential treatment for adults that has been adapted for the treatment of adolescents, and is regarded as the best known residential treatment model (University of Georgia, 2008). The TC approach views addiction holistically, as the external behavioral expression of a complex combination of personal and developmental problems. Adaptations of the approach for an adolescent population include "increased emphasis on recreation, a less confrontational stance than is found in adult programs, more supervision and evaluation by staff members, assessment of psychological disorders, a greater role for family members in treatment, and more frequent use of psychotropic medication for emotional disorders" (Morral, Jaycox, Smith, Becker, & Ebener, 2003, p. 215). Residential treatment utilizing this model calls for 6–12 planned months of stay (University of Georgia, 2008). An evaluation without random assignment showed that the Phoenix Academy TC approach was superior to matched controls receiving treatment as usual on measures of substance use and psychological adjustment (Morral, McCaffery, & Ridgeway, 2004). TC has been found to be an effective treatment for substance use disorders, but still is lacking a high amount of randomized controlled trials to be fully understood as an evidence-based practice (De Leon, 2010).

Interventions That Work—Features of Successful Programs

Although there is tremendous variation in the approach taken to the residential treatment of adolescent substance abuse, researchers have begun to identify common key elements and features most often related to positive outcomes. Kaminer (1994, p. 208) listed the common elements of adolescent alcohol and drug treatment programs including "individual counseling, individual therapy, self-help groups, substance abuse education, random urinalysis for psychoactive substances, breathalyzer testing, family therapy or involvement or both, relapse prevention techniques, educational or vocational counseling, legal assistance, various types of group activities or therapies, contingency contracting, medications, and pencil-and-paper assignments relating to the recovery process."

Research has consistently demonstrated a positive association between longer duration of residential treatment and positive posttreatment outcome (Latimer, Newcomb, Winters, & Stinchfield, 2000), although short length of treatment is often confounded with premature treatment termination. In one evaluation of residential treatment,

treatment completers were 3–4 times more likely to show improvement than were noncompleters (Winters et al., 2000). In an investigation of the role of client factors in treatment retention, Edelen et al. (2007) reported that positive self-attitude, problem recognition, and having a strong social network predicted retention in care for 90 days or more (a known predictor of better outcome post discharge). Hair's summary of the treatment literature emphasizes the need for programs to be "multimodal, holistic, and ecological" in order to achieve maximum effectiveness (Hair, 2005, p. 551). Family involvement has consistently been cited as a key factor in achieving positive outcomes and post treatment maintenance of gains (Frensch & Cameron, 2002).

Despite significant evidence that family contact and involvement in treatment are positively associated with improved response to treatment, a survey of parents with children in residential care found that most programs restrict parent–child contact during initial adjustment periods to care, and treat contact as a privilege that must be earned through point or level systems (Robinson, Kruzich, Friesen, Jivanjee, & Pullman, 2005). The authors argue that policy, licensing, and accreditation standards should be written to support the value and need for early, frequent, and meaningful contact with family during residential care.

In a survey evaluation of 144 highly regarded adolescent substance abuse treatment programs (Brannigan, Schackman, Falco, & Millman, 2004), a panel of 22 experts identified 9 key elements of effective treatment programs. The nine features they identified included (1) proper assessment and treatment matching, (2) a comprehensive integrated treatment approach, (3) family involvement in treatment, (4) a developmentally appropriate approach, (5) engagement and retention in treatment, (6) employing qualified staff, (7) providing gender-specific and culturally competent care, (8) continuity of care, and (9) assessment of treatment outcome.

Interventions That Might Work—Application of Evidence-Based Practices in Residential Settings

Given the inherent complexity and heterogeneity of residential treatment, efforts have been made to incorporate and/or integrate those evidence-based practices that have shown success in adolescent substance use treatment in general. The National Institute on Drug Abuse (NIDA) has identified several specific treatment models that are evidence-based for adolescent substance abuse treatment. These include, cognitive behavioral therapy (CBT) and CBT-based approaches, motivational enhancement therapy (MET), adolescent community reinforcement approach (ACRA), contingency management (CM), multi-systemic therapy (MST), brief strategic family therapy (BSFT), family behavior therapy (FBT), functional family therapy (FFT), and multidimensional family therapy (MDFT) (National Institute on Drug Abuse, 2014). In addition to these interventions, group therapy and psychoeducational sessions are consistently used in a variety of treatment settings with adolescents (University of Georgia, 2008). While these treatments are considered evidence based, since they are not empirically supported by research in residential settings we have put them under this "might work" section.

CBT is a broadly utilized model of care that has been adapted for the treatment of adolescent substance abuse and other psychiatric disorders. Cognitive behavioral approaches are, as the name suggests, a combination of behavioral and cognitive therapies. These therapies view addictive behavior as shaped by a combination of environmental reinforcements, thoughts, emotions, and expectations. CBT for drug and alcohol abuse involves the identification of environmental triggers of behavioral and affective sequences, rehearsal and utilization of alternative responses to raving and/or drug-seeking behavior, identification and manipulation of new sources of reinforcement, and learning of coping skills.

In the treatment of addictions, CBT has been combined with MET, as a complementary treatment approach that focuses on enhancing client motivation by facilitating movement across stages of change (Prochaska & DiClemente, 1992) from precontemplation through active and sustained change. MET is particularly focused on the role of self-determination in making behavioral change. Given the developmental significance of autonomy during adolescence, it is believed that MET is particularly suited to the treatment of this population.

MET combined with cognitive behavioral treatment (MET/CBT) has been successful in the treatment of adult substance abuse, has been adapted for adolescent development, and has been manualized (Sampl & Kadden, 2001). MET/CBT has been shown to be cost-effective.

ACRA is an intervention that focuses mainly on reinforcers and influences on drug use. These negative reinforcers are identified and positive, healthy replacements are sought, such as vocational, social, or educational reinforcers. Once replacements have been achieved, the clinician selects one of the 17 ACRA procedures to address the client's communication, coping, and problem-solving skills and thus, to promote the client's participation in positive activities. Role-playing is also utilized in this model and the caregiver is encouraged to participate in the treatment in both individual and joint sessions (Winters et al., 2014).

CM uses minor incentives for successful attendance and achievement in substance abuse treatment. These incentives can include items such as movie tickets, personal gifts, or even cash vouchers in exchange for successes and the discontinuation of drug use. This practice works in hope of diminishing the impact of drug use reinforcement on the adolescent and replacing it with more positive reinforcements. This approach can also be continued within the home after treatment if parents are trained on its use.

In addition to these behavioral approaches, family therapies have been shown to be effective as well. To begin, MST addresses the family and the adolescent's characteristics in regard to the drug use; such as the family's conflicts or other members' substance abuse and the adolescent's viewpoint because of each. Community characteristics are also addressed in regard to the adolescent's substance abuse, such as his or her peer group, school environment, and neighborhood culture. The therapist will work with the family as a whole but also conducts individual sessions with members and the adolescent.

BSFT focuses more on the family interactions in general, and less on specific characteristics of the family or community. The therapist in this model would build rapport with each individual member and takes note of the interactions between all members. After conducting observations of the family as a whole as well as individual sessions with members, the therapist helps the family with habitual negative interactions. This therapy is labeled as brief because it lasts on average 12–16 weeks.

FBT uses CM in combination with a behavior contract to address substance abuse as well as other problematic behaviors in partnership with a parent or caregiver. Behavioral strategies are selected by the adolescent and a caregiver, which are then taught by the therapist to them to use at home. Then, behavior goals are set and reinforced with rewards at sessions for completing them.

FFThighlights unhealthy family behaviors that underlie the adolescent's problematic behaviors. This model engages family members in treatment and uses behavioral techniques to modify the family's communication, conflict, and behavioral issues to interact in a healthier manner. Strategies used in this therapy include behavior contracts, teaching of problem-solving and communication skills, and CM.

MDFT is a family and community based therapy for adolescents with high-risk behaviors and substance abuse, especially ones with severe abuse. The main goal of this therapy is to educate the family on the adolescent's issue as well as assist in the family's collaboration and communication with other relevant systems involved, such as the school or the juvenile justice system (National Institute on Drug Abuse, 2014).

Family-based treatments have been proven effective with substance use disorders, externalizing disorders, school and behavior problems associated with attention deficit/hyperactivity disorder (ADHD), and as adjuncts in the cognitive-behavioral treatment of anxiety disorders and depression (Diamond & Josephson, 2005). Family treatment can also help to improve compliance, retention, engagement, and, maintenance of treatment gains. In part, because of their focus on family relationships and social ecology, family approaches have been slow to be incorporated into residential settings where, by design, children and youth are separated from their families and live apart in an artificially constructed "therapeutic" social environment.

According to some, outpatient family therapy appears to be superior to other forms of treatment for adolescent behavior problems and substance abuse (Rowe & Liddle, 2003; Williams & Chang, 2000). The American Academy of Child and Adolescent Psychiatry Practice Parameter on Adolescent Substance Abuse agrees with this assessment citing the superiority of outpatient family approaches, including FFT, MST, BSFT, and MDFT (AACAP, 2005). However, some evidence suggests that other approaches to care may be just as effective. In an evaluation of family-based and group treatment of substance abuse, Hall and colleagues (Hall, Smith, Williams, & Delaney, 2005) found both approaches to be effective at reducing substance abuse and related problems. They could not find an advantage of one approach versus another. Many of the family therapy approaches are based in theories of adolescent development, developmental psychopathology, and structural and strategic family therapy. These approaches recognize that adolescent substance abuse often involves difficulty in regulating emotions and disturbed communication patterns within the family.

Pumariega (2006b) argues that the prolonged separation and reduced family contact that is typical of many placement experiences contributes to problems with reunification due to families reorganizing into new roles and modes of relating that exclude the child in treatment. Incorporating effective family treatment models into residential care could reduce the likelihood of this occurring by increasing regular meaningful contact and maintaining the child's "place" in the family. Others have recommended modifications of policy to promote increased family contact (Leichtman, 2006). These changes include removing family contact from the list of privileges that must be earned, inviting the family into the milieu, and awarding milieu privileges based on improvements in behavior with family.

Policy Changes Pertaining to Health Care

Since the first publication of this book in 2008, there has been a significant change in the field of mental health and substance use legislation, funding, treatment and its accessibility. While the back ground for mental health parity policy began with the Mental Health Parity Act of 1996 (MHPA) which stated that large group health plans could not impose annual or lifetime dollar limits on mental health benefits that were less favorable than any such limits imposed on medical/surgical benefits), it was through the Paul Wellstone and Pete Domenici Mental Health Parity and Addiction Equity Act of 2008 (MHPAEA) and the Affordable Care Act (ACA) of 2010, that led to major strides in the mental health and substance use treatment world. MHPAEA is a federal law that has preserved the MHPA protections and added new protections, such as extending parity requirements to substance use disorders. MHPAEA was amended by the ACA to also apply to individual health insurance coverage. This new law requires parity for individuals with mental and/or substance use disorders. It requires that the coverage of mental health and substance use disorder services be a part of one of the ten essential health benefit (EHB) categories in non-grandfathered plans (individual and small group plans) (Center for Consumer Information & Insurance Oversight, 2016). There are some caveats to plans and their use of MHPAEA—to access more information on the regulations and additional changes made by MHPAEA and the ACA you can access more information through the Centers for Medicare and Medicaid Services (CMS) Website: *https://www.cms.gov/cciio/programs-and-initiatives/other-insurance-protections/mhpaea_factsheet.html#Summary of MHPAEA Protections*.

The expansion of the ACA has some beneficial implications for the populations addressed in this book. The ACA expanded coverage to young adults by allowing them to remain on their parent's health insurance up to the age of 26 years. The implications of this expansion on inpatient hospitalizations, specifically for mental health care were seen in a study by Antwi, Moriya, and Simon (2015) who found that compared to individuals aged 27–29 years, young adults who had been treated aged 19–25 years had increased their mental health related visits by 9%. And the percentage of those uninsured young adults who had been hospitalized decreased by 12.5%.

These are important findings when understanding youth and young adult treatment and accessibility issues, and have further implications for providers, family members, hospitals, and individuals needing inpatient treatment (Antwi et al., 2015).

Data from the 2015 National Survey of Substance Abuse Treatment Services (NSSATS) indicates that the substance use disorder treatment system is at capacity. Over 100% of beds (for substance use treatment) in residential treatment facilities, and inpatient hospitals were occupied. A percentage greater than 100 indicates that nondesignated beds for substance use treatment were also being used (SAMHSA, 2015b). This may be an implication of the increased accessibility, and coverage of substance use treatment disorders through insurance.

The Medicaid Institutions for Mental Diseases (IMD) exclusion (part of Section 1905 (a)(B) of the Social Security Act) dated 1965, prohibits "payments with respect to care or services for any individual who has not attained 65 years of age and who is a patient in an institution for mental diseases" except for "inpatient psychiatric hospital services for individuals under age 21." Because this exclusion is focused on states paying for inpatient psychiatric services, rather than the federal government, it has been a cause for concern, especially recently given the rapidly growing need for funding and accessibility to mental and substance use disorder treatment services. Because of this, CMS has been encouraging state Medicaid agencies to apply for Section 1115 waivers to allow them to use federal funds to provide substance use treatment services. Additionally since 2016, CMS made changes to the Medicaid managed care rules to allow Medicaid managed care organizations (MCOs) to pay for SUD treatment in an IMD. Since March of 2017, Secretary Tom Price of the Department of Health and Human Services has mentioned that CMS will support Section 1115 waiver applications related to SUD treatment. As of 2017, legislation has been proposed to allow Medicaid beneficiaries to be eligible for up to 60 days of residential services in an IMD facility. This includes extended the number of beds in these facilities to 40 or more.

Best Practice Recommendations

Despite the relative lack of quality research and compelling empirical evidence in favor of residential treatment, it is clear that many children and youth benefit from this level of care. The likelihood of positive outcomes can be increased by understanding the features and characteristics of the target population, borrowing from successful programs, and incorporating evidence-based practices that can be adapted to residential substance abuse programs. Even the most effective community-based practices fail to achieve positive outcomes with 20% of the youth served and there remains a compelling need for residential treatment. The following recommendations are offered.

Treatment Recommendations

- *Screening and Assessment*: Few programs do an adequate job screening and assessing the youth who enter care. Youth should be screened for psychiatric conditions, trauma, drug and alcohol use, and health conditions often associated with drug and alcohol abuse (hepatitis, HIV-AIDS, STDs, etc.). Assessment should be comprehensive, including assessments of strengths, inclusion of collateral sources of information, measures of quantity, frequency and age of first substance use, and assessment in the following domains, Developmental History, Educational/Vocational History, Social/Interpersonal History, Family History, Medical History, Legal History, Substance Abuse History, Recreational History, Trauma History, Psychiatric History, Sexual History, Mental Status, Functional Assessment and Activities of Daily Living, Objective Measures of Functioning and Symptomology, Cultural/Language Assessment, Summary and Clinical Formulation, Individual and Family Strengths and Problems, DSM-V Diagnosis, Recommendations & Initial Plan of Care. Programs should also utilize objective measures of key outcomes administered throughout treatment and utilized in real time to inform practice.
- *Engagement and Retention*: Programs must develop methods of actively engaging adolescents and their families in treatment and promoting treatment retention. Engagement and retention should be measured and tracked as part of quality improvement activities and programs should adopt methods, such as MET and family-based approaches, that emphasize engagement. Promotion of autonomy and active involvement of youth and families in treatment planning are also recommended to improve engagement.
- *Family Involvement*: Active involvement of families in treatment should occur whenever possible. Policies and procedures should be family friendly and active outreach is required. Specifically, family contact should not be contingent on program performance, families should be invited to participate in the milieu, and programs should consider making program privileges contingent on appropriate behavior with family. The families role in supporting the youth's treatment should be explicitly addressed as well as family members own use or abuse of, substances. Families should be encouraged (when safe and appropriate) to be, involved in treatment and visit youth even when reunification is not the goal at discharge. Therapists should be trained in family-based approaches and receive appropriate supervision from a qualified supervisor. Consider adopting variations of evidence-based family approaches (e.g., MST, FFT, MDFT, and BSFT) that have proven success in community settings.
- *Cultural and Linguistic Competence*: Minorities are overrepresented in residential care and programs must deliver care in a manner that is culturally and linguistically competent. Special care should be taken in making admission, decisions to avoid bias leading to disproportionate representation. Staff composition, policies and procedures, training, assessment, and treatment approaches, should be evaluated in terms of cultural and linguistic competence.

- *Discharge Planning and Aftercare*: Discharge planning should be comprehensive and consider the educational, social, and recreational needs of the youth as well as clinical and family issues. Discharge planning should be followed up with a formal aftercare and a follow-up program with specific goals and expectations. Discharge planning should begin early on in residential treatment. Connecting families, in addition, to youth to community-based services and supports is critical.
- *Telehealth or Telemedicine*: Telehealth encompasses a broad variety of technologies and tactics to deliver virtual medical, health, and education services. Telehealth is not a specific service, but a collection of means to enhance care. Specific to residential settings telehealth could be used a way to engage and involve families in the treatment process while the adolescent is in care. Telehealth could also be used to engage community providers that will in discharge planning early in the process so the transition can happen seamlessly. Finally, telehealth can be used to compensate for workforce issues that may be in issue in residential settings (e.g., not having a psychiatrist, nurse, or peer support specialists on site).
- *Trauma*: The majority of youth treated in RSAT have experienced trauma. Programs should screen for the presence of trauma and trauma-related symptoms, create a trauma-sensitive environment, train staff in the impact of trauma, and offer trauma treatment, either directly or through referral relationships with allied providers.
- *Strengths Based*: RSAT programs should borrow a page from the system of care and family-based approaches that recognize client and family strengths and use them to support the goals of treatment.
- *Drug Screens and Breathalyzers*: Drugs screens and breathalyzers are useful as ongoing supports for sobriety.
- *Medications*: RSAT programs should consider psychiatric medication when appropriate for co-occurring psychiatric conditions and must also guard against over medication and overuse of substances to contain behavior. Use of psychotropic medications should for treatment of specific substance abuse disorders should be considered, especially Buprenorphine for the treatment of opioid dependence. Appropriate stimulant therapy for ADHD should be viewed as protective against substance abuse; however, the potential for abuse or sale to other should be addressed.
- *Naloxone injection*: RSAT programs specifically for opioid addiction should have Naloxone injection and naloxone prefilled autoinjection device (Evzio) on hand. These are used along with emergency medical treatment to reverse the life-threatening effects of a known or suspected opiate (narcotic) overdose.
- *Avoid Punitive Approaches*: Programs that are overly rule-oriented and focus on compliance rather than treatment progress do not produce positive outcomes. Beware of the deterioration of point and level systems into a punitive staff culture and do not confuse behavioral containment with treatment.
- *Harm Reduction*: A focus on harm reduction that emphasizes the primary risks associated with drug and alcohol abuse and strategies to reduce those risks is warranted.

Organizational Recommendations

- *Multidisciplinary Staff*: The complex and diverse needs of youth entering RSAT requires a multimodal approach and multiple specialties. Staff should be prepared to provide assistance with education, vocation, legal issues, health and wellness, psychiatric needs, recreation and socialization, family, and general life skills.
- *Quality Improvement*: Internal standards should be set and monitored through a comprehensive quality improvement program. Benchmarking against past performance and other programs is highly recommended.
- *Standards of Care*: Licensing, accrediting, and other regulatory standards can improve the overall quality and consistency of care. Higher standards should be encouraged and pursued.
- *Appropriate Reimbursement*: Policymakers should be certain that rate setting methodologies take into consideration all the costs associated with delivering high-quality care. Rates should be sufficient to support the elements of care known to contribute to successful outcomes.

References

American Academy of Child and Adolescent Psychiatry. (2005). Practice parameter for the assessment and treatment of children and adolescents with substance abuse disorders. *Journal of the American Academy of Child and Adolescent Psychiatry, 44*(6), 609–621.

Antwi, Y. A., Moriya, A. S., & Simon, K. I. (2015). Access to health insurance and the use of inpatient medical care: Evidence from the affordable care act young adult mandate. *Journal of Health Economics, 39*(C), 171–187.

Blau, G. M., Caldwell, B., & Lieberman, R. (Eds.). (2014). *Residential interventions for children adolescents and families: A best practice guide*. New York, NY: Routledge Press.

Bracken, B. K., Rodolico, J., & Hill, K. P. (2013). Sex, age, and progression of drug use in adolescents admitted for substance use disorder treatment in the northeastern United States: Comparison with a national survey. *Substance Abuse: Official Publication of the Association for Medical Education and Research in Substance Abuse, 34*(3), 263–272. Retrieved from https://doi.org/10.1080/08897077.2013.770424.

Brannigan, R., Schackman, B. R., Falco, M., & Millman, R. B. (2004). The quality of highly regarded adolescent substance abuse treatment programs: Results of an in-depth national survey. *Archives of Pediatric Adolescent Medicine, 158*(9), 904–909.

Brown, S. A., Myers, M., Abrantes, A., & Kahler, C. W. (2008). Social recovery model: An 8-year investigation of adolescent 12-step group involvement following inpatient treatment. *Alcoholism: Clinical & Experimental Research (ACER), 31*(8), 1468–1478.

Center for Consumer Information & Insurance Oversight. (2016). *The mental health parity and addiction equity act: Summary of MHPAEA protections*. Retrieved from https://www.cms.gov/cciio/programs-and-initiatives/other-insurance-protections/mhpaea_factsheet.html#Summary of MHPAEA Protections.

Chan, Y., Dennis, M. L., & Funk, R. R. (2008). Prevalence and comorbidity of major internalizing and externalizing problems among adolescents and adults presenting to substance abuse treatment. *Journal of Substance Abuse Treatment, 34*(1), 14–24.

Child Welfare League of America (CWLA). (2005). Position statement on residential services. Washington, DC: Retrieved from http://www.cwla.org/programs/group-care/rgcposition-statement.pdf.

Connor, D. F., Miller, K. P., Cunningham, J. A., & Melloni, R. H. (2002). What does getting better mean? Child improvement and measure of outcome in residential treatment. *American Journal of Orthopsychiatry, 72*(1), 110–117.
Daughters, S. B., Lejuez, C. W., Bornovalova, M. A., Kahler, C. W., Strong, D. R., & Brown, R. A. (2005). Distress tolerance as a predictor of early treatment dropout in a residential substance abuse treatment facility. *Journal of Abnormal Psychology, 114*(4), 729–734.
Dennis, M. L., & Kaminer, Y. (2006). Introduction to special issue on advances in the assessment and treatment of adolescent substance use disorders. *American Journal on Addictions, 15*(S1), 1–3.
Diamond, G., & Josephson, A. (2005). Family-based treatment research: A 10-year update. *Journal of the American Academy of Child and Adolescent Psychiatry, 44*(9), 872–887.
Edelen, M. O., Tucker, J. S., Wenzel, S. L., Paddock, S. M., Ebener, P., Dahl, J., & Mandell, W. (2007). Treatment process in the therapeutic community: Associations with retention and outcomes among adolescent residential clients. *Journal of Substance Abuse Treatment, 32*(4), 415–421.
Fishman, M., Clemmey, P., & Hoover, A. (2003). Mountain manor treatment center: Residential adolescent addictions treatment program. In S. J. Stevens & A. R. Morral (Eds.), *Adolescent substance abuse treatment in the United States: Exemplary models from a national evaluation study* (pp. 135–153). New York, NY: The Haworth Press.
French, M. T., Salome, H. J., & Carney, M. (2002). Using the DATCAP and ASI to estimate the costs and benefits of residential addiction treatment in the State of Washington. *Journal of Substance Abuse Treatment, 23*(1), 21–32.
Frensch, K. M., & Cameron, G. (2002). Treatment of choice or a last resort? A review of residential mental health placements for children and youth. *Child and Youth Forum, 31*(5), 307–339.
Garrett, C. J. (1985). Effects of residential treatment on adjudicated delinquents: A meta-analysis. *Journal of Research in Crime and Delinquency, 22*(4), 287–308.
Governing the States and Localities. (2017). *Data: State marijuana laws in 2017 map*. Retrieved from http://www.governing.com/gov-data/state-marijuana-laws-map-medical-recreational.html.
Hair, H. J. (2005). Outcomes for children and adolescents after residential treatment: A review of research from 1993 to 2003. *Journal of Child and Family Studies, 14*(4), 551–575.
Hall, J. A., Smith, D. C., Williams, J. K., & Delaney, P. J. (2005). *Comparison of family and group based treatment for adolescent substance abuse* (pp. 1–47) [PowerPoint presentation]. Rockville, MD: Center for Substance Abuse Treatment.
Hawkins, E. H. (2009). A tale of two systems: Co-occurring mental health and substance abuse disorders treatment for adolescents. *Annual Review of Psychology, 60*, 197–220.
Hoagwood, K., Burns, B., Kiser, L., Ringeisen, H., & Schoenwald, S. (2001). Evidence-based practice in child and adolescent mental health services. *Psychiatric Services, 52*(9), 1179–1189.
Hooper, S. R., Murphy, J., Devaney, A., & Hultman, T. (2000). Ecological outcomes of adolescents in a psycho-educational residential treatment facility. *American Journal of Orthopsychiatry, 70*(4), 491–500.
Hulvershorn, L. A., Quinn, P. D., & Scott, E. L. (2015). Treatment of adolescent substance use disorders and co-occurring internalizing disorders: A critical review and proposed model. *Current Drug Abuse Review, 8*(1), 41–49.
Jaycox, L. H., Ebener, R., Damesek, L., & Becker, K. (2004). Trauma exposure and retention in adolescent substance abuse treatment. *Journal of Traumatic Stress, 17*(2), 113–121.
Johnston, L. D., O'Malley, P. M., Miech, R. A., Bachman, J. G., & Schulenberg, J. E. (2017). *Monitoring the future national survey results on drug use, 1975–2016: Overview, key findings on adolescent drug use*. Ann Arbor, MI: Institute for Social Research, The University of Michigan.
Kaminer, Y. (1994). *Adolescent substance abuse: A comprehensive guide to theory and practice*. New York, NY: Plenum Medical Book Company.
Kaminer, Y., Blitz, C., Burleson, J. A., Kadden, R. M., & Rounsaville, B. J. (1998). Measuring treatment process in cognitive-behavioral and interactional group therapies for adolescent substance abusers. *Journal of Nervous and Mental Disorders, 186*(7), 407–413.
Latimer, W. L., Newcomb, M., Winters, K. C., & Stinchfield, R. D. (2000). Adolescent substance treatment outcome: The role of substance abuse problem severity, psychosocial, and treatment factors. *Journal of Consulting and Clinical Psychology, 68*(4), 684–696.

Leichtman, M. (2006). Residential treatment of children and adolescents: Past, present, and future. *American Journal of Orthopsychiatry, 76*(3), 285–294.
Leichtman, M., Leichtman, M. L., Barber, C. C., & Neese, D. T. (2001). Effectiveness of intensive short-term residential treatment with severely disturbed adolescents. *American Journal of Orthopsychiatry, 71*(2), 227–235.
De Leon, G. (2010). Is the therapeutic community an evidence based treatment? What the evidence says. *International Journal of Therapeutic Communities, 31*(2), 104–128.
Lyons, J. S., & McCulloch, J. R. (2006). Monitoring and managing outcomes in residential treatment: Practice-based evidence in search of evidence-based practice. *Journal of the American Academy of Child and Adolescent Psychiatry, 45*(2), 247–251.
Miech, R. A., Johnston, L. D., O'Malley, P. M., Bachman, J. G., Schulenberg, J. E., & Patrick, M. E. (2017). Monitoring the future national survey results on drug use, 1975–2016: Vol. I. *Secondary school students*. Ann Arbor, MI: Institute for Social Research, The University of Michigan.
Morral, A. R., Jaycox, L. H., Smith, W., Becker, K., & Ebener, P. (2003). An evaluation of substance abuse treatment services provided to juvenile probationers at Phoenix Academy of Los Angeles. In S. J. Stevens & A. R. Morral (Eds.), *Adolescent substance abuse treatment in the United States: Exemplary models from a national evaluation study* (pp. 213–232). Binghamton, NY: Haworth Press.
Morral, A. R., McCaffery, D. F., & Ridgeway, G. (2004). Effectiveness of community based treatment for substance-abusing adolescents: 12 month outcomes of youths entering Phoenix Academy or alternative probation dispositions. *Psychology of Addictive Behaviors, 18*(3), 257–268.
Muck, R., Zempolich, K. A., Titus, J. C., Fishman, M., Godley, M. D., & Schwebel, R. (2001). An overview of the effectiveness of adolescent substance abuse treatment models. *Youth and Society, 33*(2), 143–168.
National Association of State Mental Health Program Directors. (2008). *Six core strategies for reducing seclusion and restraint use*. Retrieved from https://www.nasmhpd.org/sites/default/files/Consolidated%20Six%20Core%20Strategies%20Document.pdf.
National Institute on Drug Abuse. (2014). *Principles of adolescent substance use disorder: A research-based guide*. Retrieved from https://www.drugabuse.gov/publications/principles-adolescent-substance-use-disorder-treatment-research-based-guide.
Prochaska, J. O., & DiClemente, C. C. (1992). Stages of change in the modification of problem behaviors. In M. Hersen, P. M. Miller, & R. Eisler (Eds.), *Progress in behavior modification* (Vol. 28, pp. 184–218). New York, NY: Wadsworth Publishing.
Pumariega, A. J. (2006a). Residential treatment for youth: Introduction and a cautionary tale. *American Journal of Orthopsychiatry, 76*(3), 281–284.
Pumariega, A. J. (2006b). Residential treatment for children and youth: Time for reconsideration and reform. *American Journal of Orthopsychiatry, 77*(3), 343–345.
Robinson, A. D., Kruzich, J. M., Friesen, B. J., Jivanjee, P., & Pullman, M. D. (2005). Preserving family bonds: Examining parent perspectives in the light of practice standards for out-of-home treatment. *American Journal of Orthopsychiatry, 75*(4), 632–643.
Rowe, C. L., & Liddle, H. A. (2003). Substance abuse. *Journal of Marital and Family Therapy, 29*(1), 97–120.
Rudd, R. A., Seth, P., David, F., & Scholl, L. (2016). Increases in drug and opioid-involved overdose deaths: United States, 2010–2015. *MMWR, 65*(50–51), 1445–1452. Retrieved from https://doi.org/10.15585/mmwr.mm655051e1.
Sampl, S., & Kadden, R. (2001). *A 5 session motivational enhancement therapy and cognitive behavioral therapy (MET-CBT-5) for adolescent cannabis users* (DHHS Publication No. 791 SMA 01-3486), Cannabis Youth Treatment (CYT) Manual Series, Vol. 1. Rockville, MD: Center for Substance Abuse Treatment, Substance Abuse and Mental Health Services Administration.
Schulenberg, J. E., Johnston, L. D., O'Malley, P.M., Bachman, J. G., Miech, R. A., & Patrick, M. E. (2017). Monitoring the future national survey results on drug use, 1975–2016: Vol. II. *College students and adults ages 19–55*. Ann Arbor, MI: Institute for Social Research, The University of Michigan.

Schwebel, R. (2004). *The seven challenges manual*. Tuscon, AZ: Viva Press.
Sealock, M. D., Gottfredson, D. C., & Gallagher, C. A. (1997). Drug treatment for juvenile offenders: Some good and bad news. *Journal of Research in Crime and Delinquency, 34*(2), 210–236.
Subramanian, G. A., Stitzer, M. A., Clemmey, P., Kolodner, K., & Fishman, M. J. (2007). Baseline depressive symptoms predict poor substance abuse outcome following adolescent residential treatment. *Journal of the American Academy of Child and Adolescent Psychiatry, 46*(8), 1062–1069.
Substance Abuse and Mental Health Services Administration. (2015a). *Behavioral health barometer: United States, 2015*. (HHS Publication No. SMA 16–Baro–2015). Rockville, MD: Substance Abuse and Mental Health Services Administration.
Substance Abuse and Mental Health Services Administration. (2015b). National Survey of Substance Abuse Treatment Services (N-SSATS). *Data on substance abuse treatment facilities*. BHSIS Series S-88 (HHS Publication No. SMA 17-5031). Rockville, MD: Substance Abuse and Mental Health Services Administration.
The Seven Challenges. (2017). *Overview: Why seven challenges works*. Retrieved from http://www.sevenchallenges.com/overview.
Tomlinson, K. L., Brown, S. A., & Abrantes, A. (2004). Psychiatric comorbidity and substance abuse treatment outcomes of adolescents. *Psychology of Addictive Behaviors, 18*(2), 160–169.
University of Georgia. (2008, June). *Service delivery and use of evidence-based treatment practices in adolescent substance abuse treatment settings: Project report* (Grant No. 53130). Athens, GA: Institute for Behavioral Research.
Walter, U. M., & Petr, C. G. (2008). Family-centered residential treatment: Knowledge, research and values converge. *Residential Treatment for Children & Youth, 25*(1), 1–16.
Weiner, D. A., Abraham, M. E., & Lyons, J. (2001). Clinical characteristic of youths with substance use problems and implications for residential treatment. *Psychiatric Services, 52*(6), 793–799.
Williams, R. J., & Chang, S. Y. (2000). A comprehensive and comparative review of adolescent substance abuse treatment outcome. *Clinical Psychology: Science and Practice, 7*(2), 138–166.
Winters, K. C., Stinchfield, R. D., Opland, E. O., Weller, C., & Latimer, W. W. (2000). The effectiveness of the Minnesota Model approach in the treatment of adolescent drug abusers. *Addiction, 95*(4), 601–612.
Winters, K. C., Tanner-Smith, E. E., Bresani, E., & Meyers, K. (2014). Current advances in the treatment of adolescent drug use. *Adolescent Health, Medicine and Therapeutics, 5*(2014), 199–210. Retrieved from https://doi.org/10.2147/AHMT.S48053.

The Treatment and Prevention of Adolescent Opioid and Prescription Misuse and Abuse

Michelle R. Lofwall and Amy M. Yule

Introduction

The USA is in the midst of ongoing opioid epidemic that is in large part, iatrogenic, meaning that it is associated with overprescribing of opioid analgesics by health care providers (Nelson, Juurlink, & Perrone, 2015). Simultaneously, there is increasing prescribing of benzodiazepines and together, the increasing availability of these medications in American homes is adversely affecting all age groups, including adolescents (i.e., 12–21 years old) (Bachhuber, Hennessy, Cunningham, & Starrels, 2016). Unfortunately, there also has been increasing availability of heroin, an illicit opiate often first used among those with previous experience using prescription opioids. Heroin is responsible for a growing number of substance use disorder treatment admissions and overdoses, on top of already high rates of prescription opioid overdose deaths, and is often tainted with even more deadly synthetic opioids like fentanyl and carfentanyl; the latter being used to immobilize large animals in veterinary practice (Cole & Nelson, 2017; O'Donnell, Halpin, Mattson, Goldberger, & Gladden, 2017).

This chapter reviews terminology including the pharmacological effects on persons using these substances, how effects change over time and characteristic

M. R. Lofwall (✉)
Department of Behavioral Science, Straus Clinic, Center on Drug and Alcohol Research, University of Kentucky College of Medicine, Lexington, KY, USA

Department of Psychiatry, University of Kentucky College of Medicine, Lexington, KY, USA
e-mail: michelle.lofwall@uky.edu

A. M. Yule
Medical Director Addiction Recovery Management Service at Massachusetts General Hospital (MGH), Assistant Professor in Psychiatry at MGH, Instructor in Psychiatry at Harvard Medical School, Boston, MA, USA
e-mail: ayule@mgh.harvard.edu

C. G. Leukefeld, T. P. Gullotta (eds.), *Adolescent Substance Abuse*, Issues in Children's and Families' Lives, https://doi.org/10.1007/978-3-319-90611-9_8

withdrawal syndromes, epidemiology of adolescent opioid and benzodiazepine misuse, use disorder, treatment admissions, and associated morbidity such as overdose. Relevant risk factors are reviewed followed by discussion of effective preventative, harm reduction and treatment approaches. Along the way, we discuss common myths and misconceptions about prescription opioids and benzodiazepines, and heroin. Prescription stimulants, commonly prescribed to adolescents, are discussed in Chap. 8.

Terminology

This section focuses on definitions of terms used throughout the rest of this chapter. Misuse is defined as use of medications not prescribed to oneself or use of a prescribed medication in ways other than intended. For example, receiving a prescription for pain medication intended to be taken orally as one tablet up to three times a day for pain, but taking it instead for a different reason (e.g., energy, mood change, stress relief), by a different route such as crushing and snorting it or dissolving and injecting it, or taking more than prescribed all qualify as misuse. Medication diversion is defined as a misappropriation of medication to someone other than the person whom the medication is prescribed. Diversion of controlled substances is illegal, regardless whether money is exchanged or whether the underlying intent is well meaning or not (Larance, Degenhardt, Lintzeris, Winstock, & Mattick, 2011).

A substance use disorder is defined by the Diagnostic and Statistical Manual (DSM) 5 (American Psychiatric Association, 2013). The same criteria are applied for each substance because there are common brain pathways activated by all drugs of abuse such as the brain's dopamine reward system, which also helps people learn behaviors, regardless of whether the behaviors are legal or illegal or beneficial to long-term health of the individual. There are 11 criteria for a substance use disorder. These are outlined in Table 1. The more criteria present, the more severe the disorder. A severe disorder maps on to the definition of addiction, which is defined by the National Institute on Drug Abuse as a chronic relapsing brain disorder, with compulsive drug use despite harmful consequences. The brain's structure and function are altered often producing long lasting changes that can lead to harmful, self-destructive behavior (Volkow, Koob, & McLellan, 2016). A common myth is that having addiction or a use disorder is a marker of a moral failure or character flaw. Science has proven that this is not true, and these myths may only perpetuate stigma and push suffering adolescents and families away from effective treatments and preventative efforts (Wakeman & Rich, 2018).

Table 1 DSM-5 Substance use disorder definition

A problematic pattern of substance use (insert specific substance name) leading to clinically significant impairment or distress, as manifested by at least two of the following, occurring within a 12-month period:
1. Substance taken in larger amounts or over longer periods of time than intended
2. Persistent desire or unsuccessful efforts to control or cut down use of substance
3. Great deal of time spent in activities to obtain, use or recover from substance
4. Strong desire to use or craving for substance
5. Recurrent substance use causing failure to fulfill responsibilities and obligations such as at school, home or work.
6. Continued use of substance despite recurrent or persistent interpersonal or social problems caused by or exacerbated by effects of substance.
7. Important activities and roles given up or reduced because of the substance.
8. Recurrent substance use in physically hazardous situations
9. Substance use continued despite knowing that it is producing physical or psychological problems.
10. Tolerance defined as either needing more of the substance to achieve the desired effect or intoxication OR a markedly diminished effect with the same amount of substance used
11. Withdrawal defined as either a characteristic withdrawal syndrome emerges when the substance is no longer taken or decreased in amount OR substance taken in order to relieve or avoid withdrawal symptoms

Mild: 2–3 symptoms, Moderate: 4–5 symptoms, Severe: six or more symptoms
Adapted by authors Lofwall and Yule based on DSM 5 (APA, 2013).

Opioid-Specific Terms, Pharmacologic Effects, and Withdrawal

Opiates (e.g., morphine) are derived from opium, which is sourced from the poppy (*Papaver somniferum*). Opioids include opiates as well as synthetic molecules that bare little structural similarity to morphine. All opioids bind to opiate receptors present in several areas of the central and peripheral nervous system that produce a wide array of effects. While there are several types of opiate receptors in the body, the μ-opiate receptor is the one responsible for most of the medicinal and subjective effects that make opioids prone to abuse. μ-opiate receptors are located in areas of the nervous system involved with respiration, nausea and vomiting centers, pupil size, gastrointestinal motility, affect, learning, reward, and motivation.

Prescription opioids have important medicinal uses—e.g., for relief of severe acute pain and end-of-life pain, relief of diarrhea, and cough suppressant. Heroin, while now illegal, used to be a medication available through Bayer Pharmaceuticals toted to be nonaddicting. All opioids, however, also produce psychoactive effects such as euphoria, talkativeness, sedation, relief of anxiety or depression, and energy that may make them attractive for use recreationally or in other situations. Opioid intoxication is marked by pupillary constriction (dilation seen in severe overdose when the dose of opioid causes respiratory arrest and subsequent lack of oxygen to the brain) accompanied by drowsiness, slurred speech, impairment in attention or memory that cause clinically significant problematic behavioral or psychological changes that develop during or shortly after use of the opioid (APA, 2013). With repeated use over time of opioids (and benzodiazepines), physiologic dependence occurs, characterized by tolerance and withdrawal. It is important to understand that physical dependence is not the same as a substance use disorder. Opioid tolerance could be reflected by a loss in analgesia and euphoria – a higher opioid dose may be needed to produce the same effect that was initially achieved, but sometimes the initial effects cannot be achieved even with higher doses. Opioid withdrawal is similar to a bad case of the flu. It can develop minutes after an opioid antagonist is given or hours to days after cessation or reducing heavy opioid use. Three or more of the following symptoms are required to make a diagnosis of opioid withdrawal when these are causing clinically significant impairment in social, occupational, or other areas of important function: dysphoria, nausea or vomiting, muscle aches, lacrimation (watery eyes) or rhinorrhea (runny nose), diarrhea, yawning, fever, and insomnia (APA, 2013). Opioid withdrawal can vary widely between individuals, rated by severity using standardized withdrawal scales, and is often noted by patients with opioid use disorder as a reason why they continue opioid use—using to avoid withdrawal (Schuckit, 2016).

Benzodiazepine-Specific Terms, Pharmacologic Effects, and Withdrawal

Benzodiazepines are a class of substances typically categorized as a sedative, hypnotic, and anxiolytic. Other sedative, hypnotic and anxiolytic drugs include barbiturates and z-drugs (e.g., zolpidem) that also work through the GABA receptor, but these are less commonly prescribed and misused than benzodiazepines; therefore, benzodiazepines are the primary focus here.

Benzodiazepines are not naturally occurring. They are synthesized molecules that bind to specific receptor sites on the gamma-amino butyric acid (GABA) receptor complex, potentiating GABA, one of the brain's most abundant inhibitory neurotransmitters. The majority of benzodiazepine effects are due to its actions in the central nervous system where GABA receptors are located. Several brain areas such as the frontal lobes (involved in executive function such as decision making, planning, and inhibitory control) and areas also associated with memory, balance, attention, and affect contain GABA receptors (McKim, 1986).

Benzodiazepines are prescribed to treat anxiety disorders, insomnia, epilepsy, and muscle spasticity. They are also frequently given prior to surgery for their amnestic effects. Benzodiazepines, while decreasing anxiety and producing a "high" similar to alcohol also decrease attention and memory, specifically causing anterograde amnesia and impaired metamemory (Curran, 1986, 1991). This means that people will have trouble remembering things that occur after they take a benzodiazepine and that they will not realize that their memory is impaired. While this is clearly a benefit prior to surgery, benzodiazepines, such as flunitrazepam

(Rohypnol®), have been used as date-rape drugs, slipped into unknowing victims beverages at social events (e.g., raves) and are voluntarily taken by adolescents in order to ease anticipated stress in social and sexual encounters (Rickert, Wiemann, & Berenson, 2000; Schwartz, Milteer, & LeBeau, 2000).

Benzodiazepine intoxication is marked by one of the following symptoms and signs: slurred speech, incoordination, unsteady gait, nystagmus (involuntary eye movements when attempting gaze laterally or upwards), impaired cognition and stupor (or coma). The signs and symptoms must occur shortly after or during the use of a benzodiazepine and result in clinically significant and maladaptive behavioral or psychological changes (APA, 2013). Examples would include uncharacteristic sexual behavior, labile mood, and poor judgment. Repeated benzodiazepine use can result in physical dependence with a withdrawal syndrome that is very similar to alcohol withdrawal. Benzodiazepine withdrawal is marked by two or more of the following findings within hours or several days after stopping or reducing their use: autonomic hyperactivity (e.g., heart rate greater than 100 beats per minute or diaphoresis), hand tremor (seen as a fine tremor if asked to stretch arms in front of body), insomnia, nausea or vomiting, psychomotor agitation (e.g., pacing or shifting in seat—difficulty sitting still), anxiety, generalized seizures (in severe cases), and transient hallucinations (perceptions without stimuli) or illusions (misperceptions) (APA, 2013).

Epidemiology in the USA

In 2015, 12.9% of twelfth graders misused a prescription drug during the past year (Johnston, O'Malley, Miech, & Bachman, & Schulenberg, 2016), and 16.8% of high schoolers had a lifetime history of prescription drug misuse (Kann et al., 2016). Prescription opioids were the most commonly misused prescription drug among adolescents. The annual prevalence of prescription opioid misuse among twelfth graders peaked at 9.5% in 2004 and has been declining since 2009 such that in 2015, the prevalence was 5.4% (Johnston et al., 2016). Similar declining trends in the prevalence of benzodiazepine use have been reported. Among twelfth graders in 2015, 4.7% misused benzodiazepines, most commonly alprazolam (Johnston et al., 2016). Heroin use is less common than prescription opioid misuse. Annual use of heroin among twelfth graders peaked at 1.5% in 2000 and declined to 0.5% in 2015 (Johnston et al., 2016).

The prevalence of past year substance use disorder among adolescents has stayed relatively constant and low between the early 2000s to the present for prescription opioid, prescription tranquilizer (most common tranquilizer class is benzodiazepines) and heroin use disorders (0.5%, 0.3%, <0.1% respectfully) (SAMHSA, 2016a). Youth with substance use disorder less commonly present for treatment for prescription drug misuse relative to marijuana and alcohol use (SAMHSA, 2017). Among misused prescription medications, treatment for opioid use disorders is most common. The prevalence of youth presenting for primary treatment of an opioid use disorder increased from 2% between 2005 and 2008 to 3 to 4% between 2009 and 2015 (SAMHSA, 2017). The type of opioid associated with presentation for treatment shifted significantly from prescription opioids to heroin between 2010 and 2015. In 2015, 61% of youth seeking treatment for opioid use disorder primarily were using heroin and 39% were primarily using prescription opioids (SAMHSA, 2017).

Prevalence estimates for nonmedical use of prescription medications and heroin in youth vary by region, race, and gender. For example, regionally, past year heroin use among adolescents was 0.08% in the South, 0.10% in the Midwest, 0.11% in the West, and 0.14% in the Northeast (SAMHSA, 2016b). White adolescents were significantly more likely to have a lifetime history of nonmedical use of prescription opioids, benzodiazepines, or heroin when compared to Black and Hispanic adolescents (McCabe & West, 2014; Palamar, Shearston, Dawson, Mateu-Gelabert, & Ompad, 2016; Rigg & Ford, 2014). Furthermore, Cotto et al. (2010) found adolescent females were significantly more likely than same aged males to misuse prescription medication and to be dependent on prescription medication.

Risk factors for misuse of prescription opioids and benzodiazepines in youth include a history of receiving a past prescription of the medication (Boyd, Austic, Epstein-Ngo, Veliz, & McCabe, 2015; McCabe, Veliz, Wilens, & Schulenberg, 2017; Miech, Johnston, O'Malley, Keyes, & Heard, 2015). In a national study of youth, Miech, Johnston, O'Malley, Keyes, et al. (2015) found high school twelfth graders who had a history of little to no illicit drug use and strongly disapproved of marijuana were three times as likely to misuse opioids by age 23 if prescribed an opioid compared to those who were not prescribed an opioid. History of a major depressive episode has also been shown to be associated with prescription opioid misuse in adolescents (Edlund et al., 2015). Risk factors associated specifically with heroin use in youth are less known. Emerging evidence has demonstrated that most adults with heroin use disorder initiated opioid misuse with prescription opioids (Cicero, Ellis, Surratt, & Kurtz, 2014). This has been less studied in youth; however, one sample of youth with heroin use disorder found 90% of participants had a lifetime history of prescription opioid misuse (Subramaniam & Stitzer, 2009). This finding suggests youth with prescription opioid misuse should be assessed for heroin use and monitored for initiation of heroin use.

Youth often access prescription medications for misuse from friends and family (Miech, Johnston, O'Malley, Keyes, et al., 2015; Miech, Johnston, O'Malley, Bachman, & Schulenberg, 2015; Schepis & Krishnan-Sarin, 2009). The majority of twelfth graders with prescription opioid misuse in 2014 acquired them at no cost from a friend or relative (56%) or simply used their own prescription (35.1%) (Miech, Johnston, O'Malley, Bachman, et al., 2015). Among youth prescribed medication with a risk for misuse, estimates of diversion ranged from 13% to 24% (Boyd, McCabe, Cranford, & Young, 2007; McCabe et al., 2011). It is not surprising that youth can access prescription medications for free since most adolescents who are prescribed a medication with potential for misuse have unsupervised access to the medication (Ross-Durow, McCabe, & Boyd, 2013).

Prescription medication misuse and heroin use in youth is important to address because there is substantial morbidity and mortality associated with their use. Hospitalizations for opioid poisonings among adolescents increased twofold between 1997 and 2012 to an annual incidence of 10.2 youth per 100,000 (Gaither, Leventhal, Ryan, & Camenga, 2016). Injection drug use has been linked to threefold increases in hepatitis C between 2010 and 2015 (Centers for Disease Control and Prevention, 2015). Although the prevalence of hepatitis C among adolescents is low, youth who are marginally older, aged 20–29 years, have the highest incidence of acute hepatitis C relative to other age groups (CDC, 2015). In parallel to the increases in hospitalizations for opioid poisonings and the prevalence of hepatitis C, the rate of drug overdose deaths has increased threefold between 1999 and 2014 (Rudd, Seth, David, & Scholl, 2016). In 2015, 52,404 individuals died of a drug overdose (Rudd et al., 2016). Opioids including prescription opioids, heroin, methadone, and fentanyl were involved in 63.1% of overdose deaths in 2015 (Rudd et al., 2016). Benzodiazepines also are commonly involved in opioid overdose deaths (Jones & McAninch, 2015) and both contribute synergistically to respiratory depression. Although the highest rates of drug overdose deaths have been among males aged 25 to 44 years, youth also have been impacted by this epidemic (Rudd et al., 2016). The poisoning death rate among adolescents aged 15–19 years peaked in 2007 with 4.2 deaths per 100,000, largely due to prescription drug overdose (Curtin, Tejada-Vera, & Warner, 2017). After several years of a decline in poisoning death rates in older adolescents, the poisoning death rate increased in 2015 to 3.7 deaths per 100,000 (Curtin et al., 2017).

Treatment

Assessment

As described earlier in this book, a comprehensive assessment of substance use, psychiatric symptoms, and risky behaviors associated with substance use is critical to guide decisions regarding recommended level of care and the adolescent's individualized treatment plan. Assessment considerations specific to youth with prescription medication misuse and heroin use include attention to the frequency and route of use. As mentioned earlier in this chapter, youth who are regularly misusing prescription opioids, heroin, or benzodiazepines can develop physical dependence with withdrawal syndromes. Over time, youth often escalate from oral use to intranasal or intravenous use, which increases the risk for transmission of infectious diseases. Furthermore, women (including teens) using substances, particularly opioids, have high rates of unintended pregnancies (Connery, Albright, & Rodolico, 2014). One study found 47% of adult women with an opioid use disorder currently in treatment first became pregnant when they were under 18 years of age (Black, Stephens, Haber, & Lintzeris, 2012). Testing for pregnancy in females and sexual transmitted diseases in both sexes including human immunodeficiency virus and hepatitis C is an important part of the assessment process.

Collateral information is another essential component of assessment for youth who are misusing prescription medications or heroin. Urine toxicology testing is an objective marker of recent drug use, but some testing can miss detection of several types of opioids and benzodiazepines. Most qualitative toxicology screens that assess for the presence or absence of opiates (i.e., derivatives of morphine) do not detect semisynthetic or synthetic opioids such as oxycodone, hydrocodone, buprenorphine, methadone, or fentanyl. Standard qualitative benzodiazepine tests also frequently miss several benzodiazepines, such as clonazepam (Tenore, 2010). When toxicology testing is used, it is important that providers know what substances the test can assess for, and have an awareness of the specificity and sensitivity of the test that is used. Another source of collateral information includes state run electronic prescription monitoring programs, which can provide details on an individual's controlled substance prescription history.

The mortality associated with prescription drug and heroin overdoses necessitates assessment for overdose history and overdose risk factors as part of the evaluation process. Regardless of the youth's willingness to change their substance use, both adolescents and family members need to be aware of overdose risk factors (Substance Abuse and Mental Health Services Administration, 2013) including using alone, use of sedating substances like alcohol and benzodiazepines in combination with opioids, intravenous drug use, and use after a period of abstinence when the individual has a low tolerance. If an adolescent has used opioids, providers should encourage both the youth and family members to both obtain the prescription medication naloxone (in some states available without a prescription) that can reverse an opioid overdose. Naloxone is an opioid receptor antagonist that can be administered intranasally or injected intramuscularly to temporarily reverse an opioid overdose (Kerensky & Walley, 2017).

Similar to youth with other substance use disorders, youth with opioid and/or benzodiazepine use disorders often struggle early in their illness with limited insight and may be reluctant to engage in care or allow family involvement. Issues with confidentiality are complicated but nonetheless permission to communicate with a family member or legal guardian needs to be obtained given the acute risk for overdose associated with opioid and/or benzodiazepine use. Family pressure through positive and negative reinforcements may be needed to increase an adolescent's willingness to engage in care. Furthermore, some states have models of compulsory treatment for opioid and/or benzodiazepine use disorders in youth, similar to civil commitment for psychiatric illness, that are used when youth are not ready to engage in care and continue to engage in high risk behaviors.

Treatment of Opioid Use Disorders

Although the evidence base is limited, medical treatments including methadone, buprenorphine/naloxone, and extended release naltrexone should be considered for youth with an opioid use disorder (Committee on Substance, U. S. E., & Prevention,

2016). Strong evidence supports the efficacy and effectiveness of these medications in adults with opioid use disorder (US Department of Health & Human Services, 2016). Unfortunately, misconceptions about substituting one addiction for another when using a medication as treatment, assumptions that medication must be lifelong or that recovery is not possible when taking medication may contribute to low rates of medication treatment among adolescents (Bagley, Hadland, Carney, & Saitz, 2017).

Methadone is a full μ-opiate receptor agonist that is frequently used in adults for detoxification and maintenance treatment for opioid use disorders. Methadone can only be prescribed for maintenance treatment in methadone maintenance clinics that provide very structured treatment including daily in person contact until an individual is stabilized. Bell and Mutch (2006) published a retrospective review of 20 adolescent heroin users in Australia with an average age of first heroin use of 14 years and found that methadone treatment was very effective in engaging and retaining youth in substance use disorder care. Unfortunately, there is limited recent data on the use of methadone maintenance treatment in adolescents in the USA (Hopfer, Khuri, Crowley, & Hooks, 2002), and access to methadone for adolescents is restricted to severe cases of opioid use disorder. Federal guidelines specify that adolescents under 18 years of age can only receive methadone if they have had two prior unsuccessful detoxification attempts or outpatient psychosocial treatments, and additionally, have met criteria for an opioid use disorder for 1 year in duration (National Institute on Drug Abuse, 2014).

Buprenorphine is a partial μ-opiate receptor agonist and is FDA approved for use in adolescents 16 years of age and above with moderate or severe opioid use disorder. Although an additional waiver through the Drug Enforcement Agency is required to prescribe buprenorphine, it can generally be prescribed in more traditional outpatient settings with relative ease compared to methadone. The use of buprenorphine in adolescents for opioid detoxification and maintenance has been examined in three randomized controlled trials (Marsch et al., 2005, 2016; Woody et al., 2008).

Marsch et al. (2005) examined the efficacy of buprenorphine compared to clonidine for opioid detoxification over 4 weeks in 36 adolescents with opioid dependence. Clonidine is an alpha-2 adrenergic agonist that is commonly used during detoxification from opioids (Gowing, Farrell, Ali, & White, 2016). While both buprenorphine and clonidine provided relief from withdrawal symptoms, adolescents randomized to buprenorphine were significantly more likely to complete treatment compared to the clonidine group (Marsch et al., 2005). Detoxification with buprenorphine compared to clonidine was also associated with a significantly greater percentage of negative urine toxicology tests. Furthermore, participants receiving buprenorphine were more likely to transition to naltrexone maintenance for continued medication treatment after detoxification compared to those randomized to clonidine.

In a subsequent study, Woody et al. (2008) compared the use of buprenorphine/naloxone for short-term opioid detoxification versus short-term maintenance. Youth aged 16–21 years were randomized to detoxification over 2 weeks versus stabilization and maintenance for 8 weeks and subsequent taper over 4 weeks. Longer treatment with buprenorphine/naloxone when compared to detoxification over 2 weeks was associated with significantly less illicit opioid use, less injection drug use, and less need for additional addiction treatment outside of the treatment received through the study. When buprenorphine/naloxone was discontinued both groups had high rates of opioid use at 1-year follow-up that was assessed through opioid positive urine toxicology tests (mean rates 48–72%).

Another study also evaluated the effects of buprenorphine taper duration among youth aged 16–24 years with opioid dependence (Marsch et al., 2016). Youth tapered off buprenorphine/naloxone over 8 weeks were more likely to have opioid negative toxicology tests and remained engaged in treatment for a longer period compared to youth tapered off buprenorphine/naloxone over 4 weeks. These data suggest that longer treatment with buprenorphine/naloxone for adolescents is more effective than shorter-term detoxification for opioid use disorder treatment. Clinically, at a minimum, it is important to continue maintenance with buprenorphine/naloxone until the adolescent has stabilized—with opioid use disorder (OUD) in remission and adequate coping skills to manage urges, cravings, and withdrawal that can arise during a slow taper off full or partial agonist treatment.

In contrast to methadone and buprenorphine/naloxone, extended release naltrexone is an opioid receptor antagonist with no restrictions around prescribing because it is not a controlled substance. One study has been published to date describing the efficacy of extended release naltrexone in youth (Fishman, Winstanley, Curran, Garrett, & Subramaniam, 2010). Fishman et al. (2010) published a descriptive series of 16 youth, mean age 18.5 years, who received extended release naltrexone while in residential treatment and were followed over 4 months. The majority of the sample (56%) substantially reduced use of illicit opioids or was abstinent from opioids at the 4-month follow-up. One barrier to the use of naltrexone in patients with opioid use disorder is the need for a period of abstinence (e.g., 7–10 days) from opioids prior to starting the medication in order to prevent precipitating opioid withdrawal. Naltrexone is therefore a good treatment option for adolescents who present for treatment early on and are not physiologically dependent on opioids or have been engaged in treatment in a structured environment after detoxification, such as residential treatment or sober living.

The use of medication treatment has increased over the past 10 years but only 18% of adolescents admitted for treatment due to heroin in 2015 had a treatment plan that included pharmacotherapy with buprenorphine/naloxone or methadone (SAMHSA, 2017). When youth are prescribed medication, they often struggle to remain engaged in care relative to older adults. Schuman-Olivier, Claire Greene, Bergman, and Kelly (2014) found that young adults, aged 18–25 years, who were prescribed buprenorphine/naloxone relative to older adults were significantly more likely to drop out of care and more likely to test positive for illicit opioids. More research is needed to determine adolescent-specific barriers for engagement and retention with medication treatment.

As reviewed earlier in this book a large literature supports the efficacy of behavioral therapy for adolescent substance use disorders. Both randomized controlled trials that evaluated medication treatments for opioid use disorders also included therapy for all participants. Behavioral therapy is recommended for all youth with opioid use disorders in addition to medication treatment. The efficacy of different types of behavioral interventions for adolescent opioid use disorders has not been specifically compared to one another. Recently, Godley et al. (2017) evaluated the efficacy of the Adolescent Community Reinforcement Approach for adolescents with a primary opioid use problem compared to adolescents with primary marijuana or alcohol use problems. The Adolescent Community Reinforcement Approach was shown to be feasible and acceptable for adolescents with primary opioid problem use since there were no differences in treatment initiation, engagement in treatment, and satisfaction with treatment between the two groups.

Treatment of Benzodiazepine Use Disorders

There is a very limited evidence base specifically examining treatment for adolescents with benzodiazepine use disorder. There are no FDA-approved medications to treat this disorder even among adults. There is a benzodiazepine antagonist flumazenil that can be used in emergency rooms and inpatient settings for benzodiazepine overdose reversal, but it is associated with its own adverse effects including seizures. As mentioned earlier in the chapter, youth with frequent and regular use of benzodiazepines can develop physical dependence with withdrawal necessitating medical detoxification. In general, the treatment principles applied to adults are applied to adolescents (Weaver, 2015). That is, in more serious cases of withdrawal, benzodiazepines are tapered over time with close medical supervision, often with a long-acting benzodiazepine such as clonazepam that has less potential for abuse, and often in an inpatient setting. Even after withdrawal is treated, it is important to continue treatment for the benzodiazepine use disorder, which may involve individual and/or group counseling with monitoring and involvement of addiction professionals.

Effective Prevention and Harm Reduction Approaches

Prevention of illicit opioid or benzodiazepine use or receipt of inappropriate prescriptions exposing youth to these medications with abuse potential may have profound beneficial effects on delaying and/or preventing development of a use disorder or addiction. As most of the use of opioids and benzodiazepines is through medical prescriptions, family members receiving these medications should ensure their safe storage so that they are not available to youth in the home. When the medication is no longer needed, discard remaining medication through a local drug take back or dispose of it in dirty cat litter so that it is unappealing for subsequent use (Welham, Mount, & Gilson, 2015). Do not flush medication down the toilet as it then enters the water supply. In addition, parents should be alert to all prescriptions that health providers are writing for their children. Do not assume that the provider is up to date and following current recommendations for prescribing of opioids and benzodiazepines. For instance, the CDC currently recommends against opioid analgesics for chronic nonterminal pain, and benzodiazepines are not first-line treatments for mood and anxiety disorders. Educate yourself through trusted resources such as the National Institute on Drug Abuse website that has information specifically geared towards teens, teachers, and parents (https://teens.drugabuse.gov/parents).

It is critical to appreciate that initiating a prescription for an opioid in a person who is opioid naïve is a momentous, potentially life-altering decision (Frieden & Houry, 2016), particularly for an adolescent whose brain is not yet fully developed. It is not currently possible to reliably predict those who will be susceptible to the positive reinforcing effects of opioids or benzodiazepines and become addicted. No race, socioeconomic class or gender is immune. While it may be appropriate for a provider to prescribe several days of prescription opioids after a surgery for a broken bone, providers should be screening patients first for a personal or family history of substance use disorder and be discussing the risks, benefits and alternatives to the prescription. For instance, a patient getting pain relief but also reporting then that s/he has never felt better and is up all night studying or cleaning their room, may be much better off without any further access to opioids. It is not appropriate for a provider to instruct a parent to set their alarm in order to dose a sleeping adolescent with pain medication in order "to stay ahead of the pain." This is a recommendation that could potentially result in a fatal overdose.

If a prescription is agreed upon, ensure that the adolescent understands the significance of it and that it cannot be combined with other central nervous system depressants, like alcohol, because alcohol can increase risk of an overdose when used with opioids and/or benzodiazepines. Parents should hold the controlled substance medication and give it to children or adolescents, ensuring it is taken properly and that there is no temptation to give any away (this is diversion) to friends, family, bullies or other persons that may become aware of and want the prescription medication. Whenever a prescription is given, understand its purpose, have objective markers for its success, understand the monitoring plan for adverse effects and the exit strategy for if the risks are outweighing the benefits. If an opioid prescription is given, do not hesitate to request overdose prevention education and a naloxone overdose kit. This can be life-saving.

Among persons already addicted, the goal is treatment engagement as described above. However, in cases when treatment is not feasible, there are harm reduction approaches that aim to limit the consequences of untreated substance use disorder or drug injection regardless of a diagnosis. Opioid overdose education and naloxone distribution is one example of a harm reduction approach. Among persons using drugs intravenously, providing information on local needle exchanges can help to decrease risky injection drug behaviors, and prevent contracting and spreading of infectious diseases (Fernandes et al., 2017). Many needle exchanges also offer other services such as some primary care services and/or workers who engage with the clients helping to ensure a quick referral if and when the client wants to access treatment. Needle exchanges were a harm reduction approach utilized in Austin, Indiana to prevent further spread of an HIV outbreak among persons injecting prescription opioids (Strathdee & Beyrer, 2015).

Summary

In conclusion, there is increasing availability of prescription opioids and benzodiazepines, which have legitimate and effective medicinal uses. However, they also have psychoactive effects that lend them to misuse and abuse among youth. With repeated use, physical dependence develops as a normal physiologic response to repeated dosing. However, a substance use disorder or addiction may also develop, which is more than tolerance or withdrawal, whereby the brain changes in conscious and unconscious circuits involved with rewards, learning, memory, stress regulation, and affect. Prevention and treatment of these use disorders or addiction can be effective, but are currently underutilized in part because of stigma and lack of understanding. The general public, parents, teachers, and health providers are all encouraged to learn more about heroin and prescription medications as there is no current sign that their availability will decrease in the near future.

References

American Psychiatric Association (APA). (2013). *Desk reference to the diagnostic criteria from DSM-5*. Washington, DC: American Psychiatric Publishing.

Bachhuber, M. A., Hennessy, S., Cunningham, C. O., & Starrels, J. L. (2016). Increasing benzodiazepine prescriptions and overdose mortality in the United States, 1996–2013. *American Journal of Public Health, 106*(4), 686–688. https://doi.org/10.2105/AJPH.2016.303061

Bagley, S. M., Hadland, S. E., Carney, B. L., & Saitz, R. (2017). Addressing stigma in medication treatment of adolescents with opioid use disorder. *Journal of Addiction Medicine, 11*(6), 415–416. https://doi.org/10.1097/ADM.0000000000000348

Bell, J., & Mutch, C. (2006). Treatment retention in adolescent patients treated with methadone or buprenorphine for opioid dependence: A file review. *Drug Alcohol Review, 25*(2), 167–171. https://doi.org/10.1080/09595230500537670

Black, K. I., Stephens, C., Haber, P. S., & Lintzeris, N. (2012). Unplanned pregnancy and contraceptive use in women attending drug treatment services. *Australian and New Zealand Journal of Obstetrics and Gynaecology, 52*(2), 146–150. https://doi.org/10.1111/j.1479-828X.2012.01413.x

Boyd, C. J., Austic, E., Epstein-Ngo, Q., Veliz, P. T., & McCabe, S. E. (2015). A prospective study of adolescents' nonmedical use of anxiolytic and sleep medication. *Psychology of Addictive Behaviors, 29*(1), 184–191. https://doi.org/10.1037/adb0000026

Boyd, C. J., McCabe, S. E., Cranford, J. A., & Young, A. (2007). Prescription drug abuse and diversion among adolescents in a southeast Michigan school district. *Archives of Pediatrics and Adolescent Medicine, 161*(3), 276–281. https://doi.org/10.1001/archpedi.161.3.276

Centers for Disease Control and Prevention. (2015). *National notifiable diseases surveillance system. Surveillance for viral hepatitis—United States 2015*. Retrieved July 11, 2017, from https://www.cdc.gov/hepatitis/statistics/2015surveillance/index.htm.

Cicero, T. J., Ellis, M. S., Surratt, H. L., & Kurtz, S. P. (2014). The changing face of heroin use in the United States: A retrospective analysis of the past 50 years. *JAMA Psychiatry, 71*(7), 821–826. https://doi.org/10.1001/jamapsychiatry.2014.366

Cole, J. B., & Nelson, L. S. (2017). Controversies and carfentanil: We have much to learn about the present state of opioid poisoning. *American Journal of Emergency Medicine, 35*(11), 1743–1745. https://doi.org/10.1016/j.ajem.2017.08.045

Committee on Substance Use & Prevention. (2016). Medication-assisted treatment of adolescents with opioid use disorders. *Pediatrics, 138*(3), 1–6. https://doi.org/10.1542/peds.2016-1893

Connery, H. S., Albright, B. B., & Rodolico, J. M. (2014). Adolescent substance use and unplanned pregnancy: Strategies for risk reduction. *Obstetrics and Gynecology Clinics of North America, 41*(2), 191–203. https://doi.org/10.1016/j.ogc.2014.02.011

Cotto, J. H., Davis, E., Dowling, G. J., Elcano, J. C., Staton, A. B., & Weiss, S. R. (2010). Gender effects on drug use, abuse, and dependence: A special analysis of results from the National Survey on Drug Use and Health. *Gender Medicine, 7*(5), 402–413. https://doi.org/10.1016/j.genm.2010.09.004

Curran, H. V. (1986). Tranquillising memories: A review of the effects of benzodiazepines on human memory. *Biological Psychology, 23*(2), 179–213.

Curran, H. V. (1991). Benzodiazepines, memory and mood: A review. *Psychopharmacology, 105*(1), 1–8.

Curtin, S. C., Tejada-Vera, B., & Warner, M. (2017). *Drug overdose deaths among adolescents aged 15–19 in the United States: 1999–2015*. NCHS data brief, no. 282. Hyattsville, MD: National Center for Health Statistics.

Edlund, M. J., Forman-Hoffman, V. L., Winder, C. R., Heller, D. C., Kroutil, L. A., Lipari, R. N., & Colpe, L. J. (2015). Opioid abuse and depression in adolescents: Results from the National Survey on Drug Use and Health. *Drug and Alcohol Dependence, 152*(2015), 131–138. https://doi.org/10.1016/j.drugalcdep.2015.04.010

Fernandes, R. M., Cary, M., Duarte, G., Jesus, G., Alarcao, J., Torre, C., . . . Carneiro, A. V. (2017). Effectiveness of needle and syringe programmes in people who inject drugs – An overview of systematic reviews. *BMC Public Health*, 17(1), 309. doi:https://doi.org/10.1186/s12889-017-4210-2

Fishman, M. J., Winstanley, E. L., Curran, E., Garrett, S., & Subramaniam, G. (2010). Treatment of opioid dependence in adolescents and young adults with extended release naltrexone: Preliminary case-series and feasibility. *Addiction, 105*(9), 1669–1676. https://doi.org/10.1111/j.1360-0443.2010.03015.x

Frieden, T. R., & Houry, D. (2016). Reducing the risks of relief—The CDC opioid-prescribing guideline. *New England Journal of Medicine, 374*(16), 1501–1504. https://doi.org/10.1056/NEJMp1515917

Gaither, J. R., Leventhal, J. M., Ryan, S. A., & Camenga, D. R. (2016). National trends in hospitalizations for opioid poisonings among children and adolescents, 1997 to 2012. *JAMA Pediatrics, 170*(12), 1195–1201. https://doi.org/10.1001/jamapediatrics.2016.2154

Godley, M. D., Passetti, L. L., Subramaniam, G. A., Funk, R. R., Smith, J. E., & Meyers, R. J. (2017). Adolescent Community Reinforcement Approach implementation and treatment outcomes for youth with opioid problem use. *Drug and Alcohol Dependence, 174*, 9–16. https://doi.org/10.1016/j.drugalcdep.2016.12.029

Gowing, L., Farrell, M., Ali, R., & White, J. M. (2016). Alpha(2)-adrenergic agonists for the management of opioid withdrawal. *Cochrane Database of Systematic Reviews*, (5), CD002024. https://doi.org/10.1002/14651858.CD002024.pub5 Hoboken, NJ: John Wiley & Sons, Inc.

Hopfer, C. J., Khuri, E., Crowley, T. J., & Hooks, S. (2002). Adolescent heroin use: A review of the descriptive and treatment literature. *Journal of Substance Abuse Treatment, 23*(3), 231–237.

Johnston, L. D., O'Malley, P. M., Miech, R. A., Bachman, J. G., & Schulenberg, J. E. (2016). *Monitoring the Future national survey results on drug use, 1975–2015: Overview, key findings on adolescent drug use*. Ann Arbor, MI: Institute for Social Research, The University of Michigan.

Jones, C. M., & McAninch, J. K. (2015). Emergency department visits and overdose deaths from combined use of opioids and benzodiazepines. *American Journal of Preventive Medicine, 49*(4), 493–501. https://doi.org/10.1016/j.amepre.2015.03.040

Kann, L., McManus, T., Harris, W. A., Shanklin, S. L., Flint, K. H., Hawkins, J., … Zaza, S. (2016). Youth risk behavior surveillance – United States, 2015. *MMWR Surveillance Summaries, 65*(6), 1–174. https://doi.org/10.15585/mmwr.ss6506a1

Kerensky, T., & Walley, A. Y. (2017). Opioid overdose prevention and naloxone rescue kits: What we know and what we don't know. *Addiction Science & Clinical Practice, 12*(1), 1–7. https://doi.org/10.1186/s13722-016-0068-3

Larance, B., Degenhardt, L., Lintzeris, N., Winstock, A., & Mattick, R. (2011). Definitions related to the use of pharmaceutical opioids: Extramedical use, diversion, non-adherence and aberrant medication-related behaviours. *Drug Alcohol Review, 30*(3), 236–245. https://doi.org/10.1111/j.1465-3362.2010.00283.x

Marsch, L. A., Bickel, W. K., Badger, G. J., Stothart, M. E., Quesnel, K. J., Stanger, C., & Brooklyn, J. (2005). Comparison of pharmacological treatments for opioid-dependent adolescents: A randomized controlled trial. *Archives of General Psychiatry, 62*(10), 1157–1164.

Marsch, L. A., Moore, S. K., Borodovsky, J. T., Solhkhah, R., Badger, G. J., Semino, S., … Ducat, E. (2016). A randomized controlled trial of buprenorphine taper duration among opioid-dependent adolescents and young adults. *Addiction, 111*(8), 1406–1415. https://doi.org/10.1111/add.13363

McCabe, S. E., Veliz, P., Wilens, T. E., & Schulenberg, J. E. (2017). Adolescents' prescription stimulant use and adult functional outcomes: A national prospective study. *Journal of the American Academy of Child & Adolescent Psychiatry, 56*(3), 226–233.e4. https://doi.org/10.1016/j.jaac.2016.12.008

McCabe, S. E., & West, B. T. (2014). Medical and nonmedical use of prescription benzodiazepine anxiolytics among U.S. high school seniors. *Addictive Behaviors, 39*(5), 959–964. https://doi.org/10.1016/j.addbeh.2014.01.009

McCabe, S. E., West, B. T., Teter, C. J., Ross-Durow, P., Young, A., & Boyd, C. J. (2011). Characteristics associated with the diversion of controlled medications among adolescents. *Drug and Alcohol Dependence, 118*(2-3), 452–458. https://doi.org/10.1016/j.drugalcdep.2011.05.004

McKim, W. (1986). *Chapter 8: The benzodiazepines drugs and behavior: An introduction to behavioral pharmacology*. Englewood Cliffs, NJ: Prentice Hall.

Miech, R., Johnston, L., O'Malley, P. M., Keyes, K. M., & Heard, K. (2015). Prescription opioids in adolescence and future opioid misuse. *Pediatrics, 136*(5), e1169–e1177. https://doi.org/10.1542/peds.2015-1364

Miech, R. A., Johnston, L. D., O'Malley, P. M., Bachman, J. G., & Schulenberg, J. E. (2015). *Monitoring the future national survey results on drug use, 1975–2014: Vol. I. Secondary school students*. Ann Arbor, MI: Institute for Social Research, The University of Michigan.

National Institute on Drug Abuse (NIDA). (2014). Principles of adolescent substance use disorder treatment: A research-based guide. Retrieved from https://www.drugabuse.gov/publications/principles-adolescent-substance-use-disorder-treatment-research-based-guide

Nelson, L. S., Juurlink, D. N., & Perrone, J. (2015). Addressing the opioid epidemic. *JAMA, 314*(14), 1453–1454. https://doi.org/10.1001/jama.2015.12397

O'Donnell, J. K., Halpin, J., Mattson, C. L., Goldberger, B. A., & Gladden, R. M. (2017). Deaths involving fentanyl, fentanyl analogs, and U-47700 – 10 States, July–December 2016. *Morbidity Mortality Weekly Report (MMWR), 66*(43), 1197–1202. https://doi.org/10.15585/mmwr.mm6643e1

Palamar, J. J., Shearston, J. A., Dawson, E. W., Mateu-Gelabert, P., & Ompad, D. C. (2016). Nonmedical opioid use and heroin use in a nationally representative sample of us high school seniors. *Drug and Alcohol Dependence, 158*, 132–138. https://doi.org/10.1016/j.drugalcdep.2015.11.005

Rickert, V. I., Wiemann, C. M., & Berenson, A. B. (2000). Flunitrazepam: More than a date rape drug. *Journal of Pediatric & Adolescent Gynecology, 13*(1), 37–42.
Rigg, K. K., & Ford, J. A. (2014). The misuse of benzodiazepines among adolescents: Psychosocial risk factors in a national sample. *Drug and Alcohol Dependence, 137*, 137–142. https://doi.org/10.1016/j.drugalcdep.2014.01.026
Ross-Durow, P. L., McCabe, S. E., & Boyd, C. J. (2013). Adolescents' access to their own prescription medications in the home. *Journal of Adolescent Health, 53*(2), 260–264. https://doi.org/10.1016/j.jadohealth.2013.02.012
Rudd, R. A., Seth, P., David, F., & Scholl, L. (2016). Increases in drug and opioid-involved overdose deaths – United States, 2010–2015. *Morbidity Mortality Weekly Report (MMWR), 65*(5051), 1445–1452. https://doi.org/10.15585/mmwr.mm655051e1
Schepis, T. S., & Krishnan-Sarin, S. (2009). Sources of prescriptions for misuse by adolescents: Differences in sex, ethnicity, and severity of misuse in a population-based study. *Journal of the American Academy of Child & Adolescent Psychiatry, 48*(8), 828–836. https://doi.org/10.1097/CHI.0b013e3181a8130d
Schuckit, M. A. (2016). Treatment of opioid-use disorders. *New England Journal of Medicine, 375*(16), 1596–1597. https://doi.org/10.1056/NEJMc1610830
Schuman-Olivier, Z., Claire Greene, M., Bergman, B. G., & Kelly, J. F. (2014). Is residential treatment effective for opioid use disorders? A longitudinal comparison of treatment outcomes among opioid dependent, opioid misusing, and non-opioid using emerging adults with substance use disorder. *Drug and Alcohol Dependence, 144*, 178–185. https://doi.org/10.1016/j.drugalcdep.2014.09.009
Schwartz, R. H., Milteer, R., & LeBeau, M. A. (2000). Drug-facilitated sexual assault ('date rape'). *Southern Medical Journal, 93*(6), 558–561.
Strathdee, S. A., & Beyrer, C. (2015). Threading the needle—How to stop the HIV outbreak in rural Indiana. *New England Journal of Medicine, 373*(5), 397–399. https://doi.org/10.1056/NEJMp1507252
Subramaniam, G. A., & Stitzer, M. A. (2009). Clinical characteristics of treatment-seeking prescription opioid vs. heroin-using adolescents with opioid use disorder. *Drug and Alcohol Dependence, 101*(1–2), 13–19. https://doi.org/10.1016/j.drugalcdep.2008.10.015
Substance Abuse and Mental Health Services Administration (SAMHSA). (2013). *SAMHSA Opioid Overdose Prevention Toolkit*. (HHS Publication No. SMA 13-4742). Rockville, MD: Substance Abuse and Mental Health Services Administration.
Substance Abuse and Mental Health Services Administration (SAMHSA), Center for Behavioral Health Statistics and Quality. (2016a). *Key substance use and mental health indicators in the United States: Results from the 2015 national survey on drug use and health* (HHS Publication No. SMA 16-4984, NSDUH Series H-51). Retrieved from July 3, 2017, http:///www.samhsa.gov/data.
Substance Abuse and Mental Health Services Administration (SAMHSA), Center for Behavioral Health Statistics and Quality. (2016b). *2015 National survey on drug use and health: Detailed tables*. Rockville, MD: Substance Abuse and Mental Health Services Administration.
Substance Abuse and Mental Health Services Administration (SAMHSA), Center for Behavioral Health Statistics and Quality. (2017). *Treatment Episode Data Set (TEDS): 2005–2015. National admissions to substance abuse treatment services*. BHSIS Series S-91 (HHS Publication No. SMA 17-5037). Rockville, MD: Substance Abuse and Mental Health Services Administration.
Tenore, P. L. (2010). Advanced urine toxicology testing. *Journal of Addictive Diseases, 29*(4), 436–448. 927630617 [pii]. https://doi.org/10.1080/10550887.2010.509277
U.S. Department of Health & Human Services (USDHHS), Office of the Surgeon General. (2016). Facing addiction in America: The Surgeon General's report on alcohol, drugs, and health. Washington, DC: HHS.
Volkow, N. D., Koob, G. F., & McLellan, A. T. (2016). Neurobiologic advances from the brain disease model of addiction. *New England Journal of Medicine, 374*(4), 363–371. https://doi.org/10.1056/NEJMra1511480

Wakeman, S. E., & Rich, J. D. (2018). Barriers to medications for addiction treatment: How stigma kills. *Substance Use & Misuse, 53*(2), 330–333. https://doi.org/10.1080/10826084.2017.1363238

Weaver, M. F. (2015). Prescription sedative misuse and abuse. *Yale Journal of Biology and Medicine, 88*(3), 247–256.

Welham, G. C., Mount, J. K., & Gilson, A. M. (2015). Type and frequency of opioid pain medications returned for disposal. *Drugs Real World Outcomes, 2*(2), 129–135. https://doi.org/10.1007/s40801-015-0019-4

Woody, G. E., Poole, S. A., Subramaniam, G., Dugosh, K., Bogenschutz, M., Abbott, P., … Fudala, P. (2008). Extended vs short-term buprenorphine-naloxone for treatment of opioid-addicted youth: A randomized trial. *JAMA, 300*(17), 2003–2011. https://doi.org/10.1001/jama.2008.574

The Prevention and Treatment of Adolescent Stimulant and Methamphetamine Use

Justin C. Strickland and William W. Stoops

Introduction

Stimulant use remains a significant public health concern despite decades of research on prevention and treatment efforts. The use of cocaine, amphetamine, and methamphetamine produces a range of problems for the individual, specifically, and society, broadly. These costs include premature mortality, crime and lost productivity, transmission of infectious diseases, medical complications such as cardiovascular problems, and exacerbation of mental health conditions (Cavazos-Rehg et al., 2009; Havakuk, Rezkalla, & Kloner, 2017; Pasic, Russo, Ries, & Roy-Byrne, 2007; Shoptaw, King, et al., 2009; Stein, 1999). Stimulant misuse is particularly worrisome for adolescent populations because substance use can alter developmental trajectories during a period of dramatic physiological and psychological growth (Crowley & Riggs, 1995). High-risk behaviors already prominent in adolescents, such as violence, aggression, and unprotected sexual encounters, are also likely to increase under the influence of drugs (Jessor & Jessor, 1977). The pervasive impact

J. C. Strickland
Department of Psychology, University of Kentucky College of Arts and Sciences, Lexington, KY, USA

W. W. Stoops (✉)
Department of Psychology, University of Kentucky College of Arts and Sciences, Lexington, KY, USA

Department of Behavioral Science, University of Kentucky College of Medicine, Lexington, KY, USA

Department of Psychiatry, University of Kentucky College of Medicine, Lexington, KY, USA

Center on Drug and Alcohol Research, University of Kentucky College of Medicine, Lexington, KY, USA
e-mail: william.stoops@uky.edu

C. G. Leukefeld, T. P. Gullotta (eds.), *Adolescent Substance Abuse*, Issues in Children's and Families' Lives, https://doi.org/10.1007/978-3-319-90611-9_9

of illicit substance use underscores the need for evidence-based prevention and treatment strategies targeting adolescent stimulant use.

This chapter examines the history and characteristics of stimulant use and misuse, the pharmacology and clinical effects of stimulants, and expected clinical outcomes for stimulant-using adolescents. The literature is also reviewed for current primary prevention and treatment approaches targeting adolescent stimulant use. *Primary prevention* is defined to include planned actions of health promotion that help adolescents prevent predictable problems, protect existing states of health as well as healthy functioning, and promote desired goals for adolescents. *Treatment* is defined as activities that focus on helping adolescents reduce problems associated with ongoing stimulant use/misuse and that change individual stimulant use behavior. This chapter focuses on cocaine, amphetamine, and methamphetamine because these substances represent commonly used and studied psychomotor stimulants in adolescent as well as adult populations (Center for Behavioral Health Statistics and Quality, 2016; Johnston, O'Malley, Miech, Bachman, & Schulenberg, 2017).

History of Stimulant Misuse

Cocaine is an alkaloid compound derived from the naturally occurring coca plant. The leaves of the coca plant were historically used by indigenous cultures in South America for medicinal and religious purposes. Cocaine alkaloid was isolated from the coca leaf in 1800s and soon after widely utilized in medical tonics and other commercially available products (e.g., the original Coca-Cola® formulation; Grinspoon & Bakalar, 1981). Following concerns over the health effects of cocaine use, cocaine was classified as a narcotic and put under the control of the US federal government with the 1914 Harrison Narcotics Act. Today, cocaine remains a class II schedule substance in the USA regulated by the Drug Enforcement Agency and is medically used as a topical anesthetic in eye, mouth, and nasal surgery.

The amphetamines are a group of synthetic chemicals first formulated as amphetamine isomers from ephedrine in the late 1880s. The popularity of amphetamines rose throughout the early twentieth century when they were used to promote alertness, particularly among soldiers in World War II. The nonmedical use of amphetamines was outlawed following that war citing widespread misuse and their potential negative health impact. Amphetamine isomers (e.g., Dexedrine®, Adderall®) are today used medically primarily in the treatment of attention deficit disorder/attention deficit hyperactivity disorder (ADD/ADHD). However, diversion of these medications for recreational use remains a concern, particularly among adolescent populations (Garnier et al., 2010; McCabe, Teter, & Boyd, 2004; McCabe, West, Teter, & Boyd, 2014; Wilens et al., 2008).

More recently, methamphetamine has emerged as a widely misused stimulant. The rise of methamphetamine is due, in part, to the ability to simply, but dangerously, synthesize it using common household items through pseudoephedrine reduction.

Production is further simplified for manufacture by small clandestine laboratories in a process known as the "shake 'n' bake" method (Brzeczko, Leech, & Stark, 2013). These chemical reduction methods are relatively easy to learn and instructions readily accessible to adolescents through varied resources, including Internet message boards and other online forums (e.g., erowid.org; bluelight.com). Increases in domestic regulation of methamphetamine precursors and seizures of local laboratories have been offset by a corresponding growth in international methamphetamine production and trafficking into the USA (Cunningham, Finlay, & Stoecker, 2015; Shukla, Crump, & Chrisco, 2012).

Prevalence of Adolescent Stimulant Use

Stimulant use remains a significant concern for adolescents (see Fig. 1). Findings from the 2016 Monitoring the Future Study (Johnston et al., 2017) indicate that by eighth grade, 1.4% of students have tried cocaine, 5.7% have tried amphetamines not prescribed to them, and 0.6% have tried methamphetamine. These numbers grow by tenth grade to 2.1%, 8.8%, and 0.7%, respectively, and by twelfth grade to 4.0%, 10.0%, and 1.2%, respectively. Important to note is that these estimates represent a substantial decrease over the last decade (see Fig. 1), wherein 8.5% of twelfth graders reported trying cocaine, 12.4% reported trying amphetamines, and 4.4% reported trying methamphetamine in 2006. Such decreases are consistent with general trends observed for adolescent substance use across most drug classes (Johnston et al., 2017). However, the substantial number of adolescents still misusing stimulants and the potential negative health consequences of such use reinforces the need for primary prevention efforts and evidence-based treatments.

Pharmacological and Clinical Characteristics of Stimulant Misuse

The primary pharmacological effects of stimulants are mediated by actions on the central nervous system and monoamine neurotransmitters (Elliott & Beveridge, 2005; Howell & Negus, 2014; Rocha, 2003; Rothman & Baumann, 2003; Uhl, Hall, & Sora, 2002). The following section reviews these pharmacological mechanisms, characteristic patterns of use, and the short- and long-term health consequences of cocaine, amphetamines, and methamphetamine use for adolescents and emerging adults.

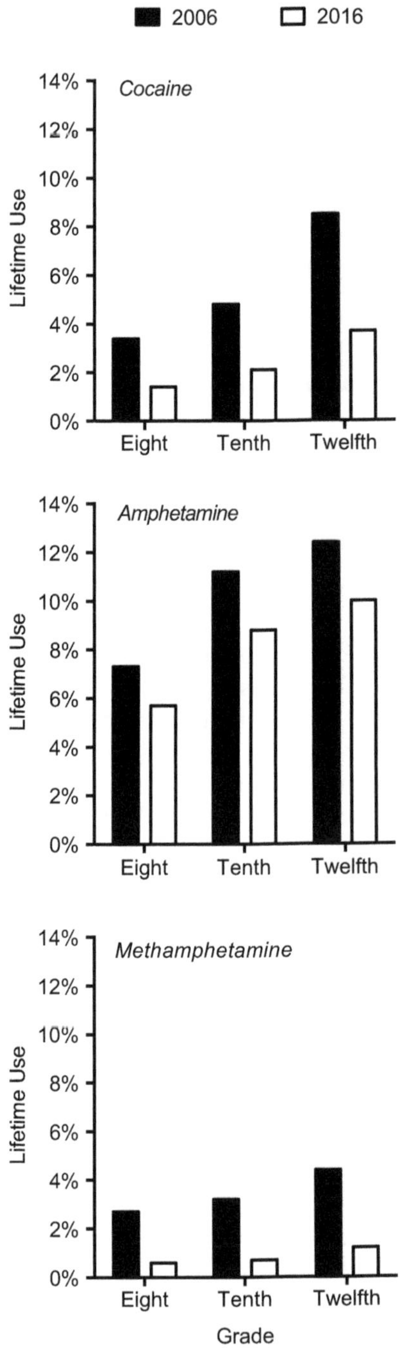

Fig. 1 Lifetime prevalence of illicit stimulant use by US adolescents. Depicted are 2006 (black bars) and 2016 (white bars) prevalence estimates of lifetime illicit cocaine (top), amphetamine (middle), and methamphetamine (bottom) use among adolescents in eight, tenth, and twelfth grade. Adapted from data in "*Monitoring the Future national survey results on drug use, 1975–2016: Overview, key findings on adolescent drug use*," by L. D. Johnston, P. M. O'Malley, R. A. Miech, J. G. Bachman, and J. E. Schulenberg, 2017, Ann Arbor, MI: Institute for Social Research, The University of Michigan

Receptor Pharmacology

Cocaine's primary mechanism of action is reuptake inhibition at monoamine transporters (i.e., dopamine, norepinephrine, and serotonin). The net effect of this reuptake inhibition is increased synaptic monoamine concentrations and sustained activation of corresponding neurotransmitter systems. Recent evidence also suggests that cocaine may produce additional passive outflow of dopamine by fixing the dopamine transporter in an outward facing confirmation (Heal, Gosden, & Smith, 2014). Cocaine acts in vitro with relative equal potency at each of the monoamine transporters (Rothman & Baumann, 2003). Research has historically focused on dopamine reuptake inhibition as the primary mediator of abuse-related effects (Nutt, Lingford-Hughes, Erritzoe, & Stokes, 2015; Wise & Bozarth, 1987). However, the last decade has witnessed an increasing focus on the importance of serotonergic systems (e.g., Cunningham & Anastasio, 2014; Howell & Cunningham, 2015; Müller, Carey, Huston, & De Souza Silva, 2007) and noradrenergic systems (e.g., Sofuoglu & Sewell, 2009; Weinshenker & Schroeder, 2007) as they relate to cocaine use and misuse.

Amphetamine and methamphetamine also act on the monoamine transporters. The primary mechanism of action for amphetamines is to encourage neurotransmitter release in contrast to the reuptake inhibition produced by cocaine (Rothman et al., 2001; Rothman & Baumann, 2003). Amphetamines brought into the cell can stimulate vesicular neurotransmitter release into the synaptic cleft through a reverse transporter mechanism. Amphetamines have high potency for dopamine and norepinephrine transporters, but are comparatively less potent at the serotonin transporter (Alexander et al., 2005; Rothman et al., 2001; Wee et al., 2005). The dextrorotary forms of amphetamines (D-amphetamine and D-methamphetamine) show greater potency for the dopamine transporter than the levorotary ones (l-amphetamine and l-methamphetamine) (Rothman et al., 2001; Rothman & Baumann, 2003) and many medical versions use varying racemic or combined formulations (e.g., Adderall® is 75% D-amphetamine and 25% L-amphetamine).

Routes of Administration and Use Patterns

Cocaine is typically administered by insufflation ("snorting") or inhalation ("smoking") when used recreationally, but is also used by oral and intravenous routes under some circumstances. Cocaine hydrochloride is a white powder salt that is water-soluble and thus may be insufflated and absorbed through the vascular region of the nasal cavity or dissolved for intravenous use. "Crack cocaine" is a freebase preparation of cocaine with a hard, rocklike appearance. The low melting point of these rock crystals means that crack cocaine may be heated and the vapors inhaled for smoked use. Cocaine is readily absorbed in the bloodstream and produces its peaks effects within 10–20 min when insufflated and within minutes when inhaled or injected (Volkow et al., 2000). Cocaine is metabolized quickly with a half-life of 30–90 min and apparent effects that diminish within an hour following administration (Isenschmid, Fischman, Foltin, & Caplan, 1992; Jeffcoat, Perez-Reyes, Hill, Sadler, & Cook, 1989; Newton, De La Garza II, Kalechstein, & Nestor, 2005). This rapid onset–offset means that recreational use may progress to binge patterns of use characterized by excessive and escalating drug intake over short periods of time (Gawin, 1991; Gawin & Kleber, 1985).

Amphetamines are typically administered for medical use by the oral route (e.g., Adderall® for ADHD). Recreationally, however, amphetamines are commonly insufflated or injected. A pure form of D-methamphetamine hydrochloride known as "crystal meth" or "ice" is also commonly used and may be melted and its vapors inhaled similar to crack cocaine. Amphetamines, and D-methamphetamine in particular, have a long duration of action due to slower metabolism and a half-life of 8–12 h depending on the compound formulation (Angrist, Corwin, Bartlik, & Cooper, 1987; Cruickshank & Dyer, 2009; Harris et al., 2003). Binge patterns exemplified by continuous intake and no sleep for multiple days are also typical for methamphetamine use (Cruickshank & Dyer, 2009; Simon et al., 2002).

Short-Term Effects

Cocaine and the amphetamines produce robust effects on the cardiovascular system, including increased heart rate, blood pressure, and respiration rate (Foltin & Fischman, 1990; Foltin, Fischman, Pedroso, & Pearlson, 1988; Marks et al., 2016; Mendelson et al., 2006; Stoops, Pike, Hays, Glaser, & Rush, 2015). Acute high doses also carry the risk of acute overdose primarily due to respiratory collapse from seizures and convulsions, stroke, or myocardial infarction. Anorectic or appetite-suppressant effects also accompany the acute administration of cocaine and amphetamines.

Acute stimulant administration also produces dose-dependent positive subjective effects, including improved mood, increased talkativeness, and decreased fatigue (Foltin & Fischman, 1991; Hart, Ward, Haney, Foltin, & Fischman, 2001; Hart et al., 2008; Kirkpatrick et al., 2012; Rush, Baker, & Wright, 1999; Stoops, Glaser, Fillmore, & Rush, 2004). Stimulants can improve performance on physical endurance and cognitive-performance tasks, although these effects often depend on the dose administered. Desirable effects related to arousal and/or cognitive-performance are a primary reason that adolescent populations report seeking out diverted stimulant medications as "study aids" (Teter, McCabe, Cranford, Boyd, & Guthrie, 2005; Vrecko, 2015; Wilens et al., 2008). Higher acute doses can also produce untoward psychotic effects, including hallucinations, paranoid delusions, and stereotyped behaviors.

Long-Term Effects

Chronic stimulant administration can result in tolerance and withdrawal upon cessation of use. Acute tolerance following repeated administration over short periods of time has also been observed for cocaine and methamphetamine (Comer et al., 2001; Ward, Haney, Fischman, & Foltin, 1997). Such tolerance to the positive subjective effects of stimulants can result in heavier and more frequent use, which exacerbates the negative effects of cardiovascular and brain function. Although withdrawal symptoms are not readily apparent compared to other substances such as opioids or alcohol, withdrawal from cocaine or amphetamine use can result in depression, anxiety, and sleep and appetite disturbances (Gossop, Bradley, & Brewis, 1982; Shoptaw, Kao, Heinzerling, & Ling, 2009). As noted earlier in this section, tolerance and withdrawal may reinforce the "crash-binge" use pattern characterized by bouts of intense and heavy use followed by several days of depressed mood and increased sleep and food intake (Cruickshank & Dyer, 2009; McGregor et al., 2005; Simon et al., 2002).

Long-term stimulant use can also disrupt physical health, particularly in adolescent populations (e.g., Mone, Gillman, Miller, Herman, & Lipshultz, 2004; Rawson, Gonzales, McCann, & Ling, 2007). Chronic cocaine and amphetamine misuse causes damage to the cardiovascular and related organ systems, including heart muscle inflammation and aortic ruptures, and increased risk of myocardial ischemia or infarction (Havakuk et al., 2017). Regular stimulant insufflation also damages the nasal vasculature and can result in the loss of smell and nasal septum inflammation (Glauser & Queen, 2007; Valencia & Castillo, 2008). Similarly, chronic inhalation of cocaine or methamphetamine can cause lung damage and aggravate existing pulmonary problems (Drent, Wijnen, & Bast, 2012; Susskind, Weber, Volkow, & Hitzemann, 1991; Tashkin et al., 1992; Wells et al., 2010). The anorexic effects of stimulants may also result in the chronic appetite loss and malnourishment. This concern is particularly troubling for adolescents who may use stimulants to engage in unhealthy weight loss behaviors or whose use may disrupt natural growth and development (e.g., Berman, Kuczenski, McCracken, & London, 2009; Dutta et al., 2006; Neale, Abraham, & Russell, 2009).

Likewise, the chronic use of stimulants during adolescents can result in neurobiological damage and changes in those brain systems associated with an increased susceptibility to other substance misuse, physical health problems, and mental health concerns (e.g., Lyoo et al., 2015; Pianca et al., 2017). Adolescent methamphetamine users exhibit greater and more widespread damage to gray and white matter, particularly in the frontostriatal region, as compared to adult users (Lyoo et al., 2015). Cocaine use during adolescence is also associated with elevated serum levels of interleukin (IL) inflammatory markers IL-6 and IL-10 as well as oxidative stress markers (Pianca et al., 2017). Notably, one study found that these increases in IL-6 and IL-10 were reduced following 20 days of abstinence suggesting possible remediation of this inflammatory damage upon treatment and use cessation (Pianca et al., 2017). Changes in central nervous and immune systems function may

Table 1 Primary prevention efforts for adolescent stimulant use

Method	Description	Example(s)	Evidence
Regulation and Law Enforcement	Actions designed to reduce the supply of and/or demand for drugs through laws and policies	*United Nations Single Convention on Narcotic Drugs*	*Weak Evidence*
Mass Media Campaigns	Campaigns typically focused on preventing illicit substance use through printed, televised, or online public service announcements (PSAs).	*The Meth Project*	*Weak Evidence*
School-Based Programs	Programs delivered in the school setting. May include didactic teaching and education and/or interactive methods (skill building, role-playing)	*Drug Abuse Resistance Education (D.A.R.E.); Project Towards No Drug Abuse (Project TND)*	*Weak Evidence (Didactic Programs) Good Evidence (Interactive Programs)*
Family-Based Programs	Family involvement to reduce pathways to initiation and improve the psychosocial development of the child	*Preparing for the Drug Free Years; Strengthening Families Program; Family Empowerment Intervention*	*Mixed Evidence/ Limited Data for Stimulant-Specific Outcomes*

Note. All evaluations represent the authors' perspective after review of the literature
Created by authors Strickland and Stoops (2017)

worsen already ongoing high rates of comorbidity between substance misuse and mental health problems in adolescents. Prospective studies, such as the ongoing Adolescent Brain Cognitive Development study (abcdstudy.org), will be essential for investigating the neurobiological mechanisms that are antecedent to and consequence of adolescent cocaine and amphetamine use.

Primary Prevention Efforts

The following section reviews primary prevention efforts designed to promote the desired goal of preventing stimulant use initiation in adolescents (see Table 1). Compared to alcohol and tobacco use, there are few studies with a primary focus on adolescent stimulant use. However, in several cases those approaches targeting alcohol or tobacco prevention have shown similar positive outcomes for preventing stimulant use.

Population and Community-Level Efforts: Regulation and Media Campaigns

Regulatory efforts include actions designed to reduce the supply of and/or demand for drugs through the laws, policies, and other enforcement measures. The nonmedical use of stimulants is prohibited under the United Nations Single Convention on Narcotic Drugs resulting in the prohibition of use in many countries, including the USA. Although strict enforcement of drug laws and sanctions is frequently noted as a primary prevention mechanism, the evidence is mixed for the utility of these policies for reducing substance use and may have the untoward effect of increasing public health harms such as market violence and risky injection practices (Kerr, Small, & Wood, 2005; Strang et al., 2012; Werb et al., 2011). Other regulatory strategies, such as minimum drinking or smoking ages and taxation efforts, have shown some positive effects for deterring alcohol and tobacco use and harms among adolescents (Botello-Harbaum et al., 2009; DiFranza, Savageau, & Fletcher, 2009; Lewit, Hyland, Kerrebrock, & Cummings, 1997; McCartt, Hellinga, & Kirley, 2010; Voas, Tippetts, & Fell, 2003). Many of those strategies (e.g., advertising regulations or bans) cannot be applied to curtail stimulant use, however, given that these drugs are only legally available through prescription and not on the commercial market.

Another commonly noted approach to prevent adolescent stimulant use is mass media campaigns (Ferri, Allara, Bo, Gasparrini, & Faggiano, 2013). These campaigns typically focus on preventing illicit substance use through printed, televised, or online public service announcements (PSAs). Some of these campaigns have specifically targeted adolescent stimulant misuse, one of the most notable being *The Montana Meth Project* and later *The Meth Project* (Siebel & Mange, 2009). Initiated in Montana and then expanded to seven other states after an apparent success, this campaign utilized a marketing strategy of television, radio, print, and social media advertising combined with community outreach to highlight the risks of methamphetamine through shocking images and slogans of use and users (e.g., "15 bucks for sex isn't normal. But on meth it is"). Minimal reductions in methamphetamine use were observed across each of the eight states adopting the program, however, after adjusting for preexisting downward trends in use (Anderson, 2010; Anderson & Elsea, 2015; Erceg-Hurn, 2008; Marsh, Copes, & Linnemann, 2017). A recent qualitative study with current and former methamphetamine users also reported that individuals found the dramatized images to be ineffective at curtailing their own drug use and that such depictions represented an inauthentic "worst-case" scenario that was not relevant to and symbolically distant from their experience (Marsh et al., 2017). These and similar depictions of substance-using populations as weak, lacking control, or "a junky" can impede recovery efforts by stigmatizing substance use or creating a symbolic boundary between oneself and a problematic user in need of help (e.g., Marsh et al., 2017; Radcliffe & Stevens, 2008; Rodner, 2005). Findings from *The Meth Project* are consistent with at least two recent systematic reviews on mass media campaigns for preventing illicit adolescent substance use (Allara, Ferri, Bo, Gasparrini, & Faggiano, 2015; Ferri et al., 2013). These reviews concluded that mass media campaigns have minimal effect on adolescent illicit substance use. They also exhort that caution should be taken for future campaign development given the potential for adverse effects, such stigmatizing substance users and/or increasing awareness of and interest in illicit substance use (i.e., the "boomerang effect" or iatrogenic effects) (e.g., Allara et al., 2015; Hornik, 2006; Marsh et al., 2017; Scheier & Grenard, 2010).

School-Based Programs

School-based interventions have received extensive attention for preventing adolescent substance and stimulant use (Carney, Myers, Louw, & Okwundu, 2016; Faggiano, Minozzi, Versino, & Buscemi, 2014). Although these interventions are limited by their inability to reach at-risk adolescents who frequently miss or have left school, they do represent a straightforward and potentially useful venue for prevention (and treatment) delivery. Many of these programs use didactic teaching and education regarding drug use and consequences. Despite the popularity of such an approach, negative outcomes have generally been reported for reducing substance use among adolescents (Paglia & Room, 1999; Tobler et al., 2000). For example, *Drug Abuse Resistance Education* (*D.A.R.E.*) is a school-based program providing information about the dangers of recreational drug use by local police officers. *D.A.R.E.* remains a popular and widely used program in the educational setting despite numerous studies and meta-analytic reviews demonstrating limited effects on long-term adolescent drug use (Clayton, Cattarello, & Johnstone, 1996; Lynam et al., 1999; Pan & Bai, 2009; West & O'Neal, 2004). Clinically useful school-based programs require varied, interactive teaching methods to enhance important life skills, including communication, coping, and assertiveness (Tobler et al., 2000). In fact, a modified version of *D.A.R.E.* *(D.A.R.E. Plus)* incorporating parental participation, skill building, and extracurricular activities resulted in better prevention of adolescent substance use (Perry et al., 2003). A meta-analysis of 207 studies found that inclusion of interactive components significantly predicted positive outcomes for school-based preventive efforts (Tobler et al., 2000). In contrast, non-interactive lectures delivering only affective development or drug knowledge demonstrated small effects.

In this respect, social competence and social norms approaches have demonstrated positive outcomes for preventing adolescent substance drug use (Faggiano et al., 2014; Thomas, McLellan, & Perera, 2013). Social competence programs are grounded in social learning theory, which posits that adolescents learn drug-use behaviors through modeling, imitation, and selective reinforcement and punishment by substance-using peers. Social norm efforts target substance use through self-management skills designed to correct incorrect beliefs about peer substance use (e.g., overestimation) and to teach skills associated with recognizing high-risk situations and refusal skills. A recent meta-analysis indicated that these programs alone and combined produce small, but consistent, protective effects for illicit drug use compared to usual curriculum (Faggiano et al., 2014). Little research exists specifically evaluating stimulant use. However, some studies have revealed positive effects on "hard drug" use (e.g., combined cocaine, hallucinogens, inhalants, stimulants, ecstasy, and "other"). For example, *Project Towards No Drug Abuse* (*Project TND*) is a classroom-based prevention program combining social competence and norm approaches to improve motivation/listening skills, provide information about the negative consequences of substance use and correct misperceptions, and teach coping, decision-making, and refusal skills to encourage health-promoting behavior. *Project TND* has shown small, but positive effects across seven cluster-randomized controlled trials for reducing and preventing "hard drug" initiation (e.g., Rohrbach, Sun, & Sussman, 2010; Sun, Skara, Sun, Dent, & Sussman, 2006; see review by Sussman, Valente, Rohrbach, Dent, & Sun, 2014). Some debate does exist, however, concerning the veracity of these findings due to inconsistent measurement and potential data analytic problems (Gorman, 2014).

Family-Based Programs

Family participation is a critical component of many successful prevention efforts. These approaches often strive to reduce pathways to drug initiation and improve the psychosocial development of the child. Successful family prevention programs typically enhance familial protective factors associated with adolescent substance use (e.g., supportive relationships with family members), provide skills training for parents, and target improvements in familial risk factors, such as poor communication or substance use among family members (Ary et al., 1999). The National Institute on Drug Abuse endorses family-based programs given this importance of family relationships as risk/protective factors and mediators of adolescent substance use (Swadi, 1999).

Some common examples of family-based programs include *Preparing for the Drug Free Years* (Park et al., 2000), *Strengthening Families Program* (Kumpfer, Alvarado, & Whiteside, 2003), and the *Family Empowerment Intervention* (Dembo, Wothke, Livingston, & Schmeidler, 2002). To this end, family-based interventions have shown good evidence for enhancing parenting skills, reducing family conflict, and improving communication across varied demographic groups (Aktan, Kumpfer, & Turner, 1996). Like other prevention efforts, the majority of family interventions targeting illicit drug use have focused on cannabis use. A recent meta-analysis supported parent–child targeted interventions for preventing the initiation of adolescent marijuana use (Vermeulen-Smit, Verdurmen, & Engels, 2015). Less support was reported for other illicit substance use, with the limited literature indicating generally small or no effect on adolescent stimulant use (e.g., Catalano, Gainey, Fleming, Haggerty, & Johnson, 1999; Haggerty, Skinner, Fleming, Gainey, & Catalano, 2008; Wu et al., 2003). However, additional and larger randomized clinical trials are needed before conclusions about the impact of family-based programs on adolescent stimulant prevention may be made.

Summary of Evidence-Based Primary Prevention Efforts

We reviewed the relative impact of population/community, school, and family-based primary prevention programs for curtailing the initiation of stimulant use in adolescent populations. Few studies have evaluated programs or outcome measures specifically targeting adolescent stimulant use despite extensive study for alcohol, cigarette, and cannabis use. The broader literature suggests that the most successful programs will likely be comprehensive ones targeting multiple dimensions of adolescent stimulant use through combinations of the methods reviewed. For example, the *Midwestern Prevention Project* was a comprehensive multi-component program targeting adolescent drug use prevention through mass media campaigns, school-based skills training, parent programming, school policy changes, and community organization to address changing local policy. Reduced rates of alcohol, cigarette, and cannabis initiation and use were observed in program relative to control students (e.g., Johnson et al., 1990; Pentz et al., 1989). Promising results were also recently reported for amphetamine and methamphetamine use with reductions in use initiation that were sustained into adulthood (Riggs, Chou, & Pentz, 2009). Such findings provide support for the continued study and implementation of multi-component prevention efforts incorporating elements from community, school, and family-level focused programs.

Evidence-Based Treatments

Treatment efforts have historically focused on adolescent alcohol, tobacco, and cannabis use much like primary prevention efforts. Recent years, however, have seen an increase in the adaptation of these evidence-based interventions for stimulant use outcomes. The following section reviews treatment strategies for managing adolescent stimulant use, including brief interventions, cognitive-behavioral therapy, contingency management, family-based approaches, and pharmacotherapies (see Table 2).

Screening and Brief Interventions

Screening and brief interventions often represent a “first-line of defense” for intervening in adolescent stimulant use disorder (Pilowsky & Wu, 2013). This strategy fits within the broader model of “Screening, Brief Interventions, and

Table 2 Evidence-based interventions for adolescent stimulant use

Method	Description	Example(s)	Evidence
Screening and Brief Interventions	Integrated identification and treatment linkage for at risk individuals. Often designed to enhance motivation for change and treatment engagement	Motivational Interviewing (MI); Motivational Enhancement Therapy (MET)	*Mixed Evidence/ Limited Data for Stimulant-Specific Outcomes*
Cognitive-Behavioral Therapy	Designed to build coping skills for craving and other temptations to use drugs, improve interpersonal relationships, and reduce risk behaviors associated with drug use (e.g., driving while intoxicated)	N/A	*Good Evidence/ Limited Data for Stimulant-Specific Outcomes*
Contingency Management	Patients are provided a non-drug reinforcer, such as money or a voucher redeemable for material items, contingent upon a clinical response, such as drug abstinence	N/A	*Good Evidence*
Family-Based Interventions	Focuses on improving adolescent social functioning in the family and other contexts, enhancing communication within the family and social system, and providing parental monitoring and other adult skills	Multidimensional Family Therapy, Functional Family Therapy, Brief Strategic Family Therapy, and Adolescent Community Reinforcement	*Good Evidence/ Limited Data for Stimulant-Specific Outcomes*
Pharmacotherapy: Substance Use	Use of pharmacological agent delivered acutely or chronically to reduce stimulant use	None successful; Bupropion tested	*Limited Data for Stimulant-Specific Outcomes*
Pharmacotherapy: Psychiatric Comorbidities	Use of pharmacological agent delivered acutely or chronically to address psychiatric comorbidity	Extended-Release Methylphenidate for ADHD	*Good Evidence for Comorbidities/ Weak Evidence for Substance Use Outcomes*

Note. All evaluations represent the authors' perspective after review of the literature
Created by authors Strickland and Stoops (2017)

Referral to Treatment" or SBIRT (Babor et al., 2007; Madras et al., 2009). SBIRT proposes a comprehensive and integrated identification and treatment linkage for individuals at risk for or suffering from a substance use disorder. Although SBIRT has only recently been applied to adolescent substance use, preliminary evidence supports its potential utility and justification for further evaluation (Mitchell et al.,

2012; Mitchell, Gryczynski, O'Grady, & Schwartz, 2013; Ozechowski, Becker, & Hogue, 2016; Sterling et al., 2015).

The most extensively researched and validated screening measure to identity substance-related problems in adolescents is the CRAFFT (named after the first letter of key words in the questionnaire; CAR, RELAX, ALONE, FORGET, FRIENDS, and TROUBLE) (Knight et al., 1999; Knight, Sherritt, Shrier, Harris, & Chang, 2002; Knight, Sherritt, Harris, Gates, & Chang, 2003; Pilowsky & Wu, 2013). The CRAFFT consists of six yes/no questions addressing potential problematic alcohol or drug use (e.g., "Do you ever use alcohol or drugs to relax, feel better about yourself, or fit in?"). Endorsing two or more items is suggestive of a substance use disorder with several studies demonstrating high specificity and sensitivity when using this cut off (Knight et al., 1999, 2002; Mitchell et al., 2014). Strong psychometric properties combined with the ease of administration (1–2 min) make it an ideal tool for rapid screening by health care professionals and primary care physicians during routine medical visits. The majority of research has evaluated the benefits of the CRAFFT in alcohol use disorder. However, some evidence indicates the utility of the CRAFFT for identifying non-medical prescription opioid use (McCabe et al., 2012) and cannabis use (Oesterle, Hitschfeld, Lineberry, & Schneekloth, 2015). Future research is needed before the ultimate utility for screening stimulant use disorders can be determined.

Brief interventions may be combined with screening assessments to provide immediate linkage to treatment and initial harm reduction. Motivational interviewing is a widely-used brief intervention characterized by short patient-centered interviewing to enhance motivation for treatment, encourage positive behavior change, and set realistic goals for recovery (Miller & Rollnick, 1991). Motivational Enhancement Therapy (MET) also uses this motivational interviewing counseling style delivery over a slightly longer intervention period (e.g., 2–4 individual treatment sessions). Patients are similarly encouraged in MET to develop internal motivation for change through a patient-oriented, non-judgmental, and non-confrontational approach. These strategies can be delivered by health care professionals in one-to-one meetings following screening and identification of a potential stimulant or other substance use disorder. Brief motivational interviewing or MET is also common prior to longer and more intense interventions (e.g., CBT) to enhance motivation for change and treatment engagement. A meta-analysis of 21 studies evaluating MI in adolescents observed small, but significant, effects sizes post-treatment as well as at 6-month or longer follow-ups (Jensen et al., 2011). Although the only study targeting stimulant use reported negative findings (Marsden et al., 2006), the positive outcomes observed for other substances and the relatively low cost and effort required for these procedures supports the continued study of MI for adolescent stimulant use.

Cognitive-Behavioral Therapy

Cognitive-behavioral therapy (CBT) is a frequently used and evidence-based psychosocial intervention for adolescent and adult substance use disorder (Carroll & Onken, 2005; Dutra et al., 2008; Waldron & Turner, 2008). CBT is designed to build coping skills for craving and other temptations to use drugs, improve interpersonal relationships, and reduce risk behaviors associated with drug use (e.g., driving while intoxicated). Modules can be selected based on the individual's needs and include teaching practice skills through individual or group therapy, behavioral modeling, and role-play. The flexibility of CBT means that it is easily incorporated into inpatient or outpatient programs and often combined with other behavioral and pharmacological interventions. One study found that adolescents with methamphetamine use history showed higher rates of substance use at treatment discharge from CBT relative to non-methamphetamine using youth (Rawson, Gonzales, Obert, McCann, & Brethen, 2005). This finding implies that adolescents presenting with methamphetamine use may need additional components or services to encourage drug use cessation. Encouragingly, similar retention rates in a 28-day inpatient CBT program were reported for youth indicating methamphetamine as their primary substance of choice and those indicating another primary substance (Callaghan, Brands, Taylor, & Lentz, 2007). Readmission patterns also did not differ between methamphetamine and cocaine-using adolescents in another study (Callaghan, Taylor, Victor, & Lentz, 2007). These findings indicate the feasibility, albeit uncertain clinical utility, of CBT for adolescent stimulant use disorders.

Contingency Management

Contingency management (CM), also known as voucher-based reinforcement therapy, is a set of procedures that encourage behavioral change through principles derived from operant psychology (see reviews by Higgins & Petry, 1999; Stitzer & Petry, 2006). Patients are provided a non-drug reinforcer, such as money or a voucher redeemable for material items, contingent upon a predetermined clinical response, such as drug abstinence. Studies in adult populations have demonstrated the robust clinical utility of CM for initiating abstinence across a range of pharmacological classes, including stimulant drugs (e.g., Farronato, Dursteler-Macfarland, Wiesbeck, & Petitjean, 2013; Lee & Rawson, 2008; Prendergast, Podus, Finney, Greenwell, & Roll, 2006; Shoptaw et al., 2006). Fewer studies have been conducted in adolescent populations, but they have generally demonstrated positive effects on health behavior change (Stanger, Lansing, & Budney, 2016; Yu et al., 2016). For example, adolescents participating in a community-based CM program showed significant reductions in illicit drug use, generally, as well as cocaine use, specifically, when compared to adolescents receiving treatment as usual (Lott & Jencius, 2009). This trial was particularly noteworthy because it used a community setting and a payment schedule that dramatically reduced direct expenditures for the program ($0.39/participant/day). Such low-cost procedures are important because perceived increases in monetary expenses are one of the greatest barriers to the widespread dissemination of CM.

Family-Based Approaches

Family participation has generally held a central role in treatment efforts consistent with its importance in prevention efforts. Commonly used programs include Multidimensional Family Therapy, Functional Family Therapy, Brief Strategic Family Therapy, and Adolescent Community Reinforcement Approach (Alexander & Parsons, 1982; Baldwin, Christian, Berkeljon, & Shadish, 2012; Godley, Godley, Dennis, Funk, & Passetti, 2002; Liddle, Rowe, Dakof, Henderson, & Greenbaum, 2009; Lindstrom, Filges, & Jorgensen, 2015; Rowe, 2012). Specific programs may differ in the extent to which the family is involved (e.g., the number of child-parent or parent only sessions). Consistent skills are provided, however, often focusing on improving adolescent social functioning in the family and other contexts, enhancing communication within the family and social system, and providing parental monitoring and other adult skills.

There is a paucity of data evaluating family-based interventions for stimulant use in adolescents, but one pilot clinical trial is of particular note. This study evaluated the Culturally Informed and Flexible Family-Based Treatment for Adolescents (CIFFTA) in Hispanic adolescents with substance use disorder (Santisteban, Mena, & McCabe, 2011). This culturally informed program was an adaptive one with flexible treatment components and manual. Adolescents assigned to the CIFFTA condition showed significant reductions in illicit drug use at an 8-month follow-up compared to those assigned to traditional family therapy. Similar, albeit not statistically significant, reductions were observed when evaluating cocaine use specifically. It is possible that this trend level for statistical significance was due to the pilot nature of the study, small sample size (n = 14/group), and/or strong comparator group (i.e., Family-Based Treatment as usual). Taken together, these findings highlight the importance of culturally informed practices in adolescent stimulant treatment.

Pharmacotherapy

Little research has evaluated pharmacological approaches for stimulant use in adolescents, particular when compared to the sizable extant literature in adult populations (Belendiuk & Riggs, 2014). To our knowledge, only one study has targeted adolescent methamphetamine use via a pharmacotherapy (Heinzerling et al., 2013). Adolescents in this parallel group study were randomly assigned to receive 150 mg bupropion SR (n = 12) or placebo (n = 7) as a part of an 8-week outpatient substance use program. Bupropion is a weak dopamine reuptake inhibitor with limited abuse potential currently indicated for depression and smoking cessation (Foley, DeSanty, & Kast, 2006; Rush, Kollins, & Pazzaglia, 1998). Adolescents receiving bupropion provided significantly fewer methamphetamine-negative urine samples (i.e., poorer treatment outcomes) and showed a trend towards poorer treatment retention. These findings are consistent with human laboratory and clinical trials of bupropion in adults that have generally reported negative findings or subgroup specific effects (i.e., individuals with lower baseline levels of methamphetamine use) as well as high rates of non-adherence (e.g., Anderson et al., 2015; Elkashef et al., 2008; Shoptaw et al., 2008; Stoops et al., 2015).

An alternative approach for addressing adolescent stimulant use is to first address psychiatric comorbidities. The majority of adolescents with substance use disorder present with at least one comorbid psychiatric condition, such as ADHD and depression. Addressing these comorbidities can improve intervention efforts because reductions in adolescent treatment retention and worse outcomes are often observed in individuals with comorbid mental illness (Warden et al., 2012). ADHD poses a particularly salient concern for adolescents with a stimulant use disorder given the high rates of comorbidity (Bukstein, 2008; Upadhyaya, 2008). Other evidence also indicates that the lifetime risk of substance use disorder is increased to over 50% in children whose ADHD persists into adulthood (Biederman et al., 1995). Symptoms may also be hard to manage because physicians are sometimes reluctant to prescribe psychostimulant medications to these comorbid populations due to potential diversion and misuse.

Other approaches, including extended-release formulations and non-stimulant medications, have been evaluated for comorbid ADHD and substance use disorder (Zaso, Park, & Antshel, 2015). Some reductions in ADHD symptoms have been reported for extended-release methylphenidate (Szobot et al., 2008; but see Riggs et al., 2011) and bupropion (Riggs, Leon, Mikulich, & Pottle, 1998; Solhkhah et al., 2005). In one crossover study, adolescents with comorbid ADHD and substance use disorder (n = 16) were assigned to receive ascending doses of spheroidal oral drug absorption system methylphenidate (0.3, 0.7, 1.2 mg/kg/day ascending each week) or placebo over 3-week periods (Szobot et al., 2008). Improvements in ADHD symptoms were observed, but changes in substance use outcomes were not observed, potentially due to the short window of treatment for each study dose. Another study evaluated an alternative formulation of extended release methylphenidate (osmotic-release) on ADHD and substance use outcomes (Riggs et al., 2011). Adolescents were assigned to receive 72 mg of osmotic-release methylphenidate/day (n = 151) and CBT or matched placebo and CBT (n = 152). Methylphenidate was well tolerated, but did not produce greater reductions in ADHD or substance use outcomes than CBT alone. The reasons for the discrepancies between these studies are unclear, but could be due to the differences in dosing regimens or treatment delivery (e.g., psychosocial intervention inclusion). The limited number of studies in this extant literature and the modest reductions observed in some studies highlights the importance of future research for this and other comorbid adolescent populations.

Summary of Evidence-Based Interventions

Consistent with prevention efforts, the ultimate impact of evidence-based treatments for stimulant use disorders will rely on the integration of multiple approaches tailored to the individual needs of the patient. Unfortunately, few studies have examined the specific effects on adolescent stimulant use for evidence-based treatments commonly used in outpatient and inpatient settings. Further research evaluating the psychosocial and pharmacological interventions noted above as well as novel formats is needed before definitive clinical recommendations may be made.

Conclusions

Cocaine, amphetamine, and methamphetamine remain a significant public health concern associated with a range of physical, psychological, and social health complications. Stimulant misuse continues to pose a particular problem for adolescents given the remaining high rates of use and potential impact on developmental trajectories during a period of dramatic physiological and psychological growth. Moreover, stimulant use has received relatively little attention in the primary prevention and treatment literature when compared to adolescent alcohol, tobacco, and cannabis use. The available literature suggests that many of those prevention and treatment efforts developed for other substance use may help deter the initiation and reduce the misuse of stimulants in adolescents. Clinically useful prevention and treatment will likely incorporate multiple approaches tailored to the individual and addressing factors at the level of the individual, peer, family, and community. More work is needed, however, to understand the ultimate utility of evidence-based and novel methods for preventing and treating adolescent stimulant use disorder.

References

Aktan, G. B., Kumpfer, K. L., & Turner, C. W. (1996). Effectiveness of a family skills training program for substance use prevention with inner city African-American families. *Substance Use & Misuse, 31*(2), 157–175.

Alexander, J. F., & Parsons, B. V. (1982). *Functional family therapy: Principles and procedures.* Carmel, CA: Brooks/Cole.

Alexander, M., Rothman, R. B., Baumann, M. H., Endres, C. J., Brasic, J. R., & Wong, D. F. (2005). Noradrenergic and dopaminergic effects of (+)-amphetamine-like stimulants in the baboon Papio anubis. *Synapse, 56*(2), 94–99. https://doi.org/10.1002/syn.20126

Allara, E., Ferri, M., Bo, A., Gasparrini, A., & Faggiano, F. (2015). Are mass-media campaigns effective in preventing drug use? A Cochrane systematic review and meta-analysis. *BMJ Open, 5*(9), e007449. https://doi.org/10.1136/bmjopen-2014-007449

Anderson, A. L., Li, S. H., Markova, D., Holmes, T. H., Chiang, N., Kahn, R., … Elkashef, A. M. (2015). Bupropion for the treatment of methamphetamine dependence in non-daily users: a randomized, double-blind, placebo-controlled trial. *Drug and Alcohol Dependence, 150*, 170–174. https://doi.org/10.1016/j.drugalcdep.2015.01.036

Anderson, D. M. (2010). Does information matter? The effect of the Meth Project on meth use among youths. *Journal of Health Economicsomics, 29*(5), 732–742. https://doi.org/10.1016/j.jhealeco.2010.06.005

Anderson, D. M., & Elsea, D. (2015). The Meth Project and teen meth use: New estimates from the National and State Youth Risk Behavior Surveys. *Health Economics, 24*(12), 1644–1650. https://doi.org/10.1002/hec.3116

Angrist, B., Corwin, J., Bartlik, B., & Cooper, T. (1987). Early pharmacokinetics and clinical effects of oral D-amphetamine in normal subjects. *Biological Psychiatry, 22*(11), 1357–1368.

Ary, D. V., Duncan, T. E., Biglan, A., Metzler, C. W., Noell, J. W., & Smolkowski, K. (1999). Development of adolescent problem behavior. *Journal of Abnormal Child Psychology, 27*(2), 141–150.

Babor, T. F., McRee, B. G., Kassebaum, P. A., Grimaldi, P. L., Ahmed, K., & Bray, J. (2007). Screening, Brief Intervention, and Referral to Treatment (SBIRT): Toward a public health approach to the management of substance abuse. *Substance Abuse, 28*(3), 7–30. https://doi.org/10.1300/J465v28n03_03

Baldwin, S. A., Christian, S., Berkeljon, A., & Shadish, W. R. (2012). The effects of family therapies for adolescent delinquency and substance abuse: A meta-analysis. *Journal of Marital and Family Therapy, 38*(1), 281–304. https://doi.org/10.1111/j.1752-0606.2011.00248.x

Belendiuk, K. A., & Riggs, P. (2014). Treatment of adolescent substance use disorders. *Current Treatment Options in Psychiatry, 1*(2), 175–188. https://doi.org/10.1007/s40501-014-0016-3

Berman, S. M., Kuczenski, R., McCracken, J. T., & London, E. D. (2009). Potential adverse effects of amphetamine treatment on brain and behavior: A review. *Molecular Psychiatry, 14*(2), 123–142. https://doi.org/10.1038/mp.2008.90

Biederman, J., Wilens, T., Mick, E., Milberger, S., Spencer, T. J., & Faraone, S. V. (1995). Psychoactive substance use disorders in adults with attention deficit hyperactivity disorder (ADHD): Effects of ADHD and psychiatric comorbidity. *American Journal of Psychiatry, 152*(11), 1652–1658. https://doi.org/10.1176/ajp.152.11.1652

Botello-Harbaum, M. T., Haynie, D. L., Iannotti, R. J., Wang, J., Gase, L., & Simons-Morton, B. (2009). Tobacco control policy and adolescent cigarette smoking status in the United States. *Nicotine & Tobacco Research, 11*(7), 875–885. https://doi.org/10.1093/ntr/ntp081

Brzeczko, A. W., Leech, R., & Stark, J. G. (2013). The advent of a new pseudoephedrine product to combat methamphetamine abuse. *The American Journal of Drug and Alcohol Abuse, 39*(5), 284–290. https://doi.org/10.3109/00952990.2013.821476

Bukstein, O. (2008). Substance abuse in patients with attention-deficit/hyperactivity disorder. *Medscape Journal of Medicine, 10*(1), 24.

Callaghan, R., Taylor, L., Victor, J. C., & Lentz, T. (2007). A case-matched comparison of readmission patterns between primary methamphetamine-using and primary cocaine-using adolescents engaged in inpatient substance-abuse treatment. *Addictive Behaviors, 32*(12), 3101–3106. https://doi.org/10.1016/j.addbeh.2007.06.007

Callaghan, R. C., Brands, B., Taylor, L., & Lentz, T. (2007). The clinical characteristics of adolescents reporting methamphetamine as their primary drug of choice: An examination of youth admitted to inpatient substance-abuse treatment in northern British Columbia, Canada, 2001–2005. *Journal of Adolescent Health, 40*(3), 286–289. https://doi.org/10.1016/j.jadohealth.2006.09.025

Carney, T., Myers, B. J., Louw, J., & Okwundu, C. I. (2016). Brief school-based interventions and behavioural outcomes for substance-using adolescents. *Cochrane Database of Systematic Reviews, 2016*(1), 1–63. https://doi.org/10.1002/14651858.CD008969.pub3

Carroll, K. M., & Onken, L. S. (2005). Behavioral therapies for drug abuse. *American Journal of Psychiatry, 162*(8), 1452–1460. https://doi.org/10.1176/appi.ajp.162.8.1452

Catalano, R. F., Gainey, R. R., Fleming, C. B., Haggerty, K. P., & Johnson, N. O. (1999). An experimental intervention with families of substance abusers: one-year follow-up of the focus on families project. *Addiction, 94*(2), 241–254.

Cavazos-Rehg, P. A., Spitznagel, E. L., Schootman, M., Strickland, J. R., Afful, S. E., Cottler, L. B., & Bierut, L. J. (2009). Risky sexual behaviors and sexually transmitted diseases: a comparison study of cocaine-dependent individuals in treatment versus a community-matched sample. *AIDS Patient Care and STDs, 23*(9), 727–734. https://doi.org/10.1089/apc.2008.0272

Center for Behavioral Health Statistics and Quality. (2016). Behavioral health trends in the United States: Results from the 2015 National Survey on Drug Use and Health (HHS Publication No. SMA 15-4927, NSDUH Series H-50). Retrieved from http://www.samhsa.gov/data/

Clayton, R. R., Cattarello, A. M., & Johnstone, B. M. (1996). The effectiveness of Drug Abuse Resistance Education (project DARE): 5-year follow-up results. *Preventive Medicine, 25*(3), 307–318. https://doi.org/10.1006/pmed.1996.0061

Comer, S. D., Hart, C. L., Ward, A. S., Haney, M., Foltin, R. W., & Fischman, M. W. (2001). Effects of repeated oral methamphetamine administration in humans. *Psychopharmacology, 155*(4), 397–404.

Crowley, T. J., & Riggs, P. D. (1995). Adolescent substance use disorder with conduct disorder and comorbid conditions. *NIDA Research Monographs, 156*, 49–111.

Cruickshank, C. C., & Dyer, K. R. (2009). A review of the clinical pharmacology of methamphetamine. *Addiction, 104*(7), 1085–1099. https://doi.org/10.1111/j.1360-0443.2009.02564.x

Cunningham, K. A., & Anastasio, N. C. (2014). Serotonin at the nexus of impulsivity and cue reactivity in cocaine addiction. *Neuropharmacology, 76*(Pt. B), 460–478. https://doi.org/10.1016/j.neuropharm.2013.06.030

Cunningham, S., Finlay, K., & Stoecker, C. (2015). Is Mississippi's prescription-only precursor control law a prescription to decrease the production and raise the price of methamphetamine? *International Journal of Drug Policy, 26*(11), 1144–1149. https://doi.org/10.1016/j.drugpo.2015.05.020

Dembo, R., Wothke, W., Livingston, S., & Schmeidler, J. (2002). The impact of a family empowerment intervention on juvenile offender heavy drinking: A latent growth model analysis. *Substance Use & Misuse, 37*(11), 1359–1390.

DiFranza, J. R., Savageau, J. A., & Fletcher, K. E. (2009). Enforcement of underage sales laws as a predictor of daily smoking among adolescents: A national study. *BMC Public Health, 9*, 107. https://doi.org/10.1186/1471-2458-9-107

Drent, M., Wijnen, P., & Bast, A. (2012). Interstitial lung damage due to cocaine abuse: Pathogenesis, pharmacogenomics and therapy. *Current Medicinal Chemistry, 19*(33), 5607–5611.

Dutra, L., Stathopoulou, G., Basden, S. L., Leyro, T. M., Powers, M. B., & Otto, M. W. (2008). A meta-analytic review of psychosocial interventions for substance use disorders. *American Journal of Psychiatry, 165*(2), 179–187. https://doi.org/10.1176/appi.ajp.2007.06111851

Dutta, S., Morton, J., Shepard, E., Peebles, R., Farrales-Nguyen, S., Hammer, L. D., & Albanese, C. T. (2006). Methamphetamine use following bariatric surgery in an adolescent. *Obesity Surgery, 16*(6), 780–782. https://doi.org/10.1381/096089206777346646

Elkashef, A. M., Rawson, R. A., Anderson, A. L., Li, S. H., Holmes, T., Smith, E. V., … Weis, D. (2008). Bupropion for the treatment of methamphetamine dependence. *Neuropsychopharmacology, 33*(5), 1162–1170. https://doi.org/10.1038/sj.npp.1301481

Elliott, J. M., & Beveridge, T. J. (2005). Psychostimulants and monoamine transporters: Upsetting the balance. *Current Opinion in Pharmacology, 5*(1), 94–100. https://doi.org/10.1016/j.coph.2004.09.005

Erceg-Hurn, D. M. (2008). Drugs, money, and graphic ads: A critical review of the Montana Meth Project. *Prevention Science, 9*(4), 256–263. https://doi.org/10.1007/s11121-008-0098-5

Faggiano, F., Minozzi, S., Versino, E., & Buscemi, D. (2014). Universal school-based prevention for illicit drug use. *Cochrane Database of Systematic Reviews, 2014*(12), 1–137. https://doi.org/10.1002/14651858.CD003020.pub3

Farronato, N. S., Dursteler-Macfarland, K. M., Wiesbeck, G. A., & Petitjean, S. A. (2013). A systematic review comparing cognitive-behavioral therapy and contingency management for cocaine dependence. *Journal of Addictive Diseases, 32*(3), 274–287. https://doi.org/10.1080/10550887.2013.824328

Ferri, M., Allara, E., Bo, A., Gasparrini, A., & Faggiano, F. (2013). Media campaigns for the prevention of illicit drug use in young people. *Cochrane Database of Systematic Reviews, 2013*(6), 1–97. https://doi.org/10.1002/14651858.CD009287.pub2

Foley, K. F., DeSanty, K. P., & Kast, R. E. (2006). Bupropion: Pharmacology and therapeutic applications. *Expert Review of Neurotherapeutics, 6*(9), 1249–1265. https://doi.org/10.1586/14737175.6.9.1249

Foltin, R. W., & Fischman, M. W. (1990). The relationship between cocaine venous blood levels and the cardiovascular and subjective effects of smoked and intravenous cocaine. *NIDA Research Monographs, 105*, 440–441.

Foltin, R. W., & Fischman, M. W. (1991). Smoked and intravenous cocaine in humans: Acute tolerance, cardiovascular and subjective effects. *Journal of Pharmacology and Experimental Therapeutics, 257*(1), 247–261.

Foltin, R. W., Fischman, M. W., Pedroso, J. J., & Pearlson, G. D. (1988). Repeated intranasal cocaine administration: Lack of tolerance to pressor effects. *Drug and Alcohol Dependence, 22*(3), 169–177.

Garnier, L. M., Arria, A. M., Caldeira, K. M., Vincent, K. B., O'Grady, K. E., & Wish, E. D. (2010). Sharing and selling of prescription medications in a college student sample. *Journal of Clinical Psychiatry, 71*(3), 262–269. https://doi.org/10.4088/JCP.09m05189ecr

Gawin, F. H. (1991). Cocaine addiction: Psychology and neurophysiology. *Science, 251*(5001), 1580–1586.

Gawin, F. H., & Kleber, H. D. (1985). Neuroendocrine findings in a chronic cocaine abusers: A preliminary report. *British Journal of Psychiatry, 147*(5), 569–573.

Glauser, J., & Queen, J. R. (2007). An overview of non-cardiac cocaine toxicity. *Journal of Emergency Medicine, 32*(2), 181–186. https://doi.org/10.1016/j.jemermed.2006.05.044

Godley, M. D., Godley, S. H., Dennis, M. L., Funk, R., & Passetti, L. L. (2002). Preliminary outcomes from the assertive continuing care experiment for adolescents discharged from residential treatment. *Journal of Substance Abuse Treatment, 23*(1), 21–32.

Gorman, D. M. (2014). Is Project Towards No Drug Abuse (Project TND) an evidence-based drug and violence prevention program? A review and reappraisal of the evaluation studies. *The Journal of Primary Prevention, 35*(4), 217–232. https://doi.org/10.1007/s10935-014-0348-1

Gossop, M. R., Bradley, B. P., & Brewis, R. K. (1982). Amphetamine withdrawal and sleep disturbance. *Drug and Alcohol Dependence, 10*(2–3), 177–183.

Grinspoon, L., & Bakalar, J. B. (1981). Coca and cocaine as medicines: An historical review. *Journal of Ethnopharmacology, 3*(2–3), 149–159.

Haggerty, K. P., Skinner, M., Fleming, C. B., Gainey, R. R., & Catalano, R. F. (2008). Long-term effects of the Focus on Families project on substance use disorders among children of parents in methadone treatment. *Addiction, 103*(12), 2008–2016. https://doi.org/10.1111/j.1360-0443.2008.02360.x

Harris, D. S., Boxenbaum, H., Everhart, E. T., Sequeira, G., Mendelson, J. E., & Jones, R. T. (2003). The bioavailability of intranasal and smoked methamphetamine. *Clinical Pharmacology & Therapeutics, 74*(5), 475–486. https://doi.org/10.1016/j.clpt.2003.08.002

Hart, C. L., Gunderson, E. W., Perez, A., Kirkpatrick, M. G., Thurmond, A., Comer, S. D., & Foltin, R. W. (2008). Acute physiological and behavioral effects of intranasal methamphetamine in humans. *Neuropsychopharmacology, 33*(8), 1847–1855. https://doi.org/10.1038/sj.npp.1301578

Hart, C. L., Ward, A. S., Haney, M., Foltin, R. W., & Fischman, M. W. (2001). Methamphetamine self-administration by humans. *Psychopharmacology, 157*(1), 75–81.

Havakuk, O., Rezkalla, S. H., & Kloner, R. A. (2017). The cardiovascular effects of cocaine. *Journal of the American College of Cardiology, 70*(1), 101–113. https://doi.org/10.1016/j.jacc.2017.05.014

Heal, D. J., Gosden, J., & Smith, S. L. (2014). Dopamine reuptake transporter (DAT) "inverse agonism"—a novel hypothesis to explain the enigmatic pharmacology of cocaine. *Neuropharmacology, 87*, 19–40. https://doi.org/10.1016/j.neuropharm.2014.06.012

Heinzerling, K. G., Gadzhyan, J., van Oudheusden, H., Rodriguez, F., McCracken, J., & Shoptaw, S. (2013). Pilot randomized trial of bupropion for adolescent methamphetamine abuse/dependence. *Journal of Adolescent Health, 52*(4), 502–505. https://doi.org/10.1016/j.jadohealth.2012.10.275

Higgins, S. T., & Petry, N. M. (1999). Contingency management. Incentives for sobriety. *Alcohol Research & Health, 23*(2), 122–127.

Hornik, R. (2006). Personal influence and the effects of the National Youth Anti-Drug Media Campaign. *The Annals of the American Academy of Political and Social Science, 608*, 282–300.

Howell, L. L., & Cunningham, K. A. (2015). Serotonin 5-HT2 receptor interactions with dopamine function: Implications for therapeutics in cocaine use disorder. *Pharmacological Reviews, 67*(1), 176–197. https://doi.org/10.1124/pr.114.009514

Howell, L. L., & Negus, S. S. (2014). Monoamine transporter inhibitors and substrates as treatments for stimulant abuse. *Advances in Pharmacology, 69*, 129–176. https://doi.org/10.1016/B978-0-12-420118-7.00004-4

Isenschmid, D. S., Fischman, M. W., Foltin, R. W., & Caplan, Y. H. (1992). Concentration of cocaine and metabolites in plasma of humans following intravenous administration and smoking of cocaine. *Journal of Analytical Toxicology, 16*(5), 311–314.

Jeffcoat, A. R., Perez-Reyes, M., Hill, J. M., Sadler, B. M., & Cook, C. E. (1989). Cocaine disposition in humans after intravenous injection, nasal insufflation (snorting), or smoking. *Drug Metabolism & Disposition, 17*(2), 153–159.

Jensen, C. D., Cushing, C. C., Aylward, B. S., Craig, J. T., Sorell, D. M., & Steele, R. G. (2011). Effectiveness of motivational interviewing interventions for adolescent substance use behavior change: A meta-analytic review. *Journal of Consulting and Clinical Psychology, 79*(4), 433–440. https://doi.org/10.1037/a0023992

Jessor, R., & Jessor, S. L. (1977). *Problem behavior and psychosocial development: A longitudinal study of youth*. New York, NY: Academic Press.

Johnson, C. A., Pentz, M. A., Weber, M. D., Dwyer, J. H., Baer, N., MacKinnon, D. P., … Flay, B. R. (1990). Relative effectiveness of comprehensive community programming for drug abuse prevention with high-risk and low-risk adolescents. *Journal of Consulting and Clinical Psychology, 58*(4), 447–456.

Johnston, L. D., O'Malley, P. M., Miech, R. A., Bachman, J. G., & Schulenberg, J. E. (2017). *Monitoring the Future national survey results on drug use, 1975–2016: Overview, key findings on adolescent drug use*. Ann Arbor, MI: Institute for Social Research, The University of Michigan.

Kerr, T., Small, W., & Wood, E. (2005). The public health and social impacts of drug market enforcement: A review of the evidence. *International Journal of Drug Policy, 16*(4), 210–220.

Kirkpatrick, M. G., Gunderson, E. W., Johanson, C. E., Levin, F. R., Foltin, R. W., & Hart, C. L. (2012). Comparison of intranasal methamphetamine and D-amphetamine self-administration by humans. *Addiction, 107*(4), 783–791. https://doi.org/10.1111/j.1360-0443.2011.03706.x

Knight, J. R., Sherritt, L., Harris, S. K., Gates, E. C., & Chang, G. (2003). Validity of brief alcohol screening tests among adolescents: A comparison of the AUDIT, POSIT, CAGE, and CRAFFT. *Alcoholism: Clinical and Experimental Research, 27*(1), 67–73. https://doi.org/10.1097/01.ALC.0000046598.59317.3A

Knight, J. R., Sherritt, L., Shrier, L. A., Harris, S. K., & Chang, G. (2002). Validity of the CRAFFT substance abuse screening test among adolescent clinic patients. *Archives of Pediatrics & Adolescent Medicine, 156*(6), 607–614.

Knight, J. R., Shrier, L. A., Bravender, T. D., Farrell, M., Vander Bilt, J., & Shaffer, H. J. (1999). A new brief screen for adolescent substance abuse. *Archives of Pediatrics & Adolescent Medicine, 153*(6), 591–596.

Kumpfer, K. L., Alvarado, R., & Whiteside, H. O. (2003). Family-based interventions for substance use and misuse prevention. *Substance Use & Misuse, 38*(11–13), 1759–1787.

Lee, N. K., & Rawson, R. A. (2008). A systematic review of cognitive and behavioural therapies for methamphetamine dependence. *Drug and Alcohol Review, 27*(3), 309–317. https://doi.org/10.1080/09595230801919494

Lewit, E. M., Hyland, A., Kerrebrock, N., & Cummings, K. M. (1997). Price, public policy, and smoking in young people. *Tobacco Control, 6*(Suppl 2), S17–S24.

Liddle, H. A., Rowe, C. L., Dakof, G. A., Henderson, C. E., & Greenbaum, P. E. (2009). Multidimensional family therapy for young adolescent substance abuse: Twelve-month outcomes of a randomized controlled trial. *Journal of Consulting and Clinical Psychology, 77*(1), 12–25. https://doi.org/10.1037/a0014160

Lindstrom, M., Filges, T., & Jorgensen, A. M. K. (2015). Brief strategic family therapy for young people in treatment for drug use. *Research on Social Work Practice, 25*(1), 61–80.

Lott, D. C., & Jencius, S. (2009). Effectiveness of very low-cost contingency management in a community adolescent treatment program. *Drug and Alcohol Dependence, 102*(1–3), 162–165. https://doi.org/10.1016/j.drugalcdep.2009.01.010

Lynam, D. R., Milich, R., Zimmerman, R., Novak, S. P., Logan, T. K., Martin, C., … Clayton, R. (1999). Project DARE: No effects at 10-year follow-up. *Journal of Consulting and Clinical Psychology, 67*(4), 590–593.

Lyoo, I. K., Yoon, S., Kim, T. S., Lim, S. M., Choi, Y., Kim, J. E., … Renshaw, P. F. (2015). Predisposition to and effects of methamphetamine use on the adolescent brain. *Molecular Psychiatry, 20*(12), 1516–1524. https://doi.org/10.1038/mp.2014.191

Madras, B. K., Compton, W. M., Avula, D., Stegbauer, T., Stein, J. B., & Clark, H. W. (2009). Screening, brief interventions, referral to treatment (SBIRT) for illicit drug and alcohol use at multiple healthcare sites: Comparison at intake and 6 months later. *Drug and Alcohol Dependence, 99*(1–3), 280–295. https://doi.org/10.1016/j.drugalcdep.2008.08.003

Marks, K. R., Lile, J. A., Stoops, W. W., Glaser, P. E., Hays, L. R., & Rush, C. R. (2016). Separate and combined effects of naltrexone and extended-release alprazolam on the reinforcing, subject-rated, and cardiovascular effects of methamphetamine. *Journal of Clinical Psychopharmacology, 36*(3), 213–221. https://doi.org/10.1097/JCP.0000000000000488

Marsden, J., Stillwell, G., Barlow, H., Boys, A., Taylor, C., Hunt, N., & Farrell, M. (2006). An evaluation of a brief motivational intervention among young ecstasy and cocaine users: No effect on substance and alcohol use outcomes. *Addiction, 101*(7), 1014–1026. https://doi.org/10.1111/j.1360-0443.2006.01290.x

Marsh, W., Copes, H., & Linnemann, T. (2017). Creating visual differences: Methamphetamine users perceptions of anti-meth campaigns. *International Journal of Drug Policy, 39*, 52–61. https://doi.org/10.1016/j.drugpo.2016.09.001

McCabe, S. E., Teter, C. J., & Boyd, C. J. (2004). The use, misuse and diversion of prescription stimulants among middle and high school students. *Substance Use & Misuse, 39*(7), 1095–1116.

McCabe, S. E., West, B. T., Teter, C. J., & Boyd, C. J. (2014). Trends in medical use, diversion, and nonmedical use of prescription medications among college students from 2003 to 2013: Connecting the dots. *Addictive Behaviors, 39*(7), 1176–1182. https://doi.org/10.1016/j.addbeh.2014.03.008

McCabe, S. E., West, B. T., Teter, C. J., Cranford, J. A., Ross-Durow, P. L., & Boyd, C. J. (2012). Adolescent nonmedical users of prescription opioids: Brief screening and substance use disorders. *Addictive Behaviors, 37*(5), 651–656. https://doi.org/10.1016/j.addbeh.2012.01.021

McCartt, A. T., Hellinga, L. A., & Kirley, B. B. (2010). The effects of minimum legal drinking age 21 laws on alcohol-related driving in the United States. *Journal of Safety Research, 41*(2), 173–181. https://doi.org/10.1016/j.jsr.2010.01.002

McGregor, C., Srisurapanont, M., Jittiwutikarn, J., Laobhripatr, S., Wongtan, T., & White, J. M. (2005). The nature, time course and severity of methamphetamine withdrawal. *Addiction, 100*(9), 1320–1329. https://doi.org/10.1111/j.1360-0443.2005.01160.x

Mendelson, J., Uemura, N., Harris, D., Nath, R. P., Fernandez, E., Jacob, P., 3rd, … Jones, R. T. (2006). Human pharmacology of the methamphetamine stereoisomers. *Clinical Pharmacology & Therapeutics, 80*(4), 403–420. https://doi.org/10.1016/j.clpt.2006.06.013

Miller, W. R., & Rollnick, S. (1991). *Motivational interviewing: Preparing people to change addictive behavior*. New York, NY: Guilford Press.

Mitchell, S. G., Gryczynski, J., Gonzales, A., Moseley, A., Peterson, T., O'Grady, K. E., & Schwartz, R. P. (2012). Screening, brief intervention, and referral to treatment (SBIRT) for substance use in a school-based program: Services and outcomes. *The American Journal on Addictions, 21*(Suppl 1), S5–S13. https://doi.org/10.1111/j.1521-0391.2012.00299.x

Mitchell, S. G., Gryczynski, J., O'Grady, K. E., & Schwartz, R. P. (2013). SBIRT for adolescent drug and alcohol use: Current status and future directions. *Journal of Substance Abuse Treatment, 44*(5), 463–472. https://doi.org/10.1016/j.jsat.2012.11.005

Mitchell, S. G., Kelly, S. M., Gryczynski, J., Myers, C. P., O'Grady, K. E., Kirk, A. S., & Schwartz, R. P. (2014). The CRAFFT cut-points and DSM-5 criteria for alcohol and other drugs: A reevaluation and reexamination. *Substance Abuse, 35*(4), 376–380. https://doi.org/10.1080/08897077.2014.936992

Mone, S. M., Gillman, M. W., Miller, T. L., Herman, E. H., & Lipshultz, S. E. (2004). Effects of environmental exposures on the cardiovascular system: Prenatal period through adolescence. *Pediatrics, 113*(4 Suppl), 1058–1069.

Müller, C. P., Carey, R. J., Huston, J. P., & De Souza Silva, M. A. (2007). Serotonin and psychostimulant addiction: Focus on 5-HT1A-receptors. *Progress in Neurobiology, 81*(3), 133–178. https://doi.org/10.1016/j.pneurobio.2007.01.001

Neale, A., Abraham, S., & Russell, J. (2009). "Ice" use and eating disorders: A report of three cases. *International Journal of Eating Disorders, 42*(2), 188–191. https://doi.org/10.1002/eat.20587

Newton, T. F., De La Garza, R., II, Kalechstein, A. D., & Nestor, L. (2005). Cocaine and methamphetamine produce different patterns of subjective and cardiovascular effects. *Pharmacology Biochemistry and Behavior, 82*(1), 90–97. https://doi.org/10.1016/j.pbb.2005.07.012

Nutt, D. J., Lingford-Hughes, A., Erritzoe, D., & Stokes, P. R. (2015). The dopamine theory of addiction: 40 years of highs and lows. *Nature Reviews Neuroscience, 16*(5), 305–312. https://doi.org/10.1038/nrn3939

Oesterle, T. S., Hitschfeld, M. J., Lineberry, T. W., & Schneekloth, T. D. (2015). CRAFFT as a substance use screening instrument for adolescent psychiatry admissions. *Journal of Psychiatric Practice, 21*(4), 259–266. https://doi.org/10.1097/PRA.0000000000000083

Ozechowski, T. J., Becker, S. J., & Hogue, A. (2016). SBIRT-A: Adapting SBIRT to maximize developmental fit for adolescents in primary care. *Journal of Substance Abuse Treatment, 62*, 28–37. https://doi.org/10.1016/j.jsat.2015.10.006

Paglia, A., & Room, R. (1999). Preventing substance use problems among youth: A literature review and recommendations. *The Journal of Primary Prevention, 20*, 3–50.

Pan, W., & Bai, H. (2009). A multivariate approach to a meta-analytic review of the effectiveness of the D.A.R.E. program. *International Journal of Environmental Research and Public Health, 6*(1), 267–277. https://doi.org/10.3390/ijerph6010267

Park, J., Kosterman, R., Hawkins, J. D., Haggerty, K. P., Duncan, T. E., Duncan, S. C., & Spoth, R. (2000). Effects of the "Preparing for the Drug Free Years" curriculum on growth in alcohol use and risk for alcohol use in early adolescence. *Prevention Science, 1*(3), 125–138.

Pasic, J., Russo, J. E., Ries, R. K., & Roy-Byrne, P. P. (2007). Methamphetamine users in the psychiatric emergency services: A case-control study. *The American Journal of Drug and Alcohol Abuse, 33*(5), 675–686. https://doi.org/10.1080/00952990701522732

Pentz, M. A., Dwyer, J. H., MacKinnon, D. P., Flay, B. R., Hansen, W. B., Wang, E. Y., & Johnson, C. A. (1989). A multicommunity trial for primary prevention of adolescent drug abuse. Effects on drug use prevalence. *Journal of the American Medical Association, 261*(22), 3259–3266.

Perry, C. L., Komro, K. A., Veblen-Mortenson, S., Bosma, L. M., Farbakhsh, K., Munson, K. A., ... Lytle, L. A. (2003). A randomized controlled trial of the middle and junior high school D.A.R.E. and D.A.R.E. Plus programs. *Archives of Pediatrics & Adolescent Medicine, 157*(2), 178–184.

Pianca, T. G., Rosa, R. L., Cereser, K. M. M., de Aguiar, B. W., de Abrahao, R. C., Lazzari, P. M., ... Szobot, C. M. (2017). Differences in biomarkers of crack-cocaine adolescent users before/after abstinence. *Drug and Alcohol Dependence, 177*, 207–213. https://doi.org/10.1016/j.drugalcdep.2017.03.043

Pilowsky, D. J., & Wu, L. T. (2013). Screening instruments for substance use and brief interventions targeting adolescents in primary care: A literature review. *Addictive Behaviors, 38*(5), 2146–2153. https://doi.org/10.1016/j.addbeh.2013.01.015

Prendergast, M., Podus, D., Finney, J., Greenwell, L., & Roll, J. (2006). Contingency management for treatment of substance use disorders: A meta-analysis. *Addiction, 101*(11), 1546–1560. https://doi.org/10.1111/j.1360-0443.2006.01581.x

Radcliffe, P., & Stevens, A. (2008). Are drug treatment services only for 'thieving junkie scumbags'? Drug users and the management of stigmatized identities. *Social Science & Medicine, 67*(7), 1065–1073.

Rawson, R. A., Gonzales, R., McCann, M., & Ling, W. (2007). Use of methamphetamine by young people: Is there reason for concern? *Addiction, 102*(7), 1021–1022. https://doi.org/10.1111/j.1360-0443.2007.01899.x

Rawson, R. A., Gonzales, R., Obert, J. L., McCann, M. J., & Brethen, P. (2005). Methamphetamine use among treatment-seeking adolescents in Southern California: Participant characteristics and treatment response. *Journal of Substance Abuse Treatment, 29*(2), 67–74. https://doi.org/10.1016/j.jsat.2005.04.001

Riggs, N. R., Chou, C. P., & Pentz, M. A. (2009). Preventing growth in amphetamine use: Long-term effects of the Midwestern Prevention Project (MPP) from early adolescence to early adulthood. *Addiction, 104*(10), 1691–1699. https://doi.org/10.1111/j.1360-0443.2009.02666.x

Riggs, P. D., Leon, S. L., Mikulich, S. K., & Pottle, L. C. (1998). An open trial of bupropion for ADHD in adolescents with substance use disorders and conduct disorder. *The American Academy of Child and Adolescent Psychiatry, 37*(12), 1271–1278. https://doi.org/10.1097/00004583-199812000-00010

Riggs, P. D., Winhusen, T., Davies, R. D., Leimberger, J. D., Mikulich-Gilbertson, S., Klein, C., ... Liu, D. (2011). Randomized controlled trial of osmotic release methylphenidate with cognitive-behavioral therapy in adolescents with attention-deficit/hyperactivity disorder and substance use disorders. *The American Academy of Child and Adolescent Psychiatry, 50*(9), 903–914. https://doi.org/10.1016/j.jaac.2011.06.010

Rocha, B. A. (2003). Stimulant and reinforcing effects of cocaine in monoamine transporter knockout mice. *European Journal of Pharmacology, 479*(1–3), 107–115.

Rodner, S. (2005). "I am not a drug abuse, I am a drug user": A discourse analysis of 44 drug users' construction of identity. *Addiction Research and Therapy, 13*(4), 333–346.

Rohrbach, L. A., Sun, P., & Sussman, S. (2010). One-year follow-up evaluation of the Project Towards No Drug Abuse (TND) dissemination trial. *Preventive Medicine, 51*(3–4), 313–319. https://doi.org/10.1016/j.ypmed.2010.07.016

Rothman, R. B., & Baumann, M. H. (2003). Monoamine transporters and psychostimulant drugs. *European Journal of Pharmacology, 479*(1–3), 23–40.

Rothman, R. B., Baumann, M. H., Dersch, C. M., Romero, D. V., Rice, K. C., Carroll, F. I., & Partilla, J. S. (2001). Amphetamine-type central nervous system stimulants release norepinephrine more potently than they release dopamine and serotonin. *Synapse, 39*(1), 32–41. https://doi.org/10.1002/1098-2396(20010101)39:1<32::AID-SYN5>3.0.CO;2-3

Rowe, C. L. (2012). Family therapy for drug abuse: review and updates 2003–2010. *Journal of Marital and Family Therapy, 38*(1), 59–81. https://doi.org/10.1111/j.1752-0606.2011.00280.x
Rush, C. R., Baker, R. W., & Wright, K. (1999). Acute physiological and behavioral effects of oral cocaine in humans: A dose-response analysis. *Drug and Alcohol Dependence, 55*(1–2), 1–12.
Rush, C. R., Kollins, S. H., & Pazzaglia, P. J. (1998). Discriminative-stimulus and participant-rated effects of methylphenidate, bupropion, and triazolam in D-amphetamine-trained humans. *Experimental and Clinical Psychopharmacology, 6*(1), 32–44.
Santisteban, D. A., Mena, M. P., & McCabe, B. E. (2011). Preliminary results for an adaptive family treatment for drug abuse in Hispanic youth. *Journal of Family Psychology, 25*(4), 610–614. https://doi.org/10.1037/a0024016
Scheier, L. M., & Grenard, J. L. (2010). Influence of a nationwide social marketing campaign on adolescent drug use. *Journal of Health Communication, 15*(3), 240–271. https://doi.org/10.1080/10810731003686580
Shoptaw, S. J., Heinzerling, K. G., Rotheram-Fuller, E., Steward, T., Wang, J., Swanson, A. N., … Ling, W. (2008). Randomized, placebo-controlled trial of bupropion for the treatment of methamphetamine dependence. *Drug and Alcohol Dependence, 96*(3), 222–232. https://doi.org/10.1016/j.drugalcdep.2008.03.010
Shoptaw, S. J., Kao, U., Heinzerling, K., & Ling, W. (2009). Treatment for amphetamine withdrawal. *Cochrane Database of Systematic Reviews, 2009*(2), 1–22. https://doi.org/10.1002/14651858.CD003021.pub2
Shoptaw, S. J., King, W. D., Landstrom, E., Bholat, M. A., Heinzerling, K., Victorianne, G. D., & Roll, J. M. (2009). Public health issues surrounding methamphetamine dependence. In J. R. Roll, W. Ling, R. A. Rawson, & S. Shoptaw (Eds.), Methamphetamine addiction: Basic science to treatment (pp. 143–156). New York, NY: Guilford Press.
Shoptaw, S. J., Klausner, J. D., Reback, C. J., Tierney, S., Stansell, J., Hare, C. B., … Dang, J. (2006). A public health response to the methamphetamine epidemic: The implementation of contingency management to treat methamphetamine dependence. *BMC Public Health, 6*, 214. https://doi.org/10.1186/1471-2458-6-214
Shukla, R. K., Crump, J. L., & Chrisco, E. S. (2012). An evolving problem: Methamphetamine production and trafficking in the United States. *International Journal of Drug Policy, 23*(6), 426–435. https://doi.org/10.1016/j.drugpo.2012.07.004
Siebel, T. M., & Mange, S. A. (2009). The Montana Meth Project: "Unselling" a dangerous drug. *Stanford Law & Policy Review, 20*, 405–416.
Simon, S. L., Richardson, K., Dacey, J., Glynn, S., Domier, C. P., Rawson, R. A., & Ling, W. (2002). A comparison of patterns of methamphetamine and cocaine use. *Journal of Addictive Diseases, 21*(1), 35–44.
Sofuoglu, M., & Sewell, R. A. (2009). Norepinephrine and stimulant addiction. *Addiction Biology, 14*(2), 119–129. https://doi.org/10.1111/j.1369-1600.2008.00138.x
Solhkhah, R., Wilens, T. E., Daly, J., Prince, J. B., Van Patten, S. L., & Biederman, J. (2005). Bupropion SR for the treatment of substance-abusing outpatient adolescents with attention-deficit/hyperactivity disorder and mood disorders. *Journal of Child and Adolescent Psychopharmacology, 15*(5), 777–786. https://doi.org/10.1089/cap.2005.15.777
Stanger, C., Lansing, A. H., & Budney, A. J. (2016). Advances in research on contingency management for adolescent substance use. *Child & Adolescent Psychiatric Clinics of North America, 25*(4), 645–659. https://doi.org/10.1016/j.chc.2016.05.002
Stein, M. D. (1999). Medical consequences of substance abuse. *Psychiatric Clinics of North America, 22*(2), 351–370.
Sterling, S., Kline-Simon, A. H., Satre, D. D., Jones, A., Mertens, J., Wong, A., & Weisner, C. (2015). Implementation of screening, brief intervention, and referral to treatment for adolescents in pediatric primary care: A cluster randomized trial. *JAMA Pediatrics, 169*(11), e153145. https://doi.org/10.1001/jamapediatrics.2015.3145

Stitzer, M., & Petry, N. (2006). Contingency management for treatment of substance abuse. *Annual Review of Clinical Psychology, 2*, 411–434. https://doi.org/10.1146/annurev.clinpsy.2.022305.095219

Stoops, W. W., Glaser, P. E., Fillmore, M. T., & Rush, C. R. (2004). Reinforcing, subject-rated, performance and physiological effects of methylphenidate and D-amphetamine in stimulant abusing humans. *Journal of Psychopharmacology, 18*(4), 534–543. https://doi.org/10.1177/0269881104047281

Stoops, W. W., Pike, E., Hays, L. R., Glaser, P. E., & Rush, C. R. (2015). Naltrexone and bupropion, alone or combined, do not alter the reinforcing effects of intranasal methamphetamine. *Pharmacology Biochemistry and Behavior, 129*, 45–50. https://doi.org/10.1016/j.pbb.2014.11.018

Strang, J., Babor, T., Caulkins, J., Fischer, B., Foxcroft, D., & Humphreys, K. (2012). Drug policy and the public good: Evidence for effective interventions. *Lancet, 379*(9810), 71–83. https://doi.org/10.1016/S0140-6736(11)61674-7

Sun, W., Skara, S., Sun, P., Dent, C. W., & Sussman, S. (2006). Project Towards No Drug Abuse: Long-term substance use outcomes evaluation. *Preventive Medicine, 42*(3), 188–192. https://doi.org/10.1016/j.ypmed.2005.11.011

Susskind, H., Weber, D. A., Volkow, N. D., & Hitzemann, R. (1991). Increased lung permeability following long-term use of free-base cocaine (crack). *Chest, 100*(4), 903–909.

Sussman, S., Valente, T. W., Rohrbach, L. A., Dent, C. W., & Sun, P. (2014). Commentary—Project Towards No Drug Abuse: An evidence-based drug abuse prevention program. *The Journal of Primary Prevention, 35*(4), 233–237. https://doi.org/10.1007/s10935-014-0353-4

Swadi, H. (1999). Individual risk factors for adolescent substance use. *Drug and Alcohol Dependence, 55*(3), 209–224.

Szobot, C. M., Rohde, L. A., Katz, B., Ruaro, P., Schaefer, T., Walcher, M., … Pechansky, F. (2008). A randomized crossover clinical study showing that methylphenidate-SODAS improves attention-deficit/hyperactivity disorder symptoms in adolescents with substance use disorder. *Brazilian Journal of Medical and Biological Research, 41*(3), 250–257.

Tashkin, D. P., Khalsa, M. E., Gorelick, D., Chang, P., Simmons, M. S., Coulson, A. H., & Gong, H., Jr. (1992). Pulmonary status of habitual cocaine smokers. *The American Review of Respiratory Disease, 145*(1), 92–100. https://doi.org/10.1164/ajrccm/145.1.92

Teter, C. J., McCabe, S. E., Cranford, J. A., Boyd, C. J., & Guthrie, S. K. (2005). Prevalence and motives for illicit use of prescription stimulants in an undergraduate student sample. *Journal of American College Health, 53*(6), 253–262. https://doi.org/10.3200/JACH.53.6.253-262

Thomas, R. E., McLellan, J., & Perera, R. (2013). School-based programs for preventing smoking. *Cochrane Database of Systematic Reviews, 2013*(4), 1–331. https://doi.org/10.1002/14651858.CD001293.pub3

Tobler, N. S., Roona, M. R., Ochshorn, P., Marshall, D. G., Streke, A. V., & Stackpole, K. M. (2000). School based adolescent drug prevention, 2 programs: 1998 meta-analysis. *The Journal of Primary Prevention, 20*(4), 275–336.

Uhl, G. R., Hall, F. S., & Sora, I. (2002). Cocaine, reward, movement and monoamine transporters. *Molecular Psychiatry, 7*(1), 21–26. https://doi.org/10.1038/sj/mp/4000964

Upadhyaya, H. P. (2008). Substance use disorders in children and adolescents with attention-deficit/hyperactivity disorder: Implications for treatment and the role of the primary care physician. *Prim Care Companion Journal of Clinical Psychiatry, 10*(3), 211–221.

Valencia, M. P., & Castillo, M. (2008). Congenital and acquired lesions of the nasal septum: A practical guide for differential diagnosis. *Radiographics, 28*(1), 205–224.; quiz 326. https://doi.org/10.1148/rg.281075049

Vermeulen-Smit, E., Verdurmen, J. E., & Engels, R. C. (2015). The effectiveness of family interventions in preventing adolescent illicit drug use: A systematic review and meta-analysis of randomized controlled trials. *Clinical Child and Family Psychology Review, 18*(3), 218–239. https://doi.org/10.1007/s10567-015-0185-7

Voas, R. B., Tippetts, A. S., & Fell, J. C. (2003). Assessing the effectiveness of minimum legal drinking age and zero tolerance laws in the United States. *Accident Analysis & Prevention, 35*(4), 579–587.

Volkow, N. D., Wang, G. J., Fischman, M. W., Foltin, R., Fowler, J. S., Franceschi, D., … Pappas, N. (2000). Effects of route of administration on cocaine induced dopamine transporter blockade in the human brain. *Life Sciences, 67*(12), 1507–1515.

Vrecko, S. (2015). Everyday drug diversions: A qualitative study of the illicit exchange and non-medical use of prescription stimulants on a university campus. *Social Science & Medicine, 131*, 297–304. https://doi.org/10.1016/j.socscimed.2014.10.016

Waldron, H. B., & Turner, C. W. (2008). Evidence-based psychosocial treatments for adolescent substance abuse. *Journal of Clinical Child & Adolescent Psychology, 37*(1), 238–261. https://doi.org/10.1080/15374410701820133

Ward, A. S., Haney, M., Fischman, M. W., & Foltin, R. W. (1997). Binge cocaine self-administration by humans: Smoked cocaine. *Behavioural Pharmacology, 8*(8), 736–744.

Warden, D., Riggs, P. D., Min, S. J., Mikulich-Gilbertson, S. K., Tamm, L., Trello-Rishel, K., & Winhusen, T. (2012). Major depression and treatment response in adolescents with ADHD and substance use disorder. *Drug and Alcohol Dependence, 120*(1–3), 214–219. https://doi.org/10.1016/j.drugalcdep.2011.08.001

Wee, S., Anderson, K. G., Baumann, M. H., Rothman, R. B., Blough, B. E., & Woolverton, W. L. (2005). Relationship between the serotonergic activity and reinforcing effects of a series of amphetamine analogs. *Journal of Pharmacology and Experimental Therapeutics, 313*(2), 848–854. https://doi.org/10.1124/jpet.104.080101

Weinshenker, D., & Schroeder, J. P. (2007). There and back again: A tale of norepinephrine and drug addiction. *Neuropsychopharmacology, 32*(7), 1433–1451. https://doi.org/10.1038/sj.npp.1301263

Wells, S. M., Buford, M. C., Porter, V. M., Brunell, H. L., Bunderson-Schelvan, M., Nevin, A. B., … Holian, A. (2010). Role of the serotonergic system in reduced pulmonary function after exposure to methamphetamine. *American Journal of Respiratory Cell and Molecular Biology, 42*(5), 537–544. https://doi.org/10.1165/rcmb.2009-0121OC

Werb, D., Rowell, G., Guyatt, G., Kerr, T., Montaner, J., & Wood, E. (2011). Effect of drug law enforcement on drug market violence: a systematic review. *International Journal of Drug Policy, 22*(2), 87–94. https://doi.org/10.1016/j.drugpo.2011.02.002

West, S. L., & O'Neal, K. K. (2004). Project D.A.R.E. outcome effectiveness revisited. *American Journal of Public Health, 94*(6), 1027–1029.

Wilens, T. E., Adler, L. A., Adams, J., Sgambati, S., Rotrosen, J., Sawtelle, R., … Fusillo, S. (2008). Misuse and diversion of stimulants prescribed for ADHD: A systematic review of the literature. *The American Academy of Child and Adolescent Psychiatry, 47*(1), 21–31. https://doi.org/10.1097/chi.0b013e31815a56f1

Wise, R. A., & Bozarth, M. A. (1987). A psychomotor stimulant theory of addiction. *Psychological Review, 94*(4), 469–492.

Wu, Y., Stanton, B. F., Galbraith, J., Kaljee, L., Cottrell, L., Li, X., … Burns, J. M. (2003). Sustaining and broadening intervention impact: A longitudinal randomized trial of 3 adolescent risk reduction approaches. *Pediatrics, 111*(1), e32–e38.

Yu, C. H., Guarna, G., Tsao, P., Jesuthasan, J. R., Lau, A. N., Siddiqi, F. S., … Advani, A. (2016). Incentivizing health care behaviors in emerging adults: A systematic review. *Patient Preference and Adherence, 10*, 371–381. https://doi.org/10.2147/PPA.S102574

Zaso, M. J., Park, A., & Antshel, K. M. (2015). Treatments for adolescents with comorbid ADHD and substance use disorder: A systematic review. *Journal of Attention Disorders*. Advance online publication. https://doi.org/10.1177/1087054715569280

Adolescent Self-Help in Substance Abuse Interventions

Sarabeth Leukefeld Biermann and Carl G. Leukefeld

"Youth is wasted on the young"

George Bernard Shaw (as cited in Cook, 1931, p. 8).

Introduction

This chapter examines the use of self-help and mutual help interventions among adolescents and youth. Illicit drug use is highlighted along with substance misuse and abuse among adolescents and youth aged 12–21 to support the need for treatment interventions, which are not payer driven and available. The chapter begins by overviewing substance use among adolescents and youth using data from the National Monitoring the Future survey for drug use among high school seniors and the National Survey on Drug Use and Health for the general US population. In addition, data from the Treatment Episode Data Set for adolescents receiving treatment in the USA are presented. After overviewing commonly used substance abuse treatment interventions, self-help/mutual help is discussed as an adjunct to adolescent treatment as well as a stand-alone intervention. The adolescent self-help literature discussion concludes that self-help/mutual help is a promising intervention for adolescents. However, since randomized and large-scale studies of effectiveness have not been completed, there is a lack of scientific rigor to support adolescent self-help/mutual help as an evidence-based practice.

S. L. Biermann (✉)
College of Social Work, University of Kentucky, Lexington, KY, USA
e-mail: sleuk00@uky.edu

C. G. Leukefeld
Department of Behavioral Science, Center on Drug and Alcohol Research, University of Kentucky, Lexington, KY, USA
e-mail: cleukef@uky.edu

C. G. Leukefeld, T. P. Gullotta (eds.), *Adolescent Substance Abuse*, Issues in Children's and Families' Lives, https://doi.org/10.1007/978-3-319-90611-9_10

Table 1 Past month alcohol, selected drug, and tobacco use for grades 8, 10, and 12 combined for the years 2014, 2015, and 2016

Substance	Percent of grade 8, 10, and 12 combined		
	2014	2015	2016
Alcohol	22.8%	21.8%	19.8%
Been drunk	11.9%	11.0%	10.1%
Any illicit drug	16.5%	15.9%	15.5%
Marijuana	14.9%	14.0%	13.7%
Crack	0.4%	0.4%	0.3%
Cocaine	0.7%	0.8%	0.9%
Inhalants	1.4%	1.3%	1.2%
Amphetamines	3.2%	2.7%	2.5%
Heroin	0.3%	0.2%	0.2%
Tranquilizers	1.5%	1.4%	1.4%
Cigarettes	8.0%	7.0%	5.9%
E-Vaporizes	–	12.8%	9.9%
Flavored Little Cigars	4.5%	4.9%	3.6%

Note. Adapted from "Monitoring the Future national survey results on drug use, 1975–2016: Overview, key findings on adolescent drug use," by L. D. Johnston, P. M. O'Malley, R. A. Miech, J. G. Bachman, and J. E. Schulenberg, 2017, Ann Arbor, MI: Institute for Social Research, The University of Michigan. Retrieved from http://www.monitoringthefuture.org//pubs/monographs/mtf-overview2016.pdf

Substance Abuse and Misuse Among US Adolescents and Youth

The following tables present information about self-reported drug use among eighth, tenth, and twelfth grade adolescents in US schools for selected drugs from the Monitoring the Future survey. Table 1 provides information about past month use for the years 2014, 2015, and 2016; Table 2 presents data for past month drug use for each of these three grades; and Table 3 presents daily use in 2016 for each of these same grades.

Table 1 shows decreases in self-reported alcohol use from 2014 to 2016 by 3% for users of alcohol, from 22.8% for 2014 to 19.8% for 2016. A decrease is also reflected in a 1.8% reduction in the number of youth self-reporting being drunk which decreased from 11.9% in 2014 to 10.1% in 2016. In addition, from 2014 to 2016, illicit drug use decreased by 1%; marijuana decreased by 1.2%; amphetamines decreased by 0.7%, 2.1% for cigarettes, and 2.9% for E-vaporizes from 2015 to 2016.

Overall, self-reported drug use decreased for most of these drugs as did binge drinking. However, there were exceptions for cocaine, which increased by 0.1% from 0.7% in 2014 to 0.8% in 2015 to 0.9% in 2016 and changed for flavored little cigars which increased from 4.5% in 2014 to 4.9% in 2015 but decreased to 3.6% in 2016.

As noted in Table 2, the self-reported use of these drugs generally increased from eighth grade to twelfth grade in 2016. The highest increases when eighth grade is

Table 2 Past month alcohol, selected drug, and tobacco use for grades 8, 10, and 12 for 2016

Substance	Percent of use by grade 8, 10, and 12 for 2016		
	Grade 8	Grade 10	Grade 12
Alcohol	7.3%	19.1%	33.2%
Been drunk	1.8%	9.0%	20.4%
Any illicit drug	6.9%	15.9%	24.4%
Marijuana	5.4%	14.0%	22.5%
Crack	0.2%	0.2%	0.5%
Cocaine	0.3%	0.4%	0.9%
Inhalants	1.8%	1.0%	0.8%
Amphetamines	1.7%	2.7%	0.4%
Heroin	0.2%	0.2%	0.2%
Tranquilizers	0.8%	1.5%	1.9%
Cigarettes	2.6%	4.9%	10.5%
E-Vaporizers	6.2%	11.0%	12.5%
Flavored little cigars	2.8%	4.9%	9.5%

Note. Adapted from "Monitoring the Future national survey results on drug use, 1975–2016: Overview, key findings on adolescent drug use," by L. D. Johnston, P. M. O'Malley, R. A. Miech, J. G. Bachman, and J. E. Schulenberg, 2017, Ann Arbor, MI: Institute for Social Research, The University of Michigan. Retrieved from http://www.monitoringthefuture.org//pubs/monographs/mtf-overview2016.pdf

Table 3 Daily use of alcohol, marijuana, and cigarettes in grades 8, 10, and 12 for 2016

Substance	Percent of daily use by grade 8, 10, and 12 for 2016		
	Grade 8	Grade 10	Grade 12
Alcohol	0.2%	0.5%	1.3%
Marijuana	0.7%	2.5%	6.0%
Cigarettes	0.9%	1.9%	4.8%

Note. Adapted from "Monitoring the Future national survey results on drug use, 1975–2016: Overview, key findings on adolescent drug use," by L. D. Johnston, P. M. O'Malley, R. A. Miech, J. G. Bachman, and J. E. Schulenberg, 2017, Ann Arbor, MI: Institute for Social Research, The University of Michigan. Retrieved from http://www.monitoringthefuture.org//pubs/monographs/mtf-overview2016.pdf

compared to twelfth grade were for alcohol at 7.3–33.2% with an associated increase in being drunk from 1.8% to 20.4%; any illicit drug use from 6.9% to 24.4%; marijuana from 5.4% to 22.5%; cigarettes from 2.6% to 10.5%; E-Vaporizers from 6.2% to 12.5% and little flavored cigars from 2.8% to 9.5%. However, there were modest decreases in self-reported use from eighth grade to twelfth grade for inhalants, from 1.8% to 0.8%, and amphetamine from 1.7% to 0.4%.

Table 3 presents daily use for the three commonly used drugs—alcohol, marijuana, and cigarettes—for eighth, tenth, and twelfth grades. When grades are compared, there are increases in each of these drugs. Specifically, from eighth grade to twelfth grade alcohol use increased from 0.2% to 1.3%, marijuana from 0.7% to 6.0% and cigarettes from 4.8%.

In addition to the Monitoring the Future school survey, the National Survey on Drug Use and Health provides estimates of US drug use in the general US population. The survey collects data through face-to-face interviews with a representative sample of the population at the respondent's place of residence. The National Survey on Drug Use and Health (NSDUH) is an annual survey of the civilian, noninstitutionalized population of the USA aged 12 years or older. NSDUH gathers information on substance use treatment need and service utilization.

The National Survey on Drug Use and Health (Substance Abuse and Mental Health Services Administration, 2014) estimated that 2.2 million US adolescents aged 12–17 were current illicit drug users. In addition, 2.2% of adolescents were nonmedical users of illicit prescription-type drugs, 1.4% of adolescents had a co-occurring major depressive episode and substance use, and 6.2% were binge users of alcohol in the past month. Using questions designed to measure dependence on or abuse of substances with the DSM-IV criteria, it was estimated that 1.3 million adolescents aged 12–17 had a substance use disorder. Although the Monitoring the Future survey and the National Survey on Drug Use and Health are the major sources for alcohol and other drug use data in the USA, there are limitations. These limitations include: the Monitoring the Future school-based surveys do not include those who dropped out of school before graduation or who were absent on the day of the survey; the National Survey on Drug Use and Health does not include persons who were inpatients or were entering inpatient treatment or those who resided in hotels, hospitals, and prisons/jails, or those without a home.

Substance Abuse and Misuse Treatment Utilization by US Adolescents and Youth

Using National Survey on Drug Use and Health data it was estimated that 1.3 million adolescents aged 12–17 needed substance use treatment in the previous year (Lipari, Park-Lee, & Van Horn, 2016). Of those who needed substance use treatment, about 80,000 adolescents (or 6.3%) received substance use treatment at a specialty facility. In other words, for those adolescents who needed substance use treatment, 93.7% of adolescents did not receive that treatment in a specialty treatment facility. However, of the estimated adolescents aged 12–17 who needed treatment but did not receive substance use treatment at a specialty facility in the past year, only 1.4% or about 17,000 adolescents said they perceived a need for substance use treatment.

Data from the Treatment Episode Data Set (TEDS), a national data system that includes information about substance abuse treatment facilities in the USA, includes treatment program admissions for 12 to 17 year olds. These data indicate that 120,239 twelve to seventeen year olds were admitted to and entered treatment in 2012 (SAMHSA, 2014). Of those admissions 71.1% were for males and 28.3% were for females. In addition, when race-ethnicity is examined for these admissions, about half (44.6%) of these admissions were White, 19.6% of these admissions were Black, 25.7% of the admissions were Hispanic, and 10.2% were Other which included American Indian/Alaska Native and Asian/Pacific Islander. When treatment referral sources were compared, the most frequent treatment referral source was the criminal justice/driving under the influence source at 44.5%, followed by self or individual at 18.3%, school at 14.6% and others including substance abuse and health care providers and community referrals at 22.6%.

When these data are examined together, it is clear that drug use among youth and adolescents has stabilized over the past 3 years. However, there are a number of adolescents and youth who do use substances. But for those who misuse and abuse substances, the amount increases as youth move into adolescence which underscores the treatment need for their substance misuse. However, the number of treatment facilities and programs are not able to meet the overall need for treatment.

Adolescent Substance Abuse and Misuse Treatment

The efficacy of adolescent substance abuse and misuse treatment approaches in a variety of settings is noteworthy considering the amount of use as noted above and which is supported by other data from the Center for Behavioral Health and Statistics at 9.4% of adolescents between the ages of 12 and 17 who reported illegal drug use and nearly 25% of individuals between 18 and 25 years of age who reported illegal drug use (Center for Behavioral Health Statistics and Quality, 2015). Treatment for adolescents is generally described as taking place in three broad areas: residential treatment, therapeutic community (TC) treatment, and community (outpatient) treatment (see Winters et al., 2018, chapter in this volume).

According to the American Society of Addiction Medicine's (2017) treatment criteria, treatment referrals are offered based on individual strength-based assessments in one of five categories: (1) Early intervention; (2) Outpatient treatment; (3) Intensive Outpatient/Partial Hospitalization; (4) Residential/Inpatient treatment; and (5) Medically Managed Intensive Inpatient treatment. However, each of these treatment interventions is not generally available in communities, but self-help groups are more common.

Among these categories of treatment, several methods and approaches including family therapy, individual therapy, group therapy, cognitive behavior therapy (CBT), motivational enhancement therapy (MET), 12 step groups, and ongoing intensive continuing care have been utilized and found to be effective in reducing substance use behaviors among adolescents (Tanner-Smith, Steinka-Fry, Kettrey, & Lipsey, 2016; Winters, Botzet, & Fahnhorst, 2011). Winters et al. (2018; in this volume) describe additional approaches to treatment including evidence-based interventions to target the negative functions within the adolescent's family; Internet and telephone therapy services; and medication to assist with sobriety. While some approaches are more effective, none of the approaches have been found to be harmful to adolescents (Tanner-Smith et al., 2016).

Group Therapy

Within the multiple approaches to adolescent substance abuse treatment, some methods have been examined more closely than others. For example, group therapy treatment orientations are most commonly used to treat substance use disorders and therefore have received a fair amount of attention from researchers. Historically, group treatment of substance use disorders has been the norm; however, as the efficacy and no-cost nature of self-help groups have become more widely understood (and accepted) among the general public, the popularity of high-cost group therapy has declined (Weiss, Jaffee, de Menil, & Cogley, 2004). Additionally, even though group therapy has been a popular methodology for substance use disorder treatment, there is a dearth of research comparing group therapy approaches to other approaches (i.e., individual therapy, residential treatment).

Therapeutic Communities

Another popular treatment approach for adolescents struggling with substance use disorders is the Therapeutic Community approach. Therapeutic Communities (TC) most often incorporate ideology that is rooted in AA (i.e., honesty, hope, faith, courage, integrity, willingness, humility, brotherly love, justice, perseverance, spirituality, and service). Additionally, TCs emphasize several points including mutual support; behavior modification and consequences for not following the rules; common practices in the group emphasizing positivity, healthy choices, strength-based change, and accountability; and giving over the self to the collective, which is responsible for the expected changes (Winters et al., 2011). Multiple studies have examined the therapeutic value of TCs (Abdel-Salam, 2013). Findings have consistently determined that TC approaches have been beneficial and have led to positive outcomes for adolescents including reduced instances of relapse, decreased criminal behaviors, and improved mental health. However, other findings have brought into question whether these positive outcomes last for the long term (Abdel-Salam, 2013; Edelen, Slaughter, McCaffrey, Becker, & Morral, 2010). For example, the process of living in a TC is stressful for adolescents. This stress is a significant precursor for adolescents to drop out of treatment. Findings indicate that the reduction of stress within the TC is essential for treatment to be effective among adolescents (Marcus et al., 2013). Thus, if the stress of the process is overwhelming, adolescents who are unable to cope with it may drop out and experience far fewer long-term benefits of the TC treatment. One study found that if adolescents were able to utilize the tools they had learned during treatment and could remain sober for 12 or more weeks post-discharge, they were likely to experience more positive outcomes (Godley, Godley, Dennis, Funk, & Passetti, 2007). However, a large part of post-treatment success is contingent upon whether or not adolescents have access to and participate in continuing care. One of the most widely available continuing care options is self-help/12-step program participation.

Self-Help

Self-help is commonly used to describe a multitude of methods for improving one's own circumstances. Since the 1960s, there have been an ever-increasing number of books written by "experts" who purport to tell us how to help ourselves learn to do anything—from finding meaning in everyday life to replacing the head gasket on a Moto Guzzi Ambassador motorcycle. Self-help has become an industry in the USA and there are entrepreneuring individuals who make a living by letting others in on their "secrets" and imparting specific types of knowledge to those who seek it. While there are often groups of individuals who seek the same kinds of information, we most often think of self-help groups as gatherings of individuals with a specific aim of sobriety.

Different from the newer self-help trends are the more traditional, tried-and-true methods of self-help. These more long-standing self-help methods are generally understood as forms of help for individuals who are experiencing a challenge to their physical and/or mental self. Specifically Alcoholics Anonymous (AA), perhaps the most enduring self-help organization, has been in existence since 1935 when Bill W. and Dr. Bob founded AA in Akron, Ohio (Alcoholics Anonymous World Services, Inc., 2017). AA fits the definition of a self-help group that is widely utilized and articulated clearly by Bekkering, Mariën, Parylo, and Hannes (2016, p. 1) as being "free of charge, ... locally available without restriction on the duration of attendance, and...available at moments of increased relapse [such as] by telephone...in the evenings or during the weekend." Humphreys et al.'s (2004, pp. 151–152) definition is even more direct in regard to self-help groups' relationships with individuals who are combating addictions: "Non-professional, peer operated organizations devoted to helping individuals who have addiction-related problems. The term 'mutual help group' is also sometimes used to reflect the fact that group members give and receive advice, encouragement, and support. Self-help groups do not charge fees and should not be equated with professional treatment services." Self-help groups differ widely from services provided by a social worker or other helping professional in a key area: availability (Kelly, Myers, & Rodolico, 2008). Whereas a helping professional is likely to keep traditional working-week hours, peers in an AA self-help group are committed to helping combat threats to sobriety whether those threats occur between 9:00 am and 5:00 pm Monday through Friday, or on a Sunday morning at 2:00 am. The benefits of this availability in regard to protecting sobriety are tantamount to the promotion of life.

Adolescent Self-Help/Mutual Help

In contrast to other adolescent and youth substance use treatment interventions, adolescent self-help has received more limited attention in the literature. A possible reason for this limited attention may be that self-help is strongly anchored in introspection, which may not be perceived as a well-developed skill among adolescents and youth by practitioners. Adolescent self-help as an approach is also more complicated with age limitations and a need to provide guidance and group leadership, frequently by adults. Consequently, we propose the following definition—Adolescent self-help/mutual help is a safe no cost group process, including 12 steps, spiritual or other grounding, in which peer youth involved in substance misuse along with sponsors and/or mentors mutually support recovering youth to deal with cravings, life stressors, and to promote change.

Adolescents do participate in self-help groups generally as part of other treatments, particularly residential treatment and therapeutic community treatment. The preponderance of self-help groups have foundations in 12-step programs, which are largely based upon the tenets of Alcoholics Anonymous (AA) (Winters et al., 2011). Those tenets are honesty, hope, faith, courage, integrity, willingness, humility, brotherly love, justice, perseverance, spirituality, and service. Specifically, adolescents have been participating in self-help groups such as Alcoholics Anonymous (AA), Narcotics Anonymous (NA), and Cocaine Anonymous (CA) over many years. For example, in 2007, 2.3% of AA members were under the age of 21 (Winters et al., 2011) while in 2014, 1% of AA members were under the age of 21 (A. A. World Services, Inc., 2014) which is a 1.3% decrease and suggests that interest among adolescents decreased significantly. Sussman (2010) has pointed out that these small percentages of youth involvement may be misleading because the overall number of adolescents in the USA with substance use problems is low (i.e., 4%) in comparison to the number of adults with substance use problems (i.e., 15%). Thus, AA participation rates among adolescents may be relatively higher than at first glance. However, while AA membership surveys show small numbers and fluctuating affiliation among adolescents, those who participate and indicate anecdotally that AA is valuable and important for their recovery.

AA is a common intervention approach that has been adopted across multiple inpatient and outpatient settings and is also used as an aftercare support and used in the absence of other treatment intervention approaches (Bekkering et al., 2016; Gonzales, Anglin, Glik, & Zavalza, 2013; Winters et al., 2011). In fact, AA self-help has been described as "the perfect aftercare"; but there is limited participation among adolescents (Kelly, Myers, & Brown, 2005). A reason for this limited participation may be the involuntary nature of many adolescent referrals to treatment interventions including AA that may impede voluntary engagement and participation (Sussman, 2010). Additionally, many adolescents have not fully formed their own ideas regarding spirituality, a key component of AA and other Anonymous groups, which may be an impediment to being comfortable in self-help groups (Sussman, 2010). This is supported by a study which reported that adolescents are less likely to participate in abstinence-only treatment programs such as AA (Gonzales et al., 2013). However, low participation rates should not be confused with the efficaciousness of the treatment. Often, when adolescents are faced with the idea of 50–70 years of sobriety, that possibility is daunting. It seems that many adolescents hesitate to fully accept the idea of total sobriety as presented by AA, NA, CA, and other Anonymous groups, and many reject the idea completely. Nevertheless, Bekkering et al. (2016), Sussman (2010), and Kelly and Myers (2007) who conducted reviews of treatment outcomes for adolescents participating in AA and NA found that despite low participation, there are multiple benefits for adolescents who participate in a 12-step self-help program.

Benefits of Self-Help/Mutual Help for Adolescents

Self-help programs, and AA in particular, are perceived to be valuable by participants and, importantly, can be effective in the treatment of substance use disorders and problems (Bekkering et al., 2016). Substance use treatment outcomes among adolescents generally parallel findings among adults: the higher the incidence of self-help group attendance, the higher the likelihood of prolonged sobriety (Bekkering et al., 2016). Despite the primary treatment (e.g., inpatient or outpatient) in which an adolescent participates, the addition of self-help group attendance can further reduce the likelihood of relapse among adolescents and increase the likelihood that the adolescent will attend treatment (Bekkering et al., 2016). Assertive aftercare/continuing care along with self-help group participation has been shown to enhance outcomes even more. Godley et al. (2007) reported that adolescents who met weekly with a case manager and who also participated in AA or another self-help group post discharge were more likely to remain abstinent for longer periods of time. Thus, the addition of a 12-step program can benefit those adolescents who have completed treatment and those adolescents who continue to participate in treatment.

Twelve-step program attendance among adolescents, while reportedly low, does prove beneficial as an adjunct to other treatments. For example, participation has been shown to increase the benefits of outpatient treatment; especially among adolescents who exhibit more symptoms of substance use (Kelly, Dow, Yeterian, & Kahler, 2011). Those adolescents who have been in treatment before and whose goal is sobriety are also more likely to fare better and have more positive outcomes when AA supplements traditional outpatient therapy (Kelly, Dow, Yeterian, & Kahler, 2011). Referrals to community AA or NA groups are the expected and usual methods of ongoing care no matter what type of treatment intervention the adolescent is receiving (e.g., group, individual, inpatient, outpatient) (Kelly, Dow, Yeterian, & Kahler, 2011; Kelly, Yeterian, & Myers, 2008; Knudsen, Ducharme, Roman, & Johnson, 2008). These referrals can be instrumental in the adolescent's perceived usefulness of self-help groups. If the adolescent's referral source (i.e., social worker, psychologist, or another helping professional) values the efficacy of self-help groups and 12-step programs, the referred adolescent is more likely to buy in to the value of the treatment method and, in turn, is more likely to attend AA or other self-help groups as part of ongoing care and/or aftercare (Kelly, Dow, Yeterian, & Kahler, 2011). In other words, the helping professional's belief in the worth of AA and other self-help groups cannot be underestimated. It is the professional's endorsement of self-help groups that influences the adolescent rather than the parent. In fact, Kelly, Dow, Yeterian, and Kahler (2011) found that an adolescent's participation in self-help groups is not contingent on a parent's approval or disapproval of self-help groups.

Barriers to Self-Help/Mutual Help Attendance

Monumental barriers to adolescent participation in self-help groups can be a lack of information and a fear of the unknown. What adolescent wants to walk into a group of anonymous strangers without knowing what to expect? Informing adolescents about AA or NA's customs, norms, and what can be expected at meetings can go a long way toward increasing attendance (Kelly, Dow, Yeterian, & Kahler, 2011) and, therefore, longer-term benefits and sobriety. Conducting orientation sessions with adolescent substance users' therapy groups and inviting current AA, NA, or other Anonymous participants to speak with them about self-help group participation and other subjects can ease fears about attending self-help groups (Kelly et al., 2016). Weekly self-help group attendance presents adolescents with the most benefits, but even more spotty attendance can still provide increases in sobriety and positive outcomes (Kelly, Dow, Yeterian, & Kahler, 2011).

Another barrier to regular AA and NA group attendance is safety. While this can be a key concern, there is very little on safety present in the literature. In fact, only one study (Kelly, Dow, Yeterian, & Myers, 2011) examined safety. Specifically, 98.9% of community AA groups are patronized by adults and adolescents may have misgivings about attending these adult dominated groups. In general, adolescents describe their well-being at meetings as "very safe," but a small minority of adolescents reported feeling that adult participants were menacing in some way (Kelly, Dow, Yeterian, & Myers, 2011). However, even negative experiences did not preclude adolescents from attending meetings. And, further, while NA meetings were perceived as more dangerous than AA meetings, professionals and parents indicated that adolescents were safe at both types of meetings. In general, little is known about the overall safety of adolescents in community self-help groups such as AA and NA. A deeper dive into the facets of safety concerning young people and anonymous groups is warranted, especially because self-help groups have been shown to be efficacious for adolescents. If we wish to break down barriers to self-help and Anonymous group attendance among adolescents, it is important to more fully examine safety and how we can more thoroughly inform youth of what to expect during AA and other community self-help groups.

Flexibility

The availability and flexibility of peer-to-peer support, which is the hallmark of Anonymous groups (e.g., AA, NA, CA) is associated with abstinence. Blonigen, Timko, Finney, Moos, and Moos (2011) found that impulsivity—a quality present in many individuals who misuse substances and prevalent among adolescents—is substantially reduced by individuals who participate in AA. The reduction in impulsivity that comes with adherence to the norms of AA is significant since individuals who begin participating in AA when they are under the age of 25 are more likely to maintain sobriety in the long-term, specifically at 1, 8, and 16 years after first attending AA (Blonigen et al., 2011). In fact, the earlier an adolescent begins to participate in self-help groups/AA, the more likely she/he is to have marked improvement in impulsivity control and other key behaviors (Timko, Billow, & DeBenedetti, 2006).

Another way in which AA and other self-help groups demonstrate flexibility is through the many opportunities the groups provide to continue to motivate adolescents to remain sober. Ongoing motivation increases possible benefits adolescents receive from AA and other Anonymous groups (Kelly & Myers, 2007). For example, Kingston, Knight, Williams, and Gordon (2015) found that adolescents who were participating in anonymous groups were motivated in multiple ways to remain sober and continue attending meetings. Sponsors were identified as important to remaining motivated to stay abstinent. In fact, some study participants said that they chose sponsors who would intervene when harmful behaviors or thinking became apparent in order to help them stay the course of sobriety. Other factors that increased or maintained motivation were having a place where everyone can understand the difficulties of remaining sober, knowing that there is hope for a sober future based on the life stories of sponsors and peers, and hearing insider tips on how to remain abstinent (Kingston et al., 2015) despite setbacks or episodes of relapse.

Relapse

Relapse is a concern for adolescents. Findings across different studies indicate that between 66% and 79% of adolescents are likely to return to substance use in 3 months to a year after completion of substance treatment, many within 2 months of treatment completion (Brown, Tapert, Tate, & Abrantes, 2000; Cornelius et al., 2003). Unlike their adult counterparts who most often relapse when they experience an impulse/urge to do so (Ramo & Brown, 2008), the majority of adolescents report situational factors as the causes for their relapses (Chung & Maisto, 2006). These factors include exposure to the same pretreatment environment in which drug use is occurring and peer pressure to use (Chung & Maisto, 2006) in order to fulfill the developmental norm of wanting to fit in with their peers (Ramo & Brown, 2008).

A complicating factor surrounding relapse is how different individuals, groups, and practitioners define the phenomenon. The way in which relapse is defined determines how it is measured. Less forgiving definitions of relapse (i.e., any substance use) were, unsurprisingly, in line with higher rates of use and earlier use after any length of sobriety among one sample of adolescents (Maisto, Pollock, Cornelius, Lynch, & Martin, 2003). Further, more use as part of relapse was predictive of long term use among the sample of adolescents. These factors are interesting when viewed in concert with the tenets of AA in which relapse is often defined as any use. Although relapse may be defined differently by others (i.e., a slip or a lapse), self-help groups can provide the support an adolescent may need to reach or expand their next period of sobriety. Clinician referrals to self-help groups may facilitate an adolescent's ongoing sobriety. One study found that clinicians are most likely to refer adolescents to 12-step-based self-help groups most often for aftercare (Passetti & Godley, 2008). Since referrals are seen as endorsements of particular ideas, many adolescents can be helped to ascertain that 12-step groups are beneficial by trusted helping professionals. These ideas may also be more likely to shape an adolescent's acceptance of a particular path to sobriety and away from relapse.

Recovery

Perhaps the major goal of any treatment intervention including self-help is recovery. However, defining recovery is fraught with problems—both temporally (months vs. years) and behaviorally (no substance use vs. some use). In order to provide clarity, the Substance Abuse and Mental Health Services Administration (SAMHSA) developed a working definition of recovery as a process of change through which individuals improve their health and wellness, live self-directed lives, and strive to reach their full potential. Recovery is built on access to evidence-based clinical treatment and recovery support services for all populations (SAMHSA, 2012).

SAMHSA also posits four dimensions that support recovery: (1) *Health*—overcoming or managing one's disease(s) or symptoms—for example, abstaining from use of alcohol, illicit drugs, and nonprescribed medications if one has an addiction problem—and, for everyone in recovery, making informed, healthy choices that support physical and emotional well-being. (2) *Home*—having a stable and safe place to live. (3) *Purpose*—conducting meaningful daily activities, such as a job, school, volunteerism, family caretaking, or creative endeavors, and the independence, income, and resources to participate in society. (4) *Community*—having relationships and social networks that provide support, friendship, love, and hope. If recovery is the process of recovering (see Marks & Leukefeld, 2018, chapter in this volume) then speculating about the process for adolescents becomes more complicated than for adults who are recovering. In our experiences, for example, adolescents generally have difficulties in making healthy choices particularly due to their young, very responsive physiology. In addition, a stable home may not be reality as well as a purpose in life which is frequently presented as "I have no idea what I want to be!" Finally, the sense of community can be particularly elusive with the dependency on social media. Perhaps, for adolescent substance misusers the focus should be immediate safety and well-being.

Concluding Remarks

After presenting select US national adolescent prevalence data for substance use and data on treatment utilization, this chapter focused on the limited use of self-help interventions by adolescents. In addition to the paucity of adolescent treatment availability in the USA, the information on adolescent self-help/mutual help was presented which complements that need. There are only a very small number of controlled adolescent research studies in this area. Specifically, the most recent review by Bekkering et al. (2016) found, after a literature search of PubMed, PsychINFO, and Web of Knowledge databases from January to March 2013, that only 12 studies met their criteria and that "[s]elf-help attendance appears to reduce alcohol and drug use, including abstinence. However, the lack of methodological rigor in these studies precludes definitive conclusions" (p. 1). They also found that "[t]here are two factors that seem to be related to higher abstinence: the number of attended meetings and the period that the adolescent engages in 12 step participation" (p. 11).

It should also be noted that a number of limitations were cited including the low percentage of adolescent subjects who attended self-help meetings, which could be a proxy of motivation and each of the studies subjects had attended treatment before attending self-help.

In summary, based on the existing research, adolescent self-help/mutual help can be considered to be a promising approach for adolescent substance misuse. However, there are a number of limitations surrounding the idea of how to help an adolescent engage in and continue to attend self-help/mutual help meetings. Further research, including controlled trials, is needed to add to our understanding of adolescent and youth self-help and as a promising and evidence-based practice. For example, research questions should go beyond "Does it work?" or "Does it not work?" and should address the question of when is self-help appropriate and effective. In addition, consideration should be given to the question of when is self-help an adjunct to other interventions and in what circumstances is self-help a stand-alone intervention. It is also important to more fully examine safety and how to prepare adolescents more thoroughly about what to expect in AA and other community self-help groups.

Acknowledgements This work was supported in part by a grant from the National Institute on Drug Abuse DA036158 (Leukefeld).

References

Abdel-Salam, S. (2013). Self-control as a predictor of relapse and recidivism in adolescent therapeutic community treatment. *Substance Use & Misuse, 48*(1–2), 157–172. https://doi.org/10.3109/10826084.2012.742544

Alcoholics Anonymous (A. A.). World Services, Inc. (2014). *Alcoholics Anonymous 2014 Membership Survey*. Retrieved from http://www.aa.org/assets/en_US/aa-literature/p-48-aa-membership-survey.

Alcoholics Anonymous (A. A.). World Services, Inc.. (2017). *Historical data: The birth of A.A. and its growth in the U.S./Canada*. Retrieved from https://www.aa.org/pages/en_US/historical-data-the-birth-of-aa-and-its-growth-in-the-uscanada.

American Society of Addiction Medicine. (2017). *What is the ASAM criteria?* Retrieved from https://www.asam.org/quality-practice/guidelines-and-consensus-documents/the-asam-criteria/about.

Bekkering, G. E., Mariën, D., Parylo, O., & Hannes, K. (2016). The effectiveness of self-help groups for adolescent substance misuse: A systematic review. *Journal of Child & Adolescent Substance Abuse, 25*(3), 229–244. https://doi.org/10.1080/1067828X.2014.981772

Blonigen, D. M., Timko, C., Finney, J. W., Moos, B. S., & Moos, R. H. (2011). Alcoholics Anonymous attendance, decreases in impulsivity and drinking and psychosocial outcomes over 16 years: Moderated-mediation from a developmental perspective. *Addiction, 106*(12), 2167–2177. https://doi.org/10.1111/j.1360-0443.2011.03522.x

Brown, S. A., Tapert, S. F., Tate, S. R., & Abrantes, A. M. (2000). The role of alcohol in adolescent relapse and outcome. *Journal of Psychoactive Drugs, 32*(1), 107–115.

Center for Behavioral Health Statistics and Quality. (2015). *Behavioral health trends in the United States: Results from the 2014 National Survey on Drug Use and Health* (HHS Publication No. SMA 15-4927, NSDUH Series H-50). Retrieved from http://www.samhsa.gov/data/sites/default/files/NSDUH-FRR1-2014/NSDUH-FRR1-2014.pdf.

Chung, T., & Maisto, S. A. (2006). Relapse to alcohol and other drug use in treated adolescents: Review and reconsideration of relapse as a change point in clinical course. *Clinical Psychology Review, 26*(2), 149–161. https://doi.org/10.1016/j.cpr.2005.11.004

Cook, T. (1931, February 14). Cook-Coos. Rockford Register-Republic, p. 8.

Cornelius, J. R., Maisto, S. A., Pollock, N. K., Martin, C. S., Salloum, I. M., Lynch, K. G., & Clark, D. B. (2003). Short communication: Rapid relapse generally follows treatment for substance use disorders among adolescents. *Addictive Behaviors, 28*(2), 381–386.

Edelen, M. O., Slaughter, M. E., McCaffrey, D. F., Becker, K., & Morral, R. (2010). Long-term effect of community-based treatment: Evidence from the adolescent outcomes project. *Drug and Alcohol Dependence, 107*(1), 62–68.

Godley, M. D., Godley, S. H., Dennis, M. L., Funk, R. R., & Passetti, L. L. (2007). The effect of assertive continuing care on continuing care linkage, adherence and abstinence following residential treatment for adolescents with substance use disorders. *Addiction, 102*(1), 81–93. https://doi.org/10.1111/j.1360-0443.2006.01648.x

Gonzales, R., Anglin, M. D., Glik, D. C., & Zavalza, C. (2013). Perceptions about recovery needs and drug-avoidance recovery behaviors among youth in substance abuse treatment. *Journal of Psychoactive Drugs, 45*(4), 297–303.

Humphreys, K., Wing, S., McCarty, D., Chappel, J., Gallant, L., Haberle, B., … Weiss, R. (2004). Self-help organizations for alcohol and drug problems: Toward evidence-based practice and policy. *Journal of Substance Abuse Treatment, 26*(3), 151–158. https://doi.org/10.1016/S0740-5472(03)00212-5

Johnston, L. D., O'Malley, P. M., Miech, R. A., Bachman, J. G., & Schulenberg, J. E. (2017). *Monitoring the future national survey results on drug use, 1975–2016: Overview, key findings on adolescent drug use*. Ann Arbor, MI: Institute for Social Research, The University of Michigan Retrieved from http://www.monitoringthefuture.org//pubs/monographs/mtf-overview2016.pdf

Kelly, J. F., Dow, S. J., Yeterian, J. D., & Kahler, C. W. (2011). Can 12-step group participation strengthen and extend the benefits of adolescent addiction treatment? A prospective analysis. *Drug and Alcohol Dependence, 110*(1–2), 117–125.

Kelly, J. F., Dow, S. J., Yeterian, J. D., & Myers, M. G. (2011). How safe are adolescents at AA and NA meetings? A prospective investigation with outpatient youth. *Journal of Substance Abuse Treatment, 40*(4), 419–425.

Kelly, J. F., & Myers, M. G. (2007). Adolescents' participation in Alcoholics Anonymous and Narcotics Anonymous: Review, implications, and future directions. *Journal of Psychoactive Drugs, 39*(3), 259–269.

Kelly, J. F., Myers, M. G., & Brown, S. A. (2005). The effects of age composition of 12-step groups and adolescent participation and substance use outcome. *Journal of Child and Adolescent Substance Abuse, 15*(1), 63–72.

Kelly, J. F., Myers, M. G., & Rodolico, J. (2008). What do adolescents exposed to Alcoholics Anonymous think about 12-step groups? *Substance Abuse, 29*(2), 53–62. https://doi.org/10.1080/08897070802093122

Kelly, J. F., Yeterian, J. D., Cristello, J. V., Kaminer, Y., Kahler, C. W., & Timko, C. (2016). Developing and testing twelve-step facilitation for adolescents with substance use disorder: Manual development and preliminary outcomes. *Substance Abuse: Research and Treatment, 10*, 55–64. https://doi.org/10.4137/SART.S39635

Kelly, J. F., Yeterian, J. D., & Myers, M. G. (2008). Treatment staff referrals, participation expectations, and perceived benefits and barriers to adolescent involvement in 12-step groups. *Alcohol Treatment Quarterly, 26*(4), 427–449. https://doi.org/10.1080/07347320802347053

Kingston, S., Knight, E., Williams, J., & Gordon, H. (2015). How do young adults view 12-step programs? A qualitative study. *Journal of Addictive Diseases, 34*(4), 311–322. https://doi.org/10.1080/10550887.2015.1074506

Knudsen, H. K., Ducharme, L. J., Roman, P. M., & Johnson, J. A. (2008). *Service delivery and use of evidence-based treatment practices in adolescent substance abuse treatment settings: Project report.* Robert Wood Johnson Foundation's Substance Abuse Policy Research Program (Grant No. 53130). Retrieved from https://ntcs.uga.edu/reports/Adolescent%20Study%20Summary%20Report.

Lipari, R. N., Park-Lee, E., & Van Horn, S. (2016). America's need for and receipt of substance treatment in 2015. *SAMHSA Short Report*. Retrieved from samhsa.gov/data/sites/default/files/report_2716ShortReport-2716.pdf-31.

Maisto, S. A., Pollock, N. K., Cornelius, J. R., Lynch, K. G., & Martin, C. S. (2003). Alcohol relapse as a function of relapse definition in a clinical sample of adolescents. *Addictive Behaviors, 28*(3), 449–459. https://doi.org/10.1016/S0306-4603(01)00267-2

Marcus, M. T., Schmitz, J., Moeller, F. G., Liehr, P., Swank, P., Cron, S. G., & Carroll, D. D. (2013). Stress and length of stay in therapeutic community treatment for adolescents with substance use disorders. *Addictive Disorders & Their Treatment, 12*(4), 175–182. https://doi.org/10.1097/ADT.0b013e31826cfd9b

Marks, K. R., & Leukefeld, C. G. (2018). Recovering among adolescents. In C. G. Leukefeld & T. P. Gullotta (Eds.), *Adolescent substance abuse: Evidence-based approaches to prevention and treatment* (2nd ed. pp. 293–307). New York, NY: Springer.

Passetti, L. L., & Godley, S. H. (2008). Adolescent substance abuse treatment clinicians' self-help meeting referral practices and adolescent attendance rates. *Journal of Psychoactive Drugs, 40*(1), 29–40.

Ramo, D. E., & Brown, S. A. (2008). Classes of substance abuse relapse situations: A comparison of adolescents and adults. *Psychology of Addictive Behaviors, 22*(3), 372–379. https://doi.org/10.1037/0893-164X.22.3.372

Substance Abuse and Mental Health Services Administration. (2012). *Working definition of recovery*. Retrieved from https://store.samhsa.gov/product/SAMHSA-s-Working-Definition-of-Recovery/PEP12-RECDEF.

Substance Abuse and Mental Health Services Administration, Center for Behavioral Health Statistics and Quality. (2014). *Treatment Episode Data Set (TEDS): 2002–2012. National admissions to substance abuse treatment services*. BHSIS Series S-71 (HHS Publication No. SMA 14-4850). Rockville, MD: Substance Abuse and Mental Health Services Administration.

Substance Abuse and Mental Health Services Administration, National Survey on Drug Use and Health, Office of Applied Studies. (2014). *Substance use and mental health estimates from the 2013 national survey on drug use and health: Overview of findings*. Rockville, MD: U.S. Department of Health and Human Services Retrieved from https://www.samhsa.gov/data/sites/default/files/NSDUH-SR200-RecoveryMonth-2014/NSDUH-SR200-RecoveryMonth-2014.htm

Sussman, S. (2010). A review of alcoholics anonymous/narcotics anonymous programs for teens. *Evaluation & the Health Professions, 33*(1), 26–55. https://doi.org/10.1177/0163278709356186

Tanner-Smith, E. E., Steinka-Fry, K. T., Kettrey, H. H., & Lipsey, M. W. (2016). *Adolescent substance abuse treatment effectiveness: A systematic review and meta-analysis*. Office of Justice Programs National Criminal Justice Reference Program. Retrieved from https://www.ncjrs.gov/pdffiles1/ojjdp/grants/250440.pdf.

Timko, C., Billow, R., & DeBenedetti, A. (2006). Determinants of 12-step group affiliation and moderators of the affiliation-abstinence relationship. *Drug & Alcohol Dependence, 83*(2), 111–121.

Weiss, R. D., Jaffee, W. B., de Menil, V. P., & Cogley, C. B. (2004). Group therapy for substance use disorders: What do we know? *Harvard Review of Psychiatry, 12*(6), 339–350. https://doi.org/10.1080/10673220490905723

Winters, K. C., Botzet, A. M., & Fahnhorst, T. (2011). Advances in adolescent substance abuse treatment. *Current Psychiatry Reports, 13*(5), 416–421. https://doi.org/10.1007/s11920-011-0214-2

Winters, K. C., Botzet, A. M., Stinchfield, R., Gonzales-Castaneda, R., Finch, A., Piehler, T., … Hemze, A. (2018). Adolescent substance abuse treatment: A review of evidence-based research. In C. G. Leukefeld & T. P. Gullotta (Eds.), *Adolescent substance abuse: Evidence-based approaches to prevention and treatment* (2nd ed. pp. 141–171). New York, NY: Springer.

Primary Prevention in Adolescent Substance Abuse

Martin Bloom and Thomas P. Gullotta

What Is Primary Prevention?

Helping is one of the oldest activities among humans, a necessary part of the great drama of species survival. Over time, this helping was aided by discovered or invented substances and methods that made helping more effective, less painful, and as a by-product, more hopeful that when problems occurred, something might be done to treat the problem and eventually bring the person back as a functioning member of society.

Primary prevention is a recent addition to the art and science of helping. Defined in the wicked spirit of Ambrose Bierce's (1911/1948) *Devil's Dictionary*, primary prevention involves a collective exercise in an ultimately personal activity, for which there is a mountain of literature and a molehill of recent hard research, in which large numbers of persons untrained in this specific field attempt to humanize abstract terms and old wives' tales through almost incomprehensible rituals that are voluntarily performed after forced indoctrination at the hands of loving family members or dedicated school personnel. Unfortunately, there are grains of truth in this formulation. However, in keeping with the optimistic spirit of this book, we offer a slightly different definition:

> **Primary prevention** involves guessing what could go wrong in a population of healthy people so as to attempt to change their ordinary and preferred behavior, by employing practitioners who have probably not been trained in this area, who follow vague theories based on limited evidence.

M. Bloom (✉)
Retired from the School of Social Work, University of Connecticut, Storrs, CT, USA
e-mail: martin.bloom@uconn.edu

T. P. Gullotta
Child and Family Agency of Southeastern Connecticut, New London, CT, USA
e-mail: tpgullotta@aol.com

C. G. Leukefeld, T. P. Gullotta (eds.), *Adolescent Substance Abuse*, Issues in Children's and Families' Lives, https://doi.org/10.1007/978-3-319-90611-9_11

Contemporary thought emphasizes the dynamic ecological perspective integrating preventive, protective, and promotive actions among persons and groups, and the settings in which they live (Durlak, 2014). Notice that primary prevention involves the persons or groups who are to be benefited by the action often perform their own helping action, hopefully guided by practitioners who are expert in the primary prevention literature offering the best available advice on achieving the positive goals. In few other modes of professional helping the clients are so directly and significantly involved for their own benefit. This dynamic perspective is seen very clearly in discussions of the prevention of substance abuse in which physiological, psychological, social, and cultural factors are actively engaged for the soul of the would-be abuser.

The background for a contemporary discussion of primary prevention emerges from the mists of folklore, which represents the ever-present hope of ordinary people that problems might be anticipated and prevented, before ever needing the substances and methods of the medical arts. Remember that for thousands of years medical treatment involved bleedings, blistering, enemas, and induced vomiting. Surgery was not considered medicine and relegated to "barbers" who undertook their tasks without effective anesthesia. No wonder people avoided getting "help" that involved voluntary torture as part of the cure.

Throughout history, people self-medicated, or more to the point, self-anesthetized their problems. Indeed, wines and beers were an early concomitant of ordinary social life, and their benefits were merely extended to extreme medical situations. For some, this self-anesthetizing became a chronic condition for a wide variety of social ills and personal problems. Often, self-anesthetizing and/or self-stimulation through substances were undertaken for recreational purposes beyond ordinary social affairs in relatively healthy individuals, which is still the case today.

History as Mirror to Today

Eventually, thoughtful people began to explore possibilities of taking informed action before problems emerged, or before desired goals had been achieved, while protecting what worked well at the moment. (This triple nature of primary prevention goals is necessary to consider, even if it makes for difficulties on sentence construction.) Following Santayana's axiom that those who ignore history are likely to repeat its errors, let us review the beginnings of primary prevention, with special reference to the prevention of intemperance. In 1817, the New York Society for the Prevention of Pauperism (NYSPP) became what might be considered the first scientifically based preventive helping in the New World (Bloom & Klein, 1995–1996). This group of mainly Quaker philanthropists broke into various study groupings that dealt with a handful of topics believed to be stemming from poverty. For example, one committee collected information on juveniles in contact with the police that led, ultimately in the Haines Report (1822), to removing them from adult prisons, and attempting to restructure and reform their lives before a fixed criminal pattern had set in. (A resulting institution, the New York House of Refuge, lasted for over 100 years.)

The NYSPP purchased firewood in the summer when it was cheap so as to sell it to the poor in winter when it was expensive. (This did not work; the poor were poor in the summer as well as in the winter.) Another committee investigated the presumed evils of pawnshops. (It found few evils, just poor people giving up whatever treasures they had to survive.) The NYSPP sent around friendly visitors anticipating social workers nearly 75 years later, and tried to encourage healthful lives, frugality, and moral lives. (These early social workers learned firsthand how difficult it was to make meaningful changes in impoverished people facing various forms of discrimination using only moral exhortations, a lesson many today still need to learn.)

But it was "intemperance" in the use of ardent spirits (whisky or gin) that was a perpetual thorn in the moral side of the NYSPP, and on which it was almost perpetually defeated in its efforts at its prevention. In its Second Annual Report (New York Society for the Prevention of Pauperism, NYSPP, 1819, p. 8), the Society's officers wrote that intemperance

> … consumes every virtue, dissolves every social tie, and destroys every noble family. It banishes industry, honesty and self-regard. It forms the nursery of crime and outrage … who can count the monuments of its desolation, in the dark valley of death!

The study group on intemperance discovered that there were 1431 persons licensed to retail liquor, which it pointed out was one "tippling house" (drinking establishment) for every 17 houses then existing in the city. In the Fourth Annual Report of the NYSPP (1821), it reports its continuing efforts, without much success. However, this report did cite a natural experiment that it hoped would be a model of action for others. It seems that a Mr. James P. Allaire, proprietor of a large foundry at Corlaer's Hook, took it upon himself to oppose a common folklore of the times, that the laboring classes could not sustain themselves under the harsh working conditions without the regular use of ardent spirits. (There was apparently no thought at this time to make the working conditions less harsh.) Mr. Allaire noticed that many of his male employees were in great debt, while others were "in easy circumstances, and their children were well provided for at school." Differences in salary did not make any difference to the level of debt—but the use or nonuse of hard liquor made all the difference. So, he took it upon himself to prohibit the use of hard liquor during working hours. This drove only 1 of his 60 employees away, and over time, he observed great changes:

> … those who, from excessive drinking, had become of but little worth to me, and in many instances, of less to their families, have now become able and steady; earn more money; and their families as well as themselves, have expressed, in a language not to be misunderstood, the many comforts and domestic happiness, which they enjoy in consequence. (pp. 9–10)

One of their few successes regarding substance use came at the city level, when the NYSPP encouraged the mayor to prohibit drinking establishments from being open on Sundays, which had a positive effect on reducing the numbers of assault and battery cases coming before the court.[1] However, all of its other proposals for legislation against intemperance were rejected.

[1]This is an example of community organization leading to a systems intervention that will be described later in this chapter.

Why spend valuable space in this chapter writing about this long-forgotten bit of American history? Let me point out that this fledgling prevention enterprise and its members dealt face to face with individuals and families, with institutions (such as savings banks for the poor and schools where they gave out selections of *Poor Richard's Almanac* to encourage the virtues of self-enterprise), and with city, state, and federal levels of social welfare policy. These were a full ecological plate of preventive activities, which does not include many other ideas that never came to fruition in the 8-year history of this society, such as centrally organizing charities to avoid duplication, job training programs (some existed at the time, so the NYSPP did not enter that field), and educational programs for the poor. It was, indeed, a moralistic enterprise, which is to say that strong public values directed its efforts at helping the poor, both materially if necessary, but with dignity throughout, so as not to encourage dependency as then-existing alms societies tended to do.

Moreover, one of the leaders of the NYSPP was John Griscom, a self-taught chemist, educator—he used the Lancasterian system of older children teaching younger children as a way of multiplying the education of large numbers of the poor—and philanthropist. He was also a one-man Campbell Collaboration, as the American correspondent for Silliman's scientific journal regarding new developments in Europe. He traveled abroad for 1 year and wrote about his visits to public institutions and creative thinkers throughout that continent. President Thomas Jefferson said that the Griscom book gave the most satisfactory view of public institutions abroad that he had ever read (Griscom, 1859, p. 152). Thus, the NYSPP, especially through its leaders, sought the best available evidence as basis for its preventive practices, using the none-too-good available demographic information to describe the scope of problems. All of these activities were in great distinction from the do-gooding philosophy of charities of the times, and bear a strong resemblance to evidence-based practice of our own day.

What is instructive about this small piece of the history of primary prevention is the difficulty to communicate effectively what are probably reasonably good suggestions for individuals, groups, and society at large. In spite of people's good intentions to be healthy, to have happy families, and to be part of a well-functioning society, things fall apart. Individuals become substance abusers harming themselves and their families. Society in turn spends enormous sums of money for ineffective methods to control the sources of drugs, the channels by which they are distributed, and the users of those substances whose addictive powers are legendary. Those early preventers of 1817 were no less enthusiastic, imaginative, and energetic than are our contemporaries. Let us hope the intervening 180 years have given us more knowledge than they had to do the good work of the primary prevention of substance abuse.

To be blunt, the USA is an alcohol-drenched society and culture, and some large-scale efforts (like prohibition) or some small-scale efforts (like Sunday closing laws) have been unsuccessful in changing people's fundamental use of alcohol and substances. This notion of an alcohol-drenched society and culture has several dimensions that recent research provides clearer understanding. Even the NYSPP recognized that alcohol was a lucrative industry. It estimated that New York drinkers paid about US $1,612,500, which should be multiplied about 100 times to get the rough equivalent contemporary dollar amount. The New York Society for the Prevention of Pauperism recognized how hedonism and greed often overcame positive feelings toward fellow creatures (including members of one's own family), and how powerful the profit motive was selling alcoholic beverages, even at the price of creating many substance abuse problems. But alcohol and drugs also affect basic physical and mental structures of the person, particularly with young substance users. In combination of the lack of future perspective of the young and their susceptibility to social pressures and indeed cultural styles and fashions involving drinking and drugs, the problems associated with preventing abusers is greatly multiplied.

On the contrary, there are many young people who do not succumb to drugs and alcohol as problematic substances, including those whose family backgrounds might predict otherwise. The issue of such resilience has only recently hit the radar screens of social science, and explorations are being made as to what constitutes the factors that make some people less vulnerable to substance abuse (Werner & Smith, 1982, 1992).

Explanatory Models of Prevention and Substance Abuse

Our prior discussion of historic background is relevant for the general and special forms of definitions of primary prevention with regard to substance abuse. Our working definition of primary prevention involves those planned actions addressing (1) predictable problems in relatively healthy individuals and groups, (2) protecting existing states of health and healthy functioning, and (3) promoting desired future states not yet attained. This general statement has to be qualified with regard to substance use and abuse.

First, efforts have to be directed toward relatively healthy and problem-free individuals. This does not mean that people will be totally free of experiences with alcohol, cigarettes, or other substances, licit and illicit. If that were a requirement, there would be few participants in these pure primary prevention programs—about 90% of Americans drink some amount of alcohol at some times in their lives (Johnston, O'Malley, Bachman, & Schulenberg, 2007), and many of these "non-drinkers" would be too young to benefit from programs delivered long in advance of the presenting challenges. It does not mean that the families of healthy young people are free of the use of any substances, because it would be hard to find families that used neither legal medications nor recreational substances, without considering any illicit ones. Yet the factual record is clear, that children coming from families that abuse alcohol, drugs, or other substances are themselves more likely to succumb to substance abuse. It does not mean that a society or culture has to be free of the use of alcohol or other substances, since the modern world seems wedded to medications and social/recreational substances that no amount of religious or moralistic sermonizing is going to change. So "relatively healthy and problem-free" individuals translate to mean those who, to some degree, use substances that do not interfere with their personal or social obligations.

We must also define primary prevention with reference to the substance use and abuse context. It might be better to define these terms in the sense of contextual outcomes, that people who are free of the problems associated with substance abuse will be fully involved in the nonsubstance world (of work, family, children, associations, etc.) and free of the stresses (personal and social/cultural) that would push them in the direction of using substances to resolve these stresses. These people will move about in a substance-drenched social environment, surrounded by media campaigns with beautiful sexy pictures promoting substances, and with friends and associates whose contacts are frequently bathed in alcohol or recreational drug smoke. They should be able to pick and choose whether or not to participate, and to what degree, recognizing the outcome of their participation on self and others. Teetotaling, while living on an isolated mountain top, is not the likely course that many contemporary people would take. So we have to place any contemporary prevention effort within a context of countervailing forces and structures of great strength.

To give some semblance of a balanced presentation, we should explore what are the benefits of substances for abuse-free people in the contemporary world. What attracts people, early in their developmental history (Leukefeld, Smiley McDonald, Stoops, Reed, & Martin, 2005), to late in their lives (Kastenbaum, 1988)? We know that a small amount of daily alcohol use has been related to preventing heart diseases, although grape juice could do the same thing.

This light use of alcohol may also be associated with reducing minor stresses of everyday life. Set within a family context of light drinking, norms are created for responsible actions that last into a child's own adulthood. This same light use of alcohol may be associated with "social fun" in settings where others are likewise less inhibited. Some people argue that marijuana is helpful in pain reduction, when other medications do not work (Grinspoon & Bakalar, 1993). Some substances are related to enhanced sexual stimulation that can be useful in some situations (some might say ecstatically wonderful), although they may lead to unanticipated consequences that could be deadly. And, let us face it, some use of substances occur just for the hell of it, because society, parents, teachers, and other goody two-shoes say we should not, which is not a bad reason in an overregulated world.

Even the second part of our working definition of primary prevention, protecting existing states of health and healthy functioning, has to be qualified in terms of preventing substance abuse. Preventers may be failing to see that people, especially young people, do not so much want to protect their current states of healthy functioning as *use* these states to attain more enjoyment in life.

People in general, but especially young people, are not well tuned to anticipate and plan for a better future. The level of saving for various desired futures is terribly low displaced by current gratifications and living for today. Piaget helped us understand this cognitive limitation in children, but this theory does not extend to adults. Eat, drink, and be merry, for tomorrow we may die—yes, this is a folk wisdom that is true as far as it goes, but it fails to note that tomorrow we may live, and yet again live into the tomorrow beyond that. And then what?

Social routines provide the structures that most people live by: "I will work, have a family, have some fun, retire into relative comfort, and die before Alzheimer's gets me (after a very brief and painless illness)." There is some truth to some of these structural assumptions, but not all of them for all people. We have to plan for that future, including alternative scenarios that are less pleasant to contemplate. Primary prevention offers some planned efforts through which individuals may shape that future to the extent that it is possible to be influenced.

So, what do adolescents (let alone their parents) know of all this? Not a lot, which is both the problem for primary preventers and a possible curriculum for delivering some solutions. Theories supply the conceptual ingredients for prevention practitioners, by identifying abstract structures and forces that can be influenced to attain desired goals. Those "desired goals" are value-loaded, which is where our balanced discussions of the pros and cons of the use of substances comes into play. Some practitioners may not like this, but we have to deliver primary prevention with regard to adolescent substance use within the real world context, not within our own pipe dreams of how reality ought to be.

Let's take the social-cognitive model of Albert Bandura (1986), whose work guides many studies across a wide range of social behaviors. Briefly, Bandura argues not only against the internal unconscious forces directing people ala Freud but also against the external forces directing people ala Skinner. Rather, Bandura proposes a multidimensional model that provides clients with relevant knowledge, skills, and motivation for obtaining a desired future, along with efforts to increase the self-efficacy of those clients, that is, the belief that they can do certain specific things. It does not matter if people have the knowledge, skill, and motivation to stop using substances; they also have to believe that they can stop using substances. To help clients reach this level of self-efficacy, preventers can use two strong tools, and two more limited ones. The first strong tool is mastery; preventers can train clients to do some specific things that are concrete steps toward the ultimate goal. Mastering these stepping-stones is a powerful inducement for self-efficacy. Likewise, showing clients how others who are like themselves are performing these steps and gaining some positive reinforcement thereby leads to vicarious learning, another powerful tool. Exhortations are more limited ways of influencing clients—"You can do it, Joe!" And physiological training, like taking a deep breath before public speaking, will reduce anxiety to some degree. We will look at how this theory is used in the prevention of adolescent substance use and abuse shortly.

Another theoretical model of many names involves the identification of risks of succumbing to substance use, along with protective factors against succumbing, in combination with promotive factors or resiliency factors that lead people in positive directions (Durlak, 2014). It is not enough not to do something negative; one must also do something positive in its place (Cowen, 2000). This general probabilistic model says that the likelihood of a person becoming involved in substance use and abuse is predictable from the *risk* factors—biological, psychological, and sociocultural—that push a person into that untoward situation such as substance abuse, reduced by the *protective* factors in the same categories that pull this person away from that untoward situation, and turned around by *promotive* factors, which move this person in some positive direction. These biological/psychological/sociocultural factors are numerous. Werner (1993) identified over one hundred factors related to resilience that can be placed into personal, interpersonal, societal, and environmental categories, from having a pleasing personality, an optimistic view of the future, and sense of humor, to finding alternative adult role models and sources of support when one's own family was lacking (see also Antonishak & Reppucci, 2008). We'll discuss how this theory can be used in prevention programming for adolescent substance use and abuse shortly.

There are also multiple systems models that involve the family, the extended family and substitutes, the relevant local social settings like schools, and the local community as well (Albee, 1983; Bloom, 1996; D'Amico, Chinman, Stern, & Wandersman, 2008). These models are closely linked to practice, and thus use as many of the real-world forces and structures that have strong influences on individuals' choices toward or against substance use and abuse. We generalize from the Sexton, Gilman, and Johnson-Erickson (2005, pp. 112–115) list of the conceptual assumptions for this kind of model (their list is made with reference to multisystemic therapy): (1) that all important social behaviors are multidetermined; (2) that primary group caregivers and educators are important for long-term developments and changes of behavior; (3) that evidence-based practice should direct interventions, along with the clinical expertise in applying this general information to the specific client; (4) that barriers to service require as much attention as the intervention itself; and (5) evaluation is an important part of practice to progress and to assess outcomes, as well as confirm the fidelity of the program when transported to new settings. These and other principles guide programs in the prevention of substance use and abuse, which we will discuss shortly.

The Tools of Primary Prevention

Gullotta (1983, 1987, 1994) and Gullotta and Bloom (2003, 2014) have described five technologies that are used to achieve illness prevention and health promotion. These technologies appear so often and in so many of the special topic areas of primary prevention that we are inclined to call them general strategies that should be considered as beginning points, and in combination, for any future preventive effort, including the prevention of substance abuse with adolescents.

Education is the first general strategy of primary prevention. It is the most often used technology that preventionists apply to reducing risk and promoting resiliency; however, it is rarely, if ever, effective when used alone. This is because clients and consumers of primary prevention usually require some knowledge about a given topic, but simple *information* alone may not affect attitudes, and probably will not change behaviors that are a product of thoughts, feelings, and external situations. For example, adolescents probably know something about the hazards of substance use (although their knowledge is often limited, fuzzy, or both). They may state their intention to stay away from these hazards or stop using substances if they are already engaged in doing so. But major behavior changes are not usually based on such cognitive factors alone. Thus, the "Just Say NO!" campaign of the 1980s was destined to failure from the outset. Education can be public, as in school lessons on the nature of substances and their effects on the body. Teachers, parents, and ministers often say to children, "do as I say" regarding substances, and "not as I do." Use of legal substances is limited to adults, and the transition period between childhood and adulthood is the perfect storm for conflict over the beginning use of substances. Rather, adults might be wiser to use information as *anticipatory guidance*, in which a nonuser (or beginning user) is informed about the immediate and long-term effects. The immediate (such as bad tobacco breath) may appeal to younger adolescents, but eventually the long-term effects of life-threatening harm to their bodies may be understood as a basis for action. This aspect of education slides into a third type, self-instruction, the *development of self-control* to achieve future goals rather than immediate gratification.

The promotion of *self-competency* is the second technology. To be socially competent involves people interacting with other people over the lifetime in mutually satisfying ways. This begins when an individual is brought into a group, such as a family, and the group values the membership of that individual who eventually comes to make meaningful contributions to the group. This circularity of mutual interactions where both individual and group benefit is learned throughout one's life, and draws on personal characteristics (e.g., a developing sense of self-esteem, an internal locus of control, and a growing sense of mastery over valued activities) and social conditions (e.g., the need for members to perform certain roles in relation to others and the need to survive against an indifferent world).

Prevention's third technology is *natural caregiving*. Gullotta (1983) identified three forms of this technology. First, there are *mutual self-help groups*. These are not led by helping professionals, but rather involve those drawn together by common experiences for which members are both caregivers and care receivers. Some members are further along in these experiences, and can guide others in preparing for what to expect. They are informal groupings where exchanges are common, sharing of small triumphs, and supporting those suffering large losses. Being human together generates support for all, by helping others and by being helped, in turn.

The second way of natural caregiving that can be found is in the way society has informally conferred on some people the expectation that they will lend a listening ear and helpful advice to others in times of need. These *trained indigenous caregivers* are ministers, teachers, police officers, coaches, youth leaders in scouting and 4H to name a few. They are not specifically trained in counseling or mental health services as such, yet their advice as caring adults is important as a first line of service for people in need. Indeed, for many, this caring enables the vast majority of individuals in society to cope and adapt when stressful demands are placed upon them.

The last form natural caregiving can take is found within the actions of each of us as individuals and can be described as *friendship*. The simple act of extending social support to another is a powerful agent for health that enables a person to receive empathy, constructive feedback, and another perspective on issues that may be either joyful or filled with sorrow.

The fourth technology of primary prevention goes beyond the individual to focus its attention on changing community behavior and institutions (community organization and systems intervention). In each of the examples that follow, a group of people have banded together to express their (common) concerns and to develop solutions for these concerns. They may work within the problematic system or from outside. Their own "organization" may be informal or formal, depending on the circumstances. To illustrate, Mothers Against Drunk Driving (MADD) began with one grief-stricken parent who had lost a loved one. Her effort was soon joined by others who too had seen a child or spouse die because of the irresponsible actions of a drunken driver. MADD spoke to the entertainment community. Their message was drunken behavior was not the stuff of comedy. MADD enlisted the law enforcement community as an ally to advocate for tougher legal repercussions against drunken driving. MADD lobbied legislators to pass laws that lowered blood alcohol rates to be considered for a driving under the influence (DUI) arrest. Collectively, these actions by citizens who have lost a loved one to a drunken driver have produced a major change in community attitudes and behavior. MADD is not alone in its success to correct societal injustice. The National Association for the Advancement of Colored People (NAACP) and its use of the legal system to achieve justice is a second example with Rosa Parks' refusal to sit at the back of the bus, an excellent illustration of this. Contrary to popular belief, Rosa Parks' action was not an unplanned refusal spurred by an "I'm mad as hell and not gonna take this anymore attitude." On the contrary, this well-educated dignified lady acted with the NAACP's knowledge to begin a process that would eventually grow to actually changing the Constitution of the USA to ensure the civil rights of all Americans.

Other community organizational activities may not be as much of a landmark as either of the two previous examples but are as equally effective. For a humorous example, with the increasing buildup of housing in many areas and a rise in lawsuits, most communities no longer permit dogs to run free in public parks, and heaven forbid they should ever stray onto a playing field even if their owner carries a pooper-scooper. The choice for a dog lover was to either buy a home with a sufficiently larger yard (cost prohibitive in Manhattan) or jettison the family canine. Both were unacceptable choices. The result—canine owners joining together on behalf of their pets to advocate for pet parks. Initially, the thought of a place for Fido to run and play with Lassie and Rin-Tin-Tin was laughed at, but with persistence and increasing members of the pet-owning community adding their howl to the call, pet parks are appearing across the country. The point of these three examples is that change to remedy a perceived injustice can and does happen when like-minded people set forth to do so.

But not all change is at the community level. Some changes happen, should happen, and can happen at the institutional level. In these instances one or more individuals identify dysfunctional practices within an institution and act to change that behavior. In her writing Tadmor (2003) has provided two outstanding examples of this. In both cases, well-meaning health care professionals in a respected hospital were providing necessary medical treatments but doing so in such a way as to increase significantly the emotional distress and depression of the patients receiving treatment. In both cases the staff were ignorant of their behavior and rejecting of the need for change. Nevertheless, persistence and courageous individual behavior forced needed changes into the delivery of services with a corresponding decrease in the emotional suffering of the client population.

The fifth technology of primary prevention focuses on the *redesign of the environment*. Ecologists and Buddhists have emphasized the interrelationship of all things, so that when we consider actions relevant to adolescents with the potential for substance use or abuse we consider not only the individuals themselves, with their complex genetic history and social psychological experiences but also the primary and secondary groups that make up their social and cultural world.

These we have discussed above, and ad nauseam everywhere else. What tends to receive far less attention is the impact of the physical environment on human beings, and the effect of human activities on the physical environment.

This is an "inconvenient truth" as Gore (2006) has vividly described, that we are harming this necessary physical environment in ways beyond our imagination and more rapidly than most pessimists had dreamed. Greed, pride, and stupidity have combined to make a crisis situation at almost every turn. American automobile manufacturers promise to reduce harmful emissions some time by the year 2020, even though European manufacturers have arrived at these lower levels now, not a decade later. Increasing percentages of Americans are growing obese, including young children who are now becoming subject to diseases at an earlier age than their (couch potato) parents, which will be putting a severe strain on the health care system that is the "best in the world" for some people, but not for the millions of uninsured others. These and other trends are worldwide conditions, rapidly increasing demands on the physical environment, such as burning down huge areas of the Amazon rain forest to grow soybeans for the exploding population of China.

Ultimately, we have to put every primary prevention question into this perspective: How will what we propose to do for some specific population of clients affect and be affected by the physical world in which we live? For example, laws against substance use in the United States affect how land will be used abroad to grow the plants used in making illicit drugs. It will also affect how third-party nations will develop factories to make chemicals to transform these plants into hard drugs. Everywhere, from the farmers, to the chemists, to the transporters, to the drug sellers, there is little concern for the effects on the physical environment and what alternative uses of land, labor, and transport there would be.

Thus, the full circle is completed—education informs, natural caregiving unites, social competency enables, social institutions create, and the physical environment supports. All are needed to institute an effective primary prevention program.

Theory-And-Evidence-Based Practice *and* Evaluation-Informed Practice in Primary Prevention

We live at the beginning of a new age in primary prevention practice where many pieces of knowledge that have been studied separately are now seen as a complex whole. This new model involves two major aspects, first the theoretical and the empirical, and second, the practical. Let us consider these and their interrelationships. First, theories or principles are needed to explain the nature of clients, problems, change agents, physical and social settings. Clearly, we need the conceptual mapping of all of these factors so that we can understand the nature of everything involved in the problem, including how the client views it. (If we don't have an understanding of all of these ingredients, then we risk diminishing our impact.) We need the available empirical evidence on what is known to influence or control the several aspects of the problem situation. (If the empirical evidence is not available, then again we risk diminishing our effectiveness.) Second, importantly, we need to understand how to translate the theoretical and empirical information into practical directions to affect positive change. (If I am able to do actions X, will positive outcomes Y occur, without negative by-products Z?) And we need to be able to measure and document how well our specific practices affected our client's real world situations (Bloom & Britner, 2012). This usually involves on-going monitoring of the X actions and the movement toward Y outcomes, without any Z problems emerging along the way. The methods to do these evaluations must be accessible to all practitioners so that the results can be comprehensible to the clients, and understandable by the funders of the service organization that these results represent positive changes in client problems.

The rules for planned actions deal with questions like what actions should I take, if I do X, will Y occur? When should I take these actions? How will I know whether the actions had their desired outcome?

Applications of These Theories/Research-Based Practices in Field Settings

As a short hand for this complex model, we have entitled this section Theory-and Evidence-Based Practice *and* Evaluation-Informed Practice in Primary Prevention. The important term in this title is the humble word *and*. It means that the two aspects (theory/research and practice) are and must be truly interrelated. If we have a conceptual sense of what the problem is and the many contextual factors in which it exists, then we have to be able to influence that conceptual sense by means of real world actions that are the operationally connected to the meaning of the problems and solutions. As a brief example, if a woman employee is not being treated fairly by her male employer in terms of career advancement, and comes to a helping professional feeling depressed, then training this woman in assertiveness skills might lead to a positive career solution (without alienating anyone in this situation) and reducing her depressed feelings. The theory being used in this situation is assertiveness training that involved learning how to put forward one's ideas and wishes, without alienating the employer. The research in this area suggests this has been an effective method of change. And the practice involves training the client to present her ideas and wishes strongly but tactfully, on being a more active and productive contributor in the business. In short, the guiding theory and supporting empirical evidence are translated into a form that the client can manage, and the employer can recognize positive outcomes of the change. One must see how these various aspects fit together as a theoretically guided and empirically supported method for changing a complex real world situation, to the benefit of all participants.

Jacobus-Kantor et al. (2014, pp. 854–864) find no interventions that meet the standard of three successful trials, but they describe a number of promising programs for children of substance-abusing parents (COSAP). We will illustrate one of these promising efforts, The Strengthening Families Program (SFP), a family-based prevention program that has been shown "to increase resilience and decrease alcohol, tobacco, and drug use among elementary-aged school children" (p. 858) whose parents are substance abusers (Kumpfer, DeMarsh, & Child, 1989). Reflecting a complex world of families with substance-abusing parents, the SFP provides participating adults with parenting skills, while also giving their children social skills training. In addition, they provided a family enhancement program involving both parents and children. The program was conducted in community settings in 2–3 h sessions, although the number of sessions involved was not discussed. Putting together all of these elements means that lessons learned in one setting by one group of participants will be reinforced and expanded with lessons learned in another setting with the same participants. This reflects the complex model we discussed above, where theory and research is smoothly combined with helping practices, while showing successful interventions over time and with various cultural groups, as we will discuss below.

The SFP is the most widely replicated program that Jacobus-Kantor, Emshoff, and Johnson discuss (2014). Long-term follow-ups with participating children shows that the positive effects persist over time. First, a 5-year follow-up demonstrated that the program was effective in reducing rates of alcohol and drug abuse among children aged 10–14 years, as well as showing an estimated cost–benefit ratio of $9.60 community benefits to $1.00 project costs (Spoth, Guyll, & Day, 2002). Then, in a 10-year follow-up, researchers report that participating children have significantly lower levels of lifetime mental health disorders, compared to a control group (Spoth & Greenberg, 2005; Trudeau, Redmond, & Spoth, 2004). Furthermore, the SFP has been modified with several cultural groups, including rural and urban African-American COSAs; Hawaiian COSAs; Hispanic COSAs, and rural preteens (Kumpfer, Pinyuchon, Teixeira de Melo, & Whiteside, 2008). Results with these groups show that the basic program with minor cultural revisions was more effective that a substantially revised program, suggesting that the core content should not be deleted when making cultural group changes. As a result of these positive outcomes, Jacobus-Kantor et al. (2014) note that NIDA has chosen SFP as a "model substance-abuse prevention program for dissemination" (p. 859).

It is important to indicate programs that do not work, or do not work as well as those cited above as promising. Meta-analyses by Tobler and her colleagues are instructive: Tobler et al. (2000, p. 275) use a detailed analysis of a large number of studies which lead to the following general conclusions: Family-based programs are less effective than school-based comprehensive life-skills programs (Schinke & Gilchrist, 1983). The effects on substance use are very weak, compared to findings on conduct disorder and aggression. Interactive programs are more effective than those that are noninteractive (solely didactic), but only for some grade levels (junior, high, and above). They recommend the use of universal school programs (targeting all students in a given grade), supplemented with some family-focused interventions (especially with selective and indicated populations that are showing more signs of emerging problems than students in general). However, they conclude with a recommendation for more community-level interventions that affect social norms and environmental determinants of individual behaviors. This last remark mirrors the conclusion of the chapter in the first edition of this book by D'Amico et al. (2008): Primary prevention at the macro level needs an interactive systems framework that includes an intervention development component, which is readied for use in a prevention synthesis and translation system, followed by a prevention delivery system in which this intervention is put into place. They note that a prevention support system is needed to link the research domain with the field practice arena, in order that all these good ideas are to be utilized in practice.

Conclusion

As we look at bouncy adolescents frolicking at local community centers in our hometowns, we wonder whether or what substances they are taking, here or elsewhere. It is difficult to differentiate "normal" adolescent behavior—if there is such a thing—from substance-enhanced behaviors, licit or illicit. These wonderful developing youths will all too soon be adults, taking their places in society, just as we did years ago. While their bounce may disturb the tranquility, but us old folks, we are glad to see them lively and engaged with life. But we worry, as a preventer, protector, promoter, that some of what they do without a whole lot of thought or anticipation of their distant future will be to their detriment, and ultimately, of ours. Reviewing the range of individual, group, institution, and community-level interventions that work, all we can do is to advocate for these effective programs with the powers that be, and hope for the best with individual members of that bouncy tribe. The good news is that we know about many things that work to prevent predictable problems, protect existing states of healthy functioning, and promote desired goals (Gullotta & Bloom, 2014). Let 'er roll!

References

Albee, G. W. (1983). Psychopathology, prevention, and the just society. *Journal of Primary Prevention, 4*(1), 5–40.

Antonishak, J., & Reppucci, N. D. (2008). Ecological and community level influences on child development. In T. P. Gullotta & G. M. Blau (Eds.), *Handbook of childhood behavioral issues: Evidence-based approaches to prevention and treatment* (pp. 69–86). New York, NY: Routledge.

Bandura, A. (1986). *Social foundations of thought and action: A social cognitive theory.* Englewood Cliffs, NJ: Prentice-Hall.

Bierce, A. (1911/1948). *Devil's dictionary.* Cleveland, OH: World Publishing Co..

Bloom, M. (1996). *Primary prevention practices.* Thousand Oaks, CA: Sage.

Bloom, M., & Britner, P. A. (2012). *Client-centered evaluation: New models for helping professionals.* Boston, MA: Allynn & Bacon.

Bloom, M., & Klein, W. C. (1995–1996). John Griscom and primary prevention at the beginning of the 19th century. *Journal of Applied Social Science, 20*(1), 15–24.

Cowen, E. L. (2000). Psychological wellness: Some hopes for the future. In D. Cicchetti, J. Rappoport, I. Sandler, & R. P. Weissberg (Eds.), *The promotion of wellness in children and adolescents* (pp. 477–503). Washington, DC: Child Welfare League of America Press.

D'Amico, E. J., Chinman, M., Stern, S. A., & Wandersman, A. (2008). Community prevention handbook on adolescent substance abuse prevention and treatment: Evidence-based practices. In C. Leukefeld, T. P. Gullotta, & M. Staton-Tindall (Eds.), *Handbook on adolescent substance abuse prevention and treatment: Evidence-based practice* (pp. 213–249). New York, NY: Springer.

Durlak, J. A. (2014). Programming for effective prevention and health promotion programming. In T. P. Gullotta & M. Bloom (Eds.), *Encyclopedia of primary prevention and health promotion* (2nd ed., pp. 102–111). New York, NY: Springer.

Gore, A. (2006). *An inconvenient truth.* Emmaus, PA: Rodale.

Grinspoon, L., & Bakalar, J. B. (1993). *Marijauna forbidden medicine.* New Haven, CT: Yale University Press.

Griscom, J. H. (1859). *Memoir of John Griscom, L.L.D., late professor of chemistry and natural philosophy; with an account of the New York High School; Society for the Prevention of Pauperism; the House of Refuge; and other institutions.* Compiled from an autobiography, and other sources. New York, NY: Robert Carter and Brothers.

Gullotta, T. P. (1983, October 25). *Prevention's developing technology.* Institute at the Annual American Orthopsychiatric Meeting, Boston, MA.

Gullotta, T. P. (1987). Prevention's technology. *Journal of Primary Prevention, 7*(4), 176–196.

Gullotta, T. P. (1994). The what, who, why, where, when, and how of primary prevention. *Journal of Primary Prevention, 15*(1), 5–14.

Gullotta, T. P., & Bloom, M. (Eds.). (2003). *Encyclopedia of primary prevention and health promotion.* New York, NY: Kluwer Academic/Plenum.

Gullotta, T. P., & Bloom, M. (Eds.). (2014). *Encyclopedia of primary prevention and health promotion* (2nd ed.). New York, NY: Springer.

Haines Report. (1822). *Report on the penitentiary system in the United States, prepared under a resolution of the Society of the Prevention of Pauperism, in the City of New York.* New York, NY: M. Day

Jacobus-Kantor, L., Emshoff, J. G., & Johnson, J. (2014). Promoting the healthy development of children whose parents are alcoholic/drug dependent. In T. P. Gullotta & M. Bloom (Eds.), *Encyclopedia of primary prevention and health promotion* (2nd ed., pp. 854–864). New York, NY: Springer.

Johnston, L. D., O'Malley, P. M., Bachman, J. G., & Schulenberg, J. E. (2007). *Monitoring the future: National survey results on drug use, 1975–2006.* Bethesda, MD: National Institute on Drug Abuse.

Kastenbaum, R. (1988). In moderation: How some older people find pleasure and meaning in alcoholic beverages. *Generations, 12*(4), 68–71.

Kumpfer, K. L., DeMarsh, J. P., & Child, W. (1989). *Strengthening families program: Children's skills training curriculum manual, parent training manual, children's skills training manual, and family skills training manual.* Salt Lake City, UT: University of Utah, Social Research Institute, Graduate School of Social Work.

Kumpfer, K. L., Pinyuchon, M., Teixeira de Melo, A., & Whiteside, H. O. (2008, June). Cultural adaptation process for international dissemination of the strengthening families program. *Evaluation & Health Professions, 31*(2), 226–239. https://doi.org/10.1177/0163278708315926

Leukefeld, C. G., Smiley McDonald, H. M., Stoops, W. W., Reed, L., & Martin, C. (2005). Substance misuse and abuse. In T. P. Gullotta & G. R. Adams (Eds.), *Handbook of adolescent behavioral problems: Evidence-based approaches to prevention and treatment* (pp. 439–465). New York, NY: Springer.

New York Society for the Prevention of Pauperism. (1819). *Second annual report.* New York, NY: E. Conrad.

New York Society for the Prevention of Pauperism. (1821). *Fourth annual report.* New York, NY: E. Conrad.

Schinke, S., & Gilchrist, L. (1983). Primary prevention of tobacco smoking. *Journal of School Health, 53*(7), 416–419.

Sexton, T. L., Gilman, L., & Johnson-Erickson, C. (2005). Evidence-based practices. In T. P. Gullotta & G. R. Adams (Eds.), *Handbook of adolescent behavioral problems: Evidence-based approaches to prevention and treatment* (pp. 101–128). New York, NY: Springer.

Spoth, R. L., & Greenberg, M. T. (2005). Toward a comprehensive strategy for effective practitioner – Scientist partnerships and larger-scale community benefits. *American Journal of Community Psychology, 35*(3–4), 107–126. Retrieved from https://www.ncbi.nlm.nih.gov/pmc/articles/PMC2848444/

Spoth, R. L., Guyll, M., & Day, S. X. (2002, March). Universal family-focused interventions in alcohol-use disorder prevention: Cost-effectiveness and cost-benefit analyses of two interventions. *Journal of Studies on Alcohol and Drugs, 63*(2), 219–228.

Streke, A., Roona, M., & Marshall, D. (2003). Substances, childhood (meta-analysis). In T. P. Gullotta & M. Bloom (Eds.), *Encyclopedia of primary prevention and health promotion* (pp. 1059–1064). New York, NY: Kluwer Academic/Plenum.

Tadmor, C. S. (2003). Perceived personal control. In T. P. Gullotta & M. Bloom (Eds.), *Encyclopedia of primary prevention and health promotion* (pp. 812–821). New York, NY: Kluwer Academic/Plenum.

Tobler, N. S., Roona, M. R., Ochshorn, P., Marshall, D. G., Streke, A. V., & Stackpole, K. M. (2000). School-based adolescent drug prevention programs: 1998 meta-analysis. *Journal of Primary Prevention, 20*(4), 275–336.

Trudeau, L., Redmond, C, & Spoth, R. (2004, May). Risk moderation of adolescent universal family and school preventive interventions. Poster presented at the Society for Prevention Research 12th annual meeting, Quebec City, Canada.

Werner, E. E. (1993). Risk, resilience, and recovery: Perspectives from the Kauai longitudinal study. *Development and Psychopathology, 5*(4), 503–515.

Werner, E. E., & Smith, R. S. (1982). *Vulnerable but invincible: A longitudinal study of resilient children and youth.* New York, NY: McGraw-Hill Book Company.

Werner, E. E., & Smith, R. S. (1992). *Overcoming the odds: High risk children from birth to adulthood.* Ithaca, NY: Cornell University Press.

Recovering to Recovery Among Adolescent Youth

Katherine R. Marks and Carl G. Leukefeld

Introduction

In 2015, it was estimated that ~1.3 million youth aged 12–17 years and 5.4 million young adults aged 18–25 years were in need of substance use treatment (Substance Abuse and Mental Health Services Administration, 2016). Of those individuals, 6.3% of youth and 7.7% of young adults received substance abuse treatment through a specialty facility in the past year (SAMHSA, 2016). Although the number of the youth who identify as recovering or in recovery through formal or informal treatment is not known, estimates of youth substance misuse, based on rates of met and unmet treatment need suggest that the number is sizeable. Despite the need, limited empirical research has been dedicated toward understanding the recovering process or recovering outcomes. This knowledge gap is not unique to the youth literature and extends to the adult literature as well.

Why Recovering Is Important

The United States Drug Control Policy now includes the promotion of recovery as a targeted area (Office of National Drug Control Policy, 2016). However, little foundational work has been conducted with recovering adolescents. Instead, the focus has generally been placed on intervention barriers and predictors of relapse. Understanding adolescent recovery, distinct from that of adults, is a paradigm shift and is important for a variety of reasons. Defining and understanding adolescent recovery is critical for growing the evidence base for both treatment and recovery

K. R. Marks (✉) · C. G. Leukefeld
Department of Behavioral Science, University of Kentucky, Lexington, KY, USA
e-mail: katie.marks@uky.edu; cleukef@uky.edu

C. G. Leukefeld, T. P. Gullotta (eds.), *Adolescent Substance Abuse*, Issues in Children's and Families' Lives, https://doi.org/10.1007/978-3-319-90611-9_12

support services as well as for research. Treatment targets can be expanded and refined through a better understanding of what adolescent recovering may or may not encompass. In addition, prevention efforts can be enhanced by understanding the skills and resources acquired while recovering and developing programs to enhance those factors in primary, secondary, and tertiary prevention programs.

This chapter provides an overview of selected factors related to adolescents recovering from substance use, a framework for thinking about recovering, a critical overview of definitions of adolescent recovery, and factors that can support recovering. Recovering is defined in this chapter as a process of change through which an individual achieves improved heath, wellness, and quality of life. This chapter also overviews selected factors, which have been found to be associated with adolescents recovering. In addition, promising recovering supports and approaches that do not work are presented.

A Common Theoretical Framework for Substance Use and Recovering

A bio/psycho/social/spiritual theoretical framework (Leukefeld & Leukefeld, 1999) proposes a way of thinking about substance use. The framework includes four possible pathways or combinations of pathways that influence the likelihood of substance misuse. Traditionally, the bio/psycho/social/spiritual framework is utilized to help organize thinking around the pathways leading to substance misuse. *Biological* pathways include genetic heritability and neurobiological factors that modulate drug-taking behavior. *Psychological* pathways incorporate individual characteristics that influence motivation such as, expectancies of rewards of substance use, personality factors such as urgency and sensation seeking, and thoughts and attitudes towards substance use. *Social and environmental* pathways include laws, culture, family norms, customs, and peer associations related to substance abuse. *Spirituality* is inversely related to substance use (Gmel et al., 2013; Staton, Webster, Hiller, Rotosky, & Leukefeld, 2003; Staton-Tindall et al., 2008) and refers to an individual's perceptions, beliefs, and feelings about a higher power, universal spirit, or ultimate purpose (Green, Fullilove, & Fullilove, 1998; Watkins, 1997).

This same framework can be applied to think about recovering pathways. *Biological recovering* pathways can include return to homeostatic neurobiology following a reduction or cessation of substance use, utilization of medication-assisted treatment when indicated (including pharmacogenetic interactions), and physical health supporting recovering outcomes (Marks & Leukefeld, 2017). *Psychological* recovering pathways incorporate individual characteristics that influence motivation such as, expectancies of rewards associated with alternative (i.e., non-substance-related) reinforcers and consequences of substance use, personality factors, mental health, as well as thoughts and attitudes about recovering. *Social and environmental* recovering pathways include laws, culture, family norms, customs, and peer associations related to recovering behavior. *Spiritual* recovering pathways can introduce a sense of purpose, life meaning, and connection with a higher power. Although the clinical literature is fairly consistent in the idea that spirituality is protective, related to recovery, and important for the process of recovering, it is not without controversy, particularly as spirituality, for some, may intersect with religiosity. Bio/psycho/social/spiritual pathways have also been expressed through the framework of recovery capital, which refers to the quantity and quality of individual and environmental factors (e.g., physical, human, social, cultural capital) that support recovering outcomes (Granfield & Cloud, 2001).

Defining Recovering

Definitions of recovering vary across stakeholders. Within the recovering community, there are many different recovering paths and such lived experience shapes each individual's understanding of what recovering looks like and what it does not look it (Kaskutas & Ritter, 2015; Laudet, 2007). Likewise, formal treatment providers, tradition-based providers, policy makers, mutual-help based, and self-help based service providers define recovering based on outcomes deemed relevant by their program and/or profession. Furthermore, definitions of recovering are bounded by factors including culture, place, and time.

The Substance Abuse and Mental Health Services Administration (SAMHSA) defines recovering as, "a process of change through which individuals improve their health and wellness, live self-directed lives, and strive to reach their full potential" (SAMHSA, 2012). In contrast, the Hazelden Betty Ford Foundation defines recovering as, "a voluntarily maintained lifestyle characterized by sobriety, personal health, and citizenship" (Schwarzlose, 2007).

Similarities and differences between definitions of recovering highlight three important points. First, common to both definitions is the subtle but critical nuance that recovering is an active and ongoing engagement in change over an undetermined period of time rather than an endpoint. Evidence supports recovering as continuing, rather than an acute care model. Second, the primary outcomes or benchmarks of recovering vary across definitions. Indeed, the only common recovering outcome between definitions is health. Third, current definitions of recovering were not developed for adolescents. As noted by Botzet, McIlvain, Winters, Fahnhorst, and Dittel (2014), this is a problem compounded by the fact that diagnostic criteria for substance use disorders were validated among adults rather than adolescents. As such, it may be that meaningful definitions of recovering cannot be established until age-appropriate criteria for substance misuse are developed.

Although definitions of recovering may be intended for broad applicability, some recovering outcomes may be developmentally inappropriate for adolescents. For example, citizenship is traditionally referencing employment; a goal that is not relevant or achievable for many youth. Living a self-directed life may also be incongruent with the developmental and environmental factors operating in youth's lives. Recovering physical health is an important outcome for recovering adults, particularly women (Marks & Leukefeld, 2017). However, it may not be the case for adolescents who have not experienced the same physical consequences of sustained, chronic use. Focus groups examining adolescents' thoughts and attitudes around recovering outcomes indicate that lifestyle improvement, personal change and growth, personal control related to substance use, and wellness are more important and salient factors (Gonzales, Anglin, Beattie, Ong, & Glik, 2012a).

Perhaps most salient in definitions of recovering is the inclusion or exclusion of abstinence. For adolescents, abstinence may not be perceived as an essential feature of recovery. For example, research on adolescents in a variety of treatment settings indicates that only 10% of adolescents would include total abstinence in their definition of recovery (Gonzales et al., 2012a). A similar study assessing adolescent's motivation for abstinence while in treatment revealed that about one fifth endorsed their motivation for total abstinence (Chung et al., 2015). Instead, nearly half the youth reported a goal of temporary abstinence, occasional use, or controlled use. This suggests an abstinence model of recovery, which is aligned with the chronic, progressive disease model, may not resonate or be useful for youth. However, Myers and Brown (1996) reported that abstinence-focused cognitions and behaviors were more predictive of subsequent problem alcohol use than perceived self-efficacy to abstain. Consequently, the extent to which adolescents include abstinence as a recovering goal may impact their long-term recovery. Harm reduction is an alternative pathway to abstinence. However, harm reduction among adolescents is complicated by factors such as the legality of any use and the demonstrated importance of protecting against the neurotoxic effects of substances during the sensitive neurodevelopmental period of adolescence. In contrast to the objective outcomes of more formal definitions, others assert that an individual is recovering when they say they are recovering (e.g., Connecticut Community for Addiction Recovery (CCAR), 2017). However, it is difficult to ascertain progress in recovery if developmentally appropriate, quantifiable outcomes are not established, understood, and used.

Relapse and Recovering

Relapse is a part of the recovering process. Rates of relapse among adolescents, like adults, are high with estimates of 66–85% returning to substance use 1 year following inpatient treatment (Brown & D'Amico, 2003; Brown, Gleghorn, Schuckit, Myers, & Mott, 1996; Kaminer, 2001; Winters, Stinchfield, Opland, Weller, & Latimer, 2000). Rather than thinking of recovering and relapse as two fixed points on a continuum, the state of recovering can be thought of as the distance between the two points (Leukefeld, 2015). Recovering can then represent a temporal distance from the last episode of relapse. As an individual is recovering, a greater temporal distance is placed between relapse and recovering. Definitions of relapse vary, particularly among adolescents (see Chung & Maisto, 2006), but total abstinence from any substance of abuse is one standard by which many assess whether a relapse has taken place (Miller, 1996). However, parameters which can impact determination of relapse include duration of recovery or abstinence, amount of substance the individual has returned to using, the negative consequences associated with that use, and the type of substance used (Chung & Maisto, 2006). Definition of relapse used can impact decisions about treatment duration, treatment effectiveness, and the mechanisms which support behavior change (Maisto, Pollock, Cornelius, Lynch, & Martin, 2003).

Adolescents are more likely to relapse when experiencing social pressure when compared with adults (Ramo & Brown, 2008). Conversely, social support is one factor associated with increased time to relapse following treatment among adolescents (Myers & Brown, 1996). This finding is consistent with the well-documented impact of peer influence, both positive and negative, on substance-use behavior during adolescence (Leukefeld et al., 1998). Research from focus groups including youth similarly report that peer pressure is one of the five most common perceived reasons for relapse (Gonzales, Anglin, Beattie, Ong, & Glik, 2012b). Other important factors include feeling unable to cope with negative emotions, negative life stressors, low motivation and confidence, craving, and environmental factors such as cues and triggers.

What Works to Support Recovering Outcomes

Pathways to recovering among adolescents vary and may not be mutually exclusive. Currently, a common, evidence-based pathway to recovering includes substance abuse treatment either in residential or outpatient settings. For many adolescents, this may begin involuntarily through the influence of parents, courts, the juvenile justice system, or school systems. A common notion of recovery is that recovering begins during or following the completion of treatment. However, as Moberg and Finch (2008) correctly point out, the majority of individuals who meet criteria for a substance use disorder do not receive treatment. The proportion of adolescents who change their substance use behavior on their own without formal intervention (i.e., "natural recovery") is unknown, but likely large (Sobell, Ellingstad, & Sobell, 2000). Thus, recovering cannot be contingent upon formal treatment.

A conceptual framework that considers recovering as a continuous process of multidimensional change is the Recovery-Oriented Systems-of-Care (ROSC; Kaplan, 2008). Adopted by the Substance Abuse and Mental Health Services Administration, ROSC provides a framework for utilizing evidence-based programs and understanding their relationship within a continuum of care. A ROSC framework is described as a coordinated network of community-based services including prevention, early intervention, treatment, and recovery support services (Kaplan, 2008). Movement within this continuum is a continuous process of multidimensional change and thus requires a wide array of individualized, person-centered services. Furthermore, programs and services are implemented to capitalize on strengths and

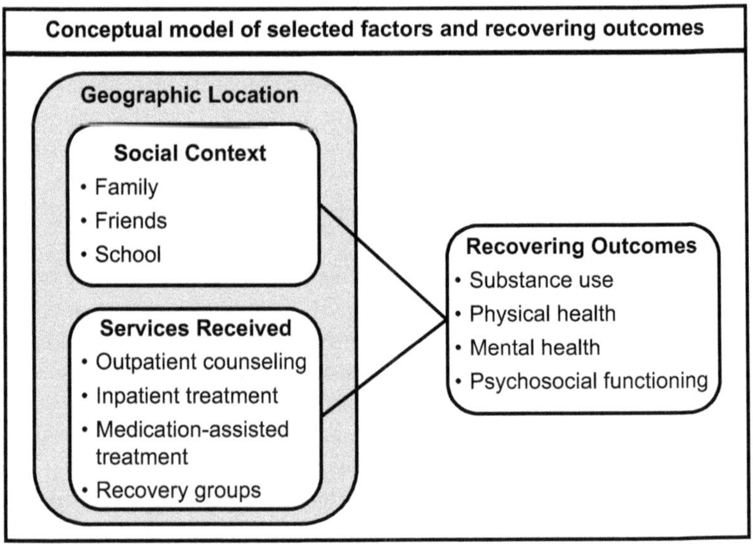

Fig. 1 Example conceptual model of selected environmental factors and recovering outcomes. Created by authors, Marks and Leukefeld (2017)

resiliencies, rather than barriers. By identifying strengths, youth along with treatment providers can build on assets to support recovering outcomes. Key to this conceptual framework is an emphasis on the variety of resources within the environment that recovering individuals can access (e.g., intervention services, social support; see Fig. 1). Examples of recovering supports within the community include recovery community centers, sober living environments, education and employment, transportation, life-skills development, and involvement in recovery groups. The ROSC framework is also based on a continuing care model in which the psychosocial supports can be accessed long-term. Although the ROSC is not evidence-based for adolescents, services and programs for adolescents within this framework should be evidence-based or evidence-informed.

Converging preclinical and clinical evidence indicates that environmental factors are critical in maintaining behavior change (Bouton, 2014). Environmental factors include places in which youth are recovering and persons with whom youth are recovering (Volkow, Koob, & Mclellan, 2016). Geographic location is a key environmental factor that can support recovering. In the USA, ~16% of youth 18 years of age and younger live in nonmetropolitan, rural areas (US Department of Health and Human Services, 2015). Substance use risk factors vary across rural and urban areas (Keyes, Cerdá, Brady, Havens, & Galea, 2014). For example, youth living in rural areas are more likely to use tobacco, smokeless tobacco, alcohol, and methamphetamine than youth living in urban areas (Gale, Lenardson, Lambert, & Hartley, 2012; Gfroerer, Larson, & Colliver, 2007; Hanson et al., 2009; Hutchison & Blakely, 2003; Zollinger, Saywell, Overgaard, Przybylski, & Dutta-Bergman, 2006; but see Hanson et al., 2009; Warren, Smalley, & Barefoot, 2016). Variation in substance use can be attributed to differences in age, region, dates of data collection, and rural context (e.g., weakening economies, decreasing isolation, and destabilization of traditional family structures (Dew, Elifson, & Dozier, 2007). Geographic location can also be associated with differential access and utilization of intervention services (Oser, Harp, O'Connell, Martine, & Leukefeld, 2012; Rosenblatt, Andrilla, Catlin, & Larson, 2015).

What Might Work to Support Recovering Outcomes

Recovery Schools

School plays a central role for adolescents and often represents the primary social venue for peer interaction and support. Among drug-using adolescents, school is often an environment with drug use and drug-using peers (Isakson & Jarvis, 1999). For recovering adolescents, returning to a drug using environment, as is often the case for adolescents who have few alternative choices, can precipitate relapse through exposure to triggers and risk factors such as school stress (Chung & Maisto, 2006; Moberg & Finch, 2008). Recovery schools or "sober schools" have emerged as a continuing care resource for high school students who are recovering from substance use and oftentimes have received specialized treatment prior to enrolling. Recovery schools, some under the accreditation of the Association of Recovery Schools, meet state educational requirements for awarding a secondary diploma.

In addition to meeting academic requirements, recovery schools can provide a therapeutic environment with wraparound services. Recovery school programming varies widely and can include services pertaining to physical heath, mental health, legal, education, family involvement, coordination of social services, and relapse prevention. Key to the rationale of recovery schools is the expectation that peer support and mutual self-help is necessary for recovering adolescents. These resources and services are key to a recovery-oriented system of care model which supports a continuum of person-centered, community-based service system (Kaplan, 2008).

Evidence based research on the effectiveness of recovery schools is lacking. This is due, in part, to the relatively low number of existing schools, the diversity of services within schools, and the rapid turnover of students within a school year (Moberg, Finch, & Lindsley, 2014).

However, evidence that recovery schools might be effective comes from studies showing significant reductions in self-reported substance use and improvements in mental health and family relationships among adolescents who remain in RC schools (Finch, Moberg, & Krupp, 2014; Moberg & Finch, 2008). Academic success is associated with school retention (Gibson, 1997), which in turn can decrease risk of relapse as well as substance misuse in adulthood. However, recovery schools currently lack racial and socioeconomic diversity and therefore results may or may not generalize to non-white students with a lower socioeconomic status and no history of formal treatment (Glaude & Torres, 2016).

Similar to high school recovery communities, collegiate recovery communities and collegiate recovery programs serve to support recovering while remaining engaged in educational pursuits. Unlike recovery high schools which are specifically designed for recovering students, collegiate recovery communities are situated within colleges and universities and provide resources and support to navigate postsecondary education while recovering in a potentially abstinence-hostile environment (Cleveland, Harris, Baker, Herbert, & Dean, 2007). Responding to the need for on-campus services (e.g., counseling), drug and alcohol-free housing, and a recovering community of peers, collegiate recovery communities such as the Association of Recovery in Higher Education (https://collegiaterecovery.org/ and Young People in Recovery (http://youngpeopleinrecovery.org) are proliferating college campuses. The evidence base for collegiate recovery programs, however, is lacking due to substantial heterogeneity in the programs and services offered across campuses (Laudet, 2008). Data collected by these programs indicate that the model is promising, with low rates of relapse and academic performance that average or above average (Laudet, Harris, Kimball, Winters, & Moberg, 2014).

Self-Help Groups

Self-help groups that may or may not be based on the 12-step model may support recovering outcomes. However, recovering support groups specifically designed for adolescents are uncommon. Rather, adult groups are utilized by adolescents. Available adolescent-specific evidence is limited both in quantity and quality, largely due to the inherent limitations of observational research and selection bias. However, existing research indicates that youth who participate in 12-step groups have better outcomes 1–2 years post-treatment (Alford, Koehler, & Leonard, 1991; Hsieh, Hoffman, & Hollister, 1998; Kelly, Myers, & Brown, 2000, 2002). For example, in a study examining rates of abstinence 8 year's post-treatment, adolescents who believed they could not use substances in moderation and those with greater addiction severity scores were more likely to attend Alcoholics Anonymous and/or Narcotics Anonymous (AA/NA) meetings (Kelly, Brown, Abrantes, Kahler, & Myers, 2008). Furthermore, self-reported abstinence was positive correlated with AA/NA attendance up to 8 years following treatment. The composition of self-help groups can also influence outcomes. Among young adults who have recently completed treatment, a more similar age composition among the 12-step attendees may enhance the positive effects of 12-step participation. However, have a more diverse age composition (i.e., older individuals with longer lengths of recovery) may be more beneficial for young adults established in a 12-step program and pursuing long-term recovery.

What Does Not Support Recovering Outcomes

Gender contributes to the risks and resiliencies that impact recovering outcomes, although the effects are complex and variable. As such, programs that are not responsive to gender-specific needs do not work. Gender-responsive treatment interventions from research on women have demonstrated promise (Bougard, Laupola, Parker-Dias, Creekmore, & Stangland, 2016; Greenfield, Back, Lawson, & Brady, 2010). For example, decreased substance use was observed in women participating in a women-only treatment program emphasizing factors such as trauma and self-esteem as compared to mixed-gender treatment program (Prendergast, Messina, Hall, & Ward, 2011). Strength-based, trauma-informed recovery support is therefore critical for recovering adolescent females.

A key factor for adolescent females is social context and evidence suggests that adolescent females may be more sensitive to social context and environmental cues than adolescent males (Kennedy, Epstein, Phillips, & Preston, 2013; Robbins, Ehrman, Childress, & O'Brien, 1999). Social context refers to the social setting in which females are recovering and includes family and friends. As posited by the Relational Model, relationships are highly significant to females and influence drug use and risk behavior (Covington, 1998; Covington & Surrey, 1997; Finkelstein & Piedade, 1993; Knudsen, Staton-Tindall, Oser, Havens, & Leukefeld, 2014). For example, having a recovery-oriented interpersonal network predicts decreased alcohol use (Granfield & Cloud, 2001; Humphreys, Moos, & Cohen, 1997; Weisner, Delucchi, Matzger, & Schmidt, 2003) and a substance-using partner predicts relapse among females (Grella, Scott, Foss, Joshi, & Hser, 2003). The interpersonal networks of recovering women are likely to be small (El-Bassel, Chen, & Cooper, 1998; Manuel, McCrady, Epstein, Cook, & Tonigan, 2007) and retain many friends and family members who actively use substances and do not provide recovery support (Greenfield et al., 2007; Grella, 2008; Laudet, Morgen, & White, 2006). Furthermore, relationships with substance-using network members increase the likelihood of substance use and do not support recovering outcomes (Rivaux, Sohn, Armour, & Bell, 2008; Warren, Stein, & Grella, 2007; Wenzel, Tucker, Golinelli, Green, & Zhou, 2010). For women who do report having family members who provide support during the treatment, emotional support, and a sense of loyalty and commitment, recovering outcomes are improved (Brown, Tracy, Jun, Park, & Min, 2015).

A network of recovering indivdiuals who can provide community, decreased isolation, an opportunity for honesty within a safe space, and peers with positive attitudes and goals are also associated with positive recovering outcomes (Brown et al., 2015). However, relationships that do not support recovering outcomes, often substance-using family and friends, are often retained in a woman's life. For example, Brown and colleagues (2015) reported that one strategy recovering women may use is to isolate those network members and closely manage the distance of those members within their lives. Recovering adolescent females, however, may not have the resources or capacity to control their proximity to such risky relationships and likely need the support of adults to help regulate their personal network.

Comorbid mood disorders, anxiety disorders, and serious psychological stress are also stronger predictors of substance use for women than men. Adverse childhood experiences, particularly exposure trauma, are a significant risk factor for substance use (Garland, Pettus-Davis, & Howard, 2013) and rates of physical or sexual abuse among treatment-seeking females range from 55% to 99% (Najavits, Weiss, & Shaw, 1997). Untreated psychiatric comorbidity has been associated with poor recovering outcomes and is likely to persist after successful substance abuse treatment (Bukstein, Glancy, & Kaminer, 1992; Grella, Hser, Joshi, & Rounds-Bryant, 2001; Wise, Cuffe, & Fischer, 2001). As such mental health support should also be included in the recovery support system, particularly for adolescent females (e.g., Back, Payne, Simpson, & Brady, 2010).

Summary

Recovering is an active and ongoing engagement in change over time rather than an endpoint and relapse can be part of the process. However, specific recovering definitions and outcomes (e.g., abstinence, personal growth, wellness) for adolescents have not been established. This reflects that lack of research on adolescents more broadly, as well as the broader focus on treatment outcomes rather than long-term recovering outcomes. Recovering supports include recovery community centers, sober living environments, education, transportation, and life-skills development. Recovering support groups and self-help groups are promising practices, but additional data is needed to rise to the level of evidence based. Gender contributes to the risks and resiliencies that impact recovering outcomes, although the effects are complex and variable. As such recovering supports which are not gender-responsive do not work. For recovering adolescent females, strength-based, trauma-informed recovery support is often indicated. More adolescent-centered research is essential to better understand the unmet needs of recovering adolescent and identify evidence-based recovering supports. Such research needs to be grounded in the experiences of adolescents and validated with instrumentation designed for adolescents.

References

Alford, G. S., Koehler, R. A., & Leonard, J. (1991). Alcoholics Anonymous-Narcotics Anonymous model inpatient treatment of chemically dependent adolescents: A 2-year outcome study. *Journal of Studies on Alcohol, 52*(2), 118–126.

Back, S. E., Payne, R. L., Simpson, A. N., & Brady, K. T. (2010). Gender and prescription opioids: Findings from the national survey on drug use and health. *Addictive Behaviors, 35*(11), 1001–1007.

Botzet, A. M., McIlvain, P. W., Winters, K. C., Fahnhorst, T., & Dittel, C. (2014). Data collection strategies and measurement tools for assessing academic and therapeutic outcomes in recovery schools. *Peabody Journal of Education, 89*(2), 197–213.

Bougard, K. G., Laupola, T. M. T., Parker-Dias, J., Creekmore, J., & Stangland, S. (2016). Turning the Tides: Coping with trauma and addiction through residential adolescent group therapy. *Journal of Child and Adolescent Psychiatric Nursing, 29*(4), 196–206.

Bouton, M. E. (2014). Why behavior change is difficult to sustain. *Preventative Medicine, 68*, 29–36.

Brown, S., Tracy, E. M., Jun, M., Park, H., & Min, M. O. (2015). Personal network recovery enablers and relapse risks for women with substance dependence. *Qualitative Health Research, 25*(3), 371–385.

Brown, S. A., & D'Amico, E. A. (2003). Outcomes of alcohol treatment for adolescents. In M. Galanter (Ed.), *Recent developments in alcoholism* (Vol. 16, pp. 289–312). New York, NY: Kluwer Academic/Plenum.

Brown, S. A., Gleghorn, A., Schuckit, M. A., Myers, M. G., & Mott, M. A. (1996). Conduct disorder among adolescent alcohol and drug abusers. *Journal of Studies on Alcohol, 57*(3), 314–324.

Bukstein, O. G., Glancy, L. J., & Kaminer, Y. (1992). Patterns of affective comorbidity in a clinical population of dually diagnosed adolescent substance abusers. *Journal of the American Academy of Child and Adolescent Psychiatry, 31*(6), 1041–1045.

Chung, T., & Maisto, S. A. (2006). Relapse to alcohol and other drug use in treated adolescents: Review and reconsideration of relapse as a change point in clinical course. *Clinical Psychology Review, 26*(2), 149–161.

Chung, T., Sealy, L., Abraham, M., Ruglovsky, C., Schall, J., & Maisto, S. A. (2015). Personal network characteristics of youth in substance use treatment: Motivation for and perceived difficulty of positive network change. *Substance Abuse, 36*(3), 380–388.

Cleveland, H. H., Harris, K. S., Baker, A. K., Herbert, R., & Dean, L. R. (2007). Characteristics of a collegiate recovery community: Maintaining recovery in an abstinence-hostile environment. *Journal of Substance Abuse Treatment, 33*(1), 13–23.

Connecticut Community for Addiction Recovery (CCAR). (2017). *What does CCAR do – And why do these things matter?* Retrieved from https://ccar.us/about-ccar/.

Covington, S. S. (1998). *Women in prison: Approaches in the treatment of our most invisible population. Breaking the rules: Women in prison and the feminist theory* (pp. 141–155). New York, NY: Haworth Press.

Covington, S. S., & Surrey, J. L. (1997). The relational model of women's psychological development: Implications for substance abuse. In R. W. Wilsnack & S. C. Wilsnack (Eds.), *Gender and alcohol: Individual and social perspectives* (pp. 335–351). New Brunswick, NJ: Alcohol Research Documentation.

Dew, B., Elifson, K., & Dozier, M. (2007). Social and environmental factors and their influence on drug use vulnerability and resiliency in rural populations. *The Journal of Rural Health, 23*, 16–21.

El-Bassel, N., Chen, D., & Cooper, D. (1998). Social support and social network profiles among women on methadone. *Social Service Review, 72*(3), 379–491.

Finch, A. J., Moberg, D. P., & Krupp, A. L. (2014). Continuing care in high schools: A descriptive study of recovery high school programs. *Journal of Child & Adolescent Substance Abuse, 23*(2), 116–129.

Finkelstein, N., & Piedade, E. (1993). The relational-model and the treatment of addicted females. *Counselor Magazine*, May–June, 8–11.

Gale, J. A., Lenardson, J. D., Lambert, D., & Hartley, D. (2012). *Adolescent alcohol use: Do risk and protective factors explain rural-urban differences?* Maine Rural Health Research Center (Working Paper #48). Retrieved from http://muskie.usm.maine.edu/Publications/WP48_Adolescent-Alcohol-Use-Rural-Urban.pdf.

Garland, E. L., Pettus-Davis, C., & Howard, M. O. (2013). Self-medication among traumatized youth: Structural equation modeling of pathways between trauma history, substance misuse, and psychological distress. *Journal of Behavioral Medicine, 36*(2), 175–185.

Gfroerer, J. C., Larson, S. L., & Colliver, J. D. (2007). Drug use patterns and trends in rural communities. *The Journal of Rural Health, 23*(s1), 10–15.

Gibson, J. T. (1997). Rekindling the spirits of throw-away children. *New Directions for School Leadership, 6*, 1–9.

Glaude, M., & Torres, L. R. (2016). Hispanic perspectives on recovery high schools: If we build them, will they come? *Journal of Groups in Addict and Recovery, 11*(4), 240–249.

Gmel, G., Mohler-Kuo, M., Dermota, P., Guame, J., Bertholet, N., Daeppen, J. B., & Studer, J. (2013). Religion is good, belief is better: Religion, religiosity, and substance use among young Swiss men. *Substance Use and Misuse, 48*(12), 1085–1098.

Gonzales, R., Anglin, M. D., Beattie, R., Ong, C. A., & Glik, D. C. (2012a). Perceptions of chronicity and recovery among youth in treatment for substance use problems. *Journal of Adolescent Health, 51*(2), 144–149.

Gonzales, R., Anglin, M. D., Beattie, R., Ong, C. A., & Glik, D. C. (2012b). Understanding recovery barriers: Youth perceptions about substance use relapse. *American Journal of Health Behavior, 36*(5), 602–614.

Granfield, R., & Cloud, W. (2001). Social context and "natural recovery": The role of social capital in the resolution of drug-associated problems. *Substance Use and Misuse, 36*(11), 1543–1570. PubMed PMID: 11693955.

Green, L. L., Fullilove, M. T., & Fullilove, R. E. (1998). Stories of spiritual awakening: The nature of spirituality in recovery. *Journal of Substance Abuse Treatment, 15*(4), 325–331.

Greenfield, S. F., Back, S. E., Lawson, K., & Brady, K. T. (2010). Substance abuse in women. *Psychiatric Clinics of North America, 33*(2), 339–355.

Greenfield, S. F., Brooks, A. J., Gordon, S. M., Green, C. A., Kropp, F., McHugh, R. K., & Miele, G. M. (2007). Substance abuse treatment entry, retention, and outcome in women: A review of the literature. *Drug and Alcohol Dependence, 86*(1), 1–21.

Grella, C. E. (2008). From generic to gender-responsive treatment: Changes in social policies, treatment services, and outcomes of women in substance abuse treatment. *Journal of Psychoactive Drugs, 40*(Suppl. 5), 327–343.

Grella, C. E., Hser, Y. I., Joshi, V., & Rounds-Bryant, J. (2001). Drug treatment outcomes for adolescents with comorbid mental and substance use disorders. *Journal of Nervous and Mental Disease, 189*(6), 384–392.

Grella, C. E., Scott, C. K., Foss, M. A., Joshi, V., & Hser, Y. I. (2003). Gender differences in drug treatment outcomes among participants in the Chicago Target Cities Study. *Evaluation and Program Planning, 26*(3), 297–310.

Hanson, C. L., Novilla, M. L. L. B., Barnes, M. D., Eggett, D., McKell, C., Reichman, P., & Havens, M. (2009). Using the rural-urban continuum to explore adolescent alcohol, tobacco, and other drug use in Montana. *Journal of Child and Adolescent Substance Abuse, 18*(1), 93–105.

Hsieh, S., Hoffman, N. G., & Hollister, D. C. (1998). The Relationship between pre-, during-, post-treatment factors, and adolescent substance abuse behaviors. *Addictive Behaviors, 23*(4), 477–488.

Humphreys, K., Moos, R. H., & Cohen, C. (1997). Social and community resources and long-term recovery from treated and untreated alcoholism. *Journal of Studies on Alcoholism, 58*(3), 231–238. PubMed PMID: 9130214.

Hutchison, L., & Blakely, C. (2003). Substance abuse-trends in rural areas: A literature review. In L. Gamm, L. Hutchison, B. D. Dabney, & A. M. Dorsey (Eds.), *Rural healthy people 2010: A companion document to healthy people 2010* (Vol. 2, pp. 145–154). College Station, TX: Texas A & M University System Health Science Center, School of Rural Public Health, Southwest Rural Health Research Center.

Isakson, K., & Jarvis, P. (1999). The adjustment of adolescents during the transition into high school: A short-term longitudinal study. *Journal of Youth and Adolescence, 28*(1), 1–26.

Kaminer, Y. (2001). Adolescent substance abuse treatment: Where do we go from here? *Psychiatric Services, 52*(2), 147–149.

Kaplan, L. (2008). *The role of recovery support services in recovery-oriented systems of care* (DHHS Publication No. SMA 08-4315). Rockville, MD: Center for Substance Abuse Treatment, Substance Abuse and Mental Health Services Administration.

Kaskutas, L. A., & Ritter, L. A. (2015). Consistency between beliefs and behavior regarding use of substances in recovery. *Sage Open, 5*(1), 1–22.

Kelly, J. F., Brown, S. A., Abrantes, A., Kahler, C., & Myers, M. (2008). Social recovery model: An 8-year investigation of adolescent 12-step group involvement following inpatient treatment. *Alcoholism: Clinical and Experimental Research, 32*(8), 1468–1478.

Kelly, J. F., Myers, M. G., & Brown, S. A. (2000). A multivariate process model of adolescent 12-step attendance and substance use outcome following inpatient treatment. *Psychology of Addictive Behaviors, 14*(4), 376–389.

Kelly, J. F., Myers, M. G., & Brown, S. A. (2002). Do adolescents affiliate with 12-step Groups? A multivariate process model of effects. *Journal of Studies on Alcohol, 63*(3), 293–304.

Kennedy, A. P., Epstein, D. H., Phillips, K. A., & Preston, K. L. (2013). Sex differences in cocaine/heroin uses: Drug-use triggers and craving in daily life. *Drug and Alcohol Dependence, 132*(1-2), 29–37.

Keyes, K. M., Cerdá, M., Brady, J. E., Havens, J. R., & Galea, S. (2014). Understanding the rural-urban differences in nonmedical prescription opioid use and abuse in the United States. *American Journal of Public Health, 104*(2), e52–e59.

Knudsen, H. K., Staton-Tindall, M., Oser, C. B., Havens, J. R., & Leukefeld, C. G. (2014). Reducing risky relationships: A multi-site randomized trial of a prison-based intervention for reducing HIV sexual risk behaviors among women with a history of drug use. *AIDS Care, 26*(9), 1071–1079.

Laudet, A., Harris, K., Kimball, T., Winters, K. C., & Moberg, D. P. (2014). Collegiate recovery communities programs: What do we know and what do we need to know? *Journal of Social Work Practice in the Addictions, 14*(1), 84–100.

Laudet, A. B. (2007). What does recovery mean to you? Lessons from the recovery experience for research and practice. *Journal of Substance Abuse Treatment, 33*(3), 243–256.

Laudet, A. B. (2008). The road to recovery: Where are we going and how do we get there? Empirically-driven conclusions and future directions for service development and research. *Substance Use and Misuse, 43*(12-13), 2001–2020.

Laudet, A. B., Morgen, K., & White, W. L. (2006). The role of social supports, spirituality, religiousness, life meaning and affiliation with 12-step fellowships in quality of life satisfaction among individuals in recovery from alcohol and drug problems. *Alcoholism Treatment Quarterly, 24*(1–2), 33–73.

Leukefeld, C. (2015). Recovery is a reality: But what is it? *Substance Use and Misuse, 50*(8-9), 1028–1030.

Leukefeld, C. G., & Leukefeld, S. (1999). Primary socialization theory and a bio/psycho/social/spiritual practice model for substance abuse. *Substance Use and Misuse, 37*(4), 983–991.

Leukefeld, C. G., Logan, T. K., Clayton, R. R., Martin, C., Zimmerman, R., Cattarello, A., … Lynam, D. (1998). Adolescent drug use, delinquency, and other behaviors. In T. P. Gullotta, G. R. Adams, & R. Montemayor (Eds.), *Deliquent violent youth: Theory and Interventions* (pp. 98–128). Thousand Oaks, CA: Sage.

Maisto, S. A., Pollock, N. K., Cornelius, J. R., Lynch, K. G., & Martin, C. S. (2003). Alcohol relapse as a function of relapse definition in a clinical sample of adolescents. *Addictive Behaviors, 28*(3), 449–459.

Manuel, J. K., McCrady, B. S., Epstein, E. E., Cook, S., & Tonigan, J. S. (2007). The pretreatment social networks of women with alcohol dependence. *Journal of Studies on Alcohol and Drugs, 68*(6), 871–878.

Marks, K. R., & Leukefeld, C. G. (2017). A preliminary study examining women's physical health and nonmedical prescription opioid use in a recovering framework. *Journal of Women's Health, 26*(3), 286–293.

Miller, W. R. (1996). What is a relapse? Fifty ways to leave the wagon. *Addiction, 91*, S15–S27.

Moberg, D. P., & Finch, A. J. (2008). Recovery high schools: A descriptive study of school programs and students. *Journal of Groups in Addiction and Recovery, 2*, 128–161. https://doi.org/10.1080/15560350802081314

Moberg, D. P., Finch, A. J., & Lindsley, S. M. (2014). Recovery high schools: Students and responsive academic and therapeutic services. *Peabody Journal of Education, 89*(2), 165–182.

Myers, M. G., & Brown, S. A. (1996). The adolescent relapse coping questionnaire: Psychometric validation. *Journal of Studies on Alcohol, 57*(1), 40–56.

Najavits, L. M., Weiss, R., & Shaw, S. (1997). The link between substance abuse and posttraumatic stress disorder in women: A research review. *American Journal of Addiction, 6*(4), 237–283.

Office of National Drug Control Policy. (2016, August 31). *ONDCP recovery update*. Retrieved from https://www.whitehouse.gov/ondcp/treatment-and-recovery.

Oser, C. B., Harp, K. L., O'Connell, D. J., Martine, S. S., & Leukefeld, C. G. (2012). Correlates of participation in peer recovery support groups as well as voluntary and mandated substance abuse treatment among rural and urban probationers. *Journal of Substance Abuse Treatment, 42*(1), 95–101.

Prendergast, M. L., Messina, N. P., Hall, E. A., & Ward, U. S. (2011). The relative effectiveness of women-only and mixed-gender treatment for substance-using women. *Journal of Substance Abuse Treatment, 40*(4), 336–348.

Ramo, D. E., & Brown, S. A. (2008). Classes of substance abuse relapse situations: A comparison of adolescents and adults. *Psychology of Addictive Behaviors, 22*(3), 372–379.

Rivaux, S. L., Sohn, S., Armour, M. P., & Bell, H. (2008). Women's early recovery: Managing the dilemma of substance abuse and intimate partner relationships. *Journal of Drug Issues, 38*(4), 957–979.

Robbins, S. J., Ehrman, R. N., Childress, A. R., & O'Brien, C. P. (1999). Comparing levels of cocaine cue reactivity in male and female outpatients. *Drug and Alcohol Dependence, 53*(3), 223–230.

Rosenblatt, R. A., Andrilla, C. H., Catlin, M., & Larson, E. H. (2015). Geographic and specialty distribution of US physicians trained to treat opioid use disorder. *Annals of Family Medicine, 13*(1), 23–26.

Schwarzlose, J. (2007). What is recovery? A working definition from the Betty Ford Institute. *Journal of Substance Abuse Treatment, 33*(3), 221–228.

Sobell, L. C., Ellingstad, T. P., & Sobell, M. B. (2000). Natural recovery from alcohol and drug problems: Methodological review of the research with suggestions for future directions. *Addiction, 95*(5), 749–764.

Staton, M., Webster, J. M., Hiller, M. L., Rotosky, S., & Leukefeld, C. (2003). An exploratory examination of spiritual well-being, religiosity, and drug use among incarcerated men. *Journal of Social Work Practice in the Addictions, 3*(3), 87–103.

Staton-Tindall, M., Oser, C. B., Duvall, J. L., Havens, J. R., Webster, J. M., & Booth, B. M. (2008). Male and female stimulant use among rural Kentuckians: The contribution of spirituality and religiosity. *The Journal of Drug Issues, 38*(3), 863–882.

Substance Abuse and Mental Health Services Administration (SAMHSA). (2012). *SAMHSA's working definition of recovery*. Retrieved from https://store.samhsa.gov/shin/content/PEP12-RECDEF/PEP12-RECDEF.pdf.

Substance Abuse and Mental Health Services Administration (SAMHSA), Center for Behavioral Health Statistics and Quality. (2016). *Key substance use and mental health indicators in the United States: Results from the 2015 National survey on drug use and health* (HHS Publication No. SMA 16-4984, NSDUH Series H-51). Rockville, MD: Substance Abuse and Mental Health Services Administration.

U.S. Department of Health and Human Services, Health Resources and Services Administration, Maternal and Child Health Bureau. (2015). *Child Health USA 2014*. Rockville, MD: U.S. Department of Health and Human Services.

Volkow, N. D., Koob, G. F., & Mclellan, A. T. (2016). Neurobiologic advances from the brain disease model of addiction. *The New England Journal of Medicine, 374*(4), 363–371.

Warren, J. C., Smalley, K. B., & Barefoot, K. N. (2016). Recent alcohol, tobacco, and substance use variations between rural and urban middle and high school students. *Journal of Child & Adolescent Substance, 26*(1), 60–65.

Warren, J. I., Stein, J. A., & Grella, C. E. (2007). Role of social support and self-efficacy in treatment outcomes among clients with co-occurring disorders. *Drug and Alcohol Dependence, 89*(2-3), 267–274.

Watkins, E. (1997). Essay on spirituality. *Journal of Substance Abuse Treatment, 14*(6), 581–583.

Weisner, C., Delucchi, K., Matzger, H., & Schmidt, L. (2003). The role of community services and informal support on five-year drinking trajectories of alcohol dependent and problem drinkers. *Journal of Alcohol Studies, 64*(6), 862–873.

Wenzel, S. L., Tucker, J. S., Golinelli, D., Green, H. D., Jr., & Zhou, A. (2010). Personal network correlates of alcohol, cigarette, and marijuana use among homeless youth. *Drug and Alcohol Dependence, 112*(1-2), 140–149.

Winters, K. C., Stinchfield, R. D., Opland, E., Weller, C., & Latimer, W. W. (2000). The effectiveness of the Minnesota Model approach in the treatment of adolescent drug abusers. *Addiction, 95*(4), 601–612.

Wise, B. K., Cuffe, S. P., & Fischer, T. (2001). Dual diagnosis and successful participation of adolescents in substance abuse treatment. *Journal of Substance Abuse Treatment, 21*(3), 161–165.

Zollinger, T. W., Saywell, R. M., Overgaard, A. D., Przybylski, M. J., & Dutta-Bergman, M. (2006). Antitobacco media awareness of rural youth compared to suburban and urban youth in Indiana. *Journal of Rural Health, 22*(2), 119–123.

School-Based Prevention-Evolution of Evidence-Based Strategies

Zili Sloboda

Introduction

Several important milestones have been achieved over the past several years that can and will have a profound impact on how substance use prevention will be implemented in the future, particularly as implemented in schools.

The first of these events was the publication of the Society for Prevention Research's Standards of Knowledge for the Science of Prevention. In this document the Society for Prevention Research (2011) the authors laid out the goals and content of prevention science. "The primary goal of prevention science is to improve public health by identifying malleable risk and protective factors, assessing the efficacy and effectiveness of preventive interventions and identifying optimal means for dissemination and diffusion. The field involves the study of human development and social ecology as well as the identification of factors and processes that lead to positive and negative health behaviors and outcomes. Theories of human development are used to design interventions (programs and policies) that target the reduction of risk and the enhancement of protective factors at the individual, familial, peer, community, and environmental levels. … Prevention science is the foundation for health education and health promotion as well as preventive interventions" (p. 3).

The second event was the publication at the same time, 2011, of the European Drug Prevention Quality Standards (European Monitoring Centre for Drugs and Drug Addiction, 2011) that sets out quality standards for prevention professionals in the planning for a target population, assessing needs and available resources to meet these needs, implementing appropriate interventions and monitoring and evaluating their outcomes. It also addresses sustainability, stakeholder involvement, and ethical practices.

Z. Sloboda (✉)
Applied Prevention Science International, Ontario, OH, USA
e-mail: zili.sloboda@apsintl.org

C. G. Leukefeld, T. P. Gullotta (eds.), *Adolescent Substance Abuse*, Issues in Children's and Families' Lives, https://doi.org/10.1007/978-3-319-90611-9_13

A third event was the publication of the International Standards on Drug Use Prevention by the United Nations Office on Drugs and Crime in 2013. This document established rigorous criteria for assessing research evidence of effectiveness and summarizes the scientific evidence, describing effective interventions and policies and their characteristics by the targeted age group (prenatal and infancy, early childhood, middle childhood, adolescence, and late adolescence and adulthood) and setting (family, school, workplace, community and health sector).

These milestones are important for two major reasons. First, they underscore the evolution of a new field of study, prevention science, and the significant advances made in prevention research methodologies that have provided for rigorous controlled studies that could be replicated with positive outcomes. Second, they lay out the framework for the development of a new field of science with its own lexicon, theories, methodologies, and practice (Bosworth & Sloboda, 2015).

History of Prevention Science

Until the establishment of the National Institute on Drug Abuse (NIDA) in 1974, existing prevention efforts were generally found to have limited impact. Among the advances in shaping more effective prevention programming was the extensive epidemiologic research base that was developed and sustained by NIDA. This work provided information regarding the origins and pathways of substance use that has been summarized by Hawkins, Catalano, and Miller (1992). Other important influences on the direction prevention research was to take through the 1980s and 1990s were theoretically derived behavioral models such as the Social Learning Theory and the Theory of Planned Behavior that specify those attitudes, perceptions and beliefs leading to substance use and other problem behaviors that become the target of prevention interventions (Coie et al., 1993). Other theories of social control have also played important roles in the development of environmental or policy interventions particularly for the use of tobacco and alcohol (Ashe, Jernigan, Kline, & Galaz, 2003; Holder, 2000, 2001; Liang, Chaloupka, Nichter, & Clayton, 2003; Luke, Stamatakis, & Brownson, 2000; Ross & Chaloupka, 2003). Finally are learning theories that provide the foundation for instructional strategies and implementation including cognitive theory (e.g., Renner et al., 1976), the development of relevant and appropriate educational goals (e.g., Bloom, Engelhart, Furst, Hill, & Krathwohl, 1956), and constructivism (Bruner, 1960).

In addition, the emergence of the "ecobiodevelopmental (EBD) framework" for explaining human behavior (Fishbein, Rose, Darcey, Belcher, & VanMeter, 2016; Shonkoff, 2010) has prompted a reconceptualization of prevention that builds on and more fully transforms the concepts of risk and protection to those of vulnerability and resilience (Sloboda, Glantz, & Tarter, 2012). These frameworks serve to elucidate the etiology of behavioral problems such as substance use indicating that how we develop our attitudes, beliefs, and behaviors in response to the world around us is influenced by our interface with our microlevel and macrolevel environments. Key

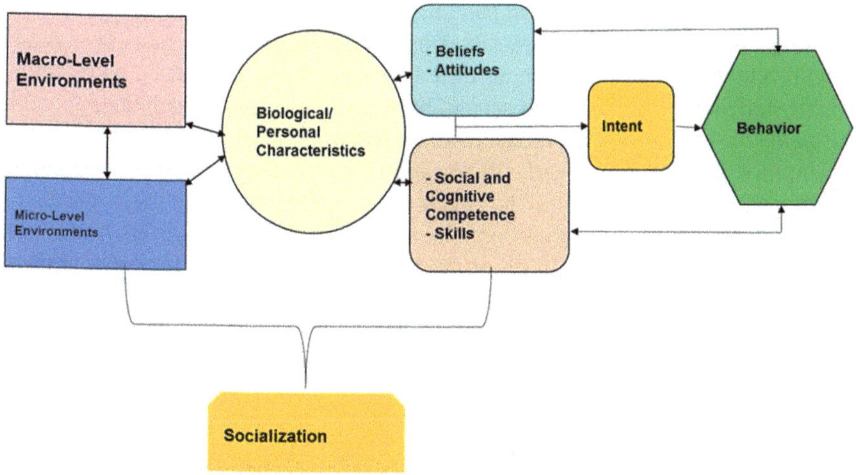

Fig. 1 The etiology model and human motivation and change process. This model shows how the various environmental levels, personal characteristics and the socialization process interact in the decision-making that takes place before the use of any substance and performance of other problem behaviors. Colombo Plan International Centre for Credentialing and Education of Addiction Professionals (ICCE). (2015). Introduction to the Universal Prevention Curriculum Series for Implementers, (p. 229). Colombo, Sri Lanka: Colombo Plan

microlevel environments include family and school. Merging this framework with the theoretical behavioral models and what we know about learning processes suggests an approach to prevention that addresses the needs of primary socialization agents: parents, teachers, peers, employers, etc., and the contexts or settings in which they function. A simplified example of such a framework is provided below in Fig. 1.

Genetic and other biological factors play a significant role in the achievement of developmental benchmarks, that is, the goal of each stage of development, from infancy to early adulthood that includes: intellectual ability, language development, cognitive, emotional, and psychological functioning, and attainment of social competency skills. The extent to which developmental benchmarks are met determines our level of vulnerability to influences from our environment. Such vulnerability can vary within an individual and across developmental periods. Children who do not reach early developmental benchmarks are most likely the most vulnerable as failure to achieve these early benchmarks signifies their difficult in reaching later ones. Environmental factors can both lessen or enhance this vulnerability. As environmental experiences are associated with heightened stress or adversity, the risk for substance use is increased. The environmental influences are viewed at two major levels, those in close proximity to the individual—microlevel environments—and those that are more distant—macrolevel environments. It is the combination of these environmental influences and personal characteristics of individuals that shapes beliefs, attitudes, and behavior. What is also important to note in this figure is that the two levels of influence—the macrolevel and microlevel—do not operate independently to influence our behavior, but they also impact one another. For instance, family stability and even parenting behaviors can be challenged when one or both caregivers are unemployed for long periods of time. This process suggests that prevention is a socialization agent in two ways. First, in working with family, school staff, and workplace and second by directly targeting populations through the media, school curricula, and the enforcement of policies, regulations and laws.

Until the late 1980s and early 1990s, substance use interventions used a public health framework to define both the targets of the interventions and the mechanisms that were applied in the interventions. However, the application of this framework that consisted of three levels of intervention: primary, secondary, and tertiary, reflecting the disease status of the individual, group, or population being addressed, did not satisfactorily meet the needs of those designing programs for substance use or mental health problems. Gordon (1983) suggested moving to a more empirically based approach, one that weighs the risk to an individual of getting a disease against the costs associated by participating in an intervention. This new model was adapted as "the mental health intervention spectrum" by the Institute of Medicine Committee on Prevention of Mental Disorders and published in the Committee's report, Reducing Risks for Mental Disorders (Mrazek & Haggerty, 1994). Three levels of prevention were defined: universal, selective, and indicated, each addressing the varying degrees of risk found in the targeted population.

Universal programs are designed to address general populations while selective programs target those segments of the population that present greater than normal risk to develop a disorder and indicated programs focus on those subgroups that exhibit signs or symptoms of developing a disorder. This nomenclature is currently in use among psychoactive substance use prevention researchers and practitioners. This designation remains in effect today and influences not only the design of interventions but also how these interventions are evaluated.

The new transactional ecological framework is useful to redefine risk and protective factors as the interface between the individual and the microlevel and macrolevel environments as well as between the two levels of environments themselves. This new way of looking at vulnerability will warrant new methods for assessing the need for prevention, identifying the target population, selecting an appropriate intervention, and then, evaluating the short-, intermediate-, and long-term outcomes of the intervention.

History of Introducing Effective Substance Use Prevention Interventions into Schools

The school as a microlevel environment is an appropriate setting for prevention strategies for several reasons. The most obvious is that the school is where children in the USA spend a great proportion of their time. In addition, the school remains a major socialization institution to reinforce societal values, norms, and acceptable behaviors. Furthermore, the school is a protective environment for children (Schaps & Solomon, 2003) where they should feel safe.

In order to learn the nature and extent of school-based activities that are provided to address a number of problem behaviors such as substance use, violence, accidents, and risky sexual behaviors, Gottfredson and Gottfredson (2001) conducted a survey of principals of a national probability sample of 848 public, private, and catholic schools. They found that the typical school offered a large range of such activities, from 0 to 66 within individual schools, with an average of 14 activities per school. These activities included rules and policies; information on topics such as substance use, health, mental health, and violence; and curriculum instruction. However, as the authors point out, the effectiveness of most of these activities in reducing or eliminating problem behaviors had not been demonstrated.

The process of translating effective prevention approaches to these problem behaviors, and specifically, psychoactive substance use, however, did not begin until the mid-1990s. Concern about moving the findings from prevention research from the research setting to the community prompted the NIDA-sponsored first National Conference of Drug Abuse Prevention Research: *Putting Research to Work for the Community* in 1996. The conference was designed to foster a dialogue between researchers and practitioners. One of the major outcomes of that conference was a booklet, *Preventing Drug Use among Children and Adolescents: A Research-Based Guide* (Sloboda & David, 1997). As Bukoski writes, "This publication clearly established the beginning of the evidence-based drug abuse prevention movement that has emerged across the country …" (Bukoski, 2003, p. 6). The guide was written to translate research for community-based practitioners including findings regarding the origins and pathways to substance use and abuse and planning prevention interventions. One part of the guide examined the consistent elements of effective prevention programming drawn from NIDA-funded research. These elements or principles set the stage for a number of other events that promoted evidence-based prevention programming. With the publication of the guide, the US Department of Education (DOE) Safe and Drug-Free Schools and Communities Act (SDFSCA) and the Center for Substance Abuse Prevention of the SAMHSA created review processes through which programs are added to lists of effective and exemplary programs. These include SAMHSA's National Registry of Evidence-Based Programs and Practices and the Department of Justice Office of Juvenile Justice and Delinquency's BluePrints. Most of these interventions are school-based, representing the history of the field that has been more school-centered, particularly when addressing psychoactive substance use issues.

Prior to this time, the SDFSCA program had come under scrutiny and criticism as to how it funded over $6 billion for school-based programming to improve school safety (Sherman, 2000). In response to such pressure and after NIDA's publication of the guide in 1997, the SDFSCA staff issued the *Principles of Prevention* in 1998. The Principles require local school districts and other recipients of SDFSCA funds to develop programs that are based on (1) an assessment of the incidence of violence and illegal drug use, (2) analysis of data regarding risk factors, (3) established set of performance measures to ensure a safe and drug-free environment, and (4) sound research that demonstrates the program is effective (either selected from SDFSCA and SAMHSA lists or with other documentation of effectiveness). In addition, school districts were expected to evaluate the extent to which these programs met established performance measures (US Department of Education, 1998).

Dissemination of information about these effective prevention interventions (EPI) by several Federal agencies, including the DOE, SAMHSA, OJJDP Model Programs Guide, and nonprofits had not been fully successful with respect to their adoption. Over time, surveys showed an increase in the availability of these EPIs in middle schools from an estimated 34.6% of schools providing EPI in 1999, to an estimated 42.6% in 2005, and 46.9% in 2008 (Ringwalt et al., 2002, 2009, 2010; US Department of Education, 1998). Among high schools, however, in the 2008 survey, only an estimated 10.3% were delivering EBI (Ringwalt et al., 2008). Sloboda and colleagues (2008) reported similar findings for middle schools with somewhat lower percentages in high schools. These studies also showed that many more middle and high schools reported that they provided "locally" developed (home-grown) or "non-EPI" curricula.

It is clear that these dissemination efforts had not been systematic, nor guided by research as to the most appropriate target audiences involved in local decision-making, nor about the most important information they need in order to make informed decisions. Crowley and colleagues (Crowley, Greenberg, Feinberg, Spoth, & Redmond, 2012) conducted one of the few studies to report on "how building stakeholders' knowledge in regard to selecting and implementing EPI was part of capacity building in the PROSPER project" (Crowley et al., 2012, p. 96). Over a 5-year period, they found that PROSPER stakeholders had increased knowledge about the standards of evidence for EPI over controls. They speculated that this was due to the fact that PROSPER staff provided the stakeholders with all the information they needed about effective interventions.

Rohrbach and colleagues (Rohrbach, Ringwalt, Ennett, & Vincus, 2005), in their national study of substance use prevention coordinators, found that the significant factors involved in district-level decisions to adopt EPI included (1) Input from a state substance use prevention group; (2) Use of information disseminated by NIDA or the Center for Substance Abuse Prevention; (3) Use of local needs assessment data; (4) Consideration of research showing which curricula are effective; and (5) A greater allocation of a prevention coordinator's time to substance use prevention activities. They also found that adoption was positively associated with large, urban schools, more administrative effort on prevention programming, and a history of organizational innovativeness. The researchers speculated that such large schools were likely to have had more resources to devote to EPI preparation. In a literature review (Durlak & DuPre, 2008) on behavioral health promotion programs in real-world settings, a number of organizational-level factors were found in successful programs, including: organizational climate (e.g., willingness to try new approaches); effective leadership; and practices that allow shared decision-making and open communication. All of these organizational factors also have an impact on adoption decisions (Sloboda, Dusenbury, & Petras, 2014).

Powers and colleagues (Powers, Bowen, & Bowen, 2010) cite multiple articles that show how few practitioners in schools are using EPI educational and social service practices. They report on the program characteristics that are likely to serve as barriers to the implementation of such practices in schools. Among 51 school-based practices, barriers appear to include: high startup costs, challenging training and staffing requirements, and a lack of easily accessible information about programs in places where school personnel are likely to find it. While the Powers et al. (2010) study detailed some of the potential barriers to implementation, their findings do not reflect "the view from the ground"—i.e., what factors do local stakeholders consider important to their decisions? For example, it is not known to what extent the recent drop in funding has had on the adoption and continuation of EBI in schools. Other factors not considered include costs, training, characteristics of the practices, time commitments, stakeholders' perceptions of the seriousness of the local problem, the types and sources of information they need, and school and district characteristics.

On the other hand, some schools do implement prevention programs effectively. Payne and associates (Payne, Gottfredson, & Gottfredson, 2006) found that implementation quality was associated with both school and program factors. Those that were found to have high-quality implementation engaged in local (within schools) program selection, integrated prevention programming into school operations, had principal support, had the organizational capacity (capacity for program development, teacher–principal communication, amenability to implementation, and no obstacles to implementation), and had the means for standardization (e.g., use of an instructor's manual). Many of these findings are supported by other studies (Ringwalt, Ennett, Vincus, Rohrbach, & Simons-Rudolph, 2004; Rohrbach et al., 2005; Wenter et al., 2002).

The Application of Prevention Science to the Development of Evidence-Based Prevention Interventions

The term "prevention science" was introduced in 1993 by Coie et al. It was not until 2011 with the online publication of Standards of Knowledge for the Science of Prevention by the US Society for Prevention Research that the term became more widely accepted by prevention professionals, both researchers and practitioners. As mentioned in the introduction to this chapter, prevention science identifies those risk and protective factors or vulnerabilities that can be addressed through interventions, provides the tools necessary to assess the efficacy and effectiveness of preventive interventions, and identifies the most optimal means for dissemination and diffusion of effective interventions. Prevention science draws from multiple scientific disciplines including psychology, neurobiology, epidemiology, sociology, developmental psychology and dissemination science. It applies theories of human development and human behavior to the development of targeted interventions and to their evaluations.

Although the question "what "works" in prevention remains an unanswered issue the process for developing effective interventions is becoming clearer. Rohrbach (2014) has laid out the stages of intervention design. Drawing on models developed in public health such as the Precede-Proceed model (Green & Kreuter, 2005), her stages of the intervention design process include Stage 1: Adopting a Theoretical Foundation that requires first identify the target population so that the appropriate theory of human development and behavior and intervention objectives can be articulated; Stage 2: Building the Intervention that is informed by age-related learning theories and strategies, conducting formative research, and tailoring the specific needs of the target population; and Stage 3: Pilot Testing to examine the feasibility of delivering the intervention and to determine if the short-term objectives of the intervention are met. The next stages include taking the intervention to scale.

Rohrbach and Dyal (2015) point out that schools face many demands on them that impede the large-scale implementation of evidence-based prevention programs. Given these barriers, they lay out an approach that was used to scale up Project To No Drug Use. Factors that are key are careful planning identifying a "home" for the program, in what subject area or class could the program be delivered. Focus should first begin with teachers who have positive attitudes and are supportive of the program. Furthermore, they found that building partnerships between schools and local social service agencies particularly those that may have funding to assist in the implementation of the program and also involving social service staff in the training and delivery of the program provided support needed to bring the program into the schools.

The International Standards on Drug Use Prevention

Until 2013, terms that were applied to effective prevention interventions continued to be "research-based" or "science-based." With the push for evidence-based medical practice in the late twentieth century (Sackett, Rosenberg, McGray, Haynes, & Richardson, 1996), it was the United Nations Office on Drugs and Crime first defined and applied the term in the Office's International Standards on Drug Use Prevention [2013/2015] (cited in the United Nations Office on Drugs and Crime, 2013). The Standards used a rating system based on the rigor of the research methods applied in the evaluation process from "excellent," "very good," and "good" ratings for effectiveness supported by meta-analyses and systematic reviews, multiple randomized controlled trials and quasi-experimental methods, primarily time series analyses. Ratings of "good" and "adequate" were used for single randomized control trials or evaluations conducted through acceptable methodologies.

The International Standards document does not advocate for a particular program but rather presents the content, structure, and delivery strategy used in the evaluated interventions. The findings are presented within development age groups (infancy and early childhood, middle childhood, early adolescence, and late adolescence and adulthood) and developmental age groups within settings in which the interventions are delivered (family, school, workplace, community and the health sector). What is presented below is an enhanced summary of the findings from the Standards document.

Evidence-Based Prevention Interventions for Schools

There are three aspects of the school environment that lend themselves specifically to substance use prevention intervention: (1) school culture, that is, norms, beliefs, and expectancies, and school bonding, that is, connecting the individual to the school experience and community; (2) school policy or social control, the most common approach establishing disciplinary policies and procedures; and (3) classroom curriculum or manualized programs.

School Culture and School Bonding

Earlier we discussed the etiology model that describes risk and protective factors associated with the initiation of substance use as an individual–environmental interaction (Fishbein et al., 2016; Sloboda, 2015; Tarter et al., 1999). Prevention programs that address this interaction intend to make the school environment more attractive to students to help students develop more prosocial attitudes and affiliations and to engage in more prosocial behaviors. The intent is to increase self-efficacy and school bonding and decrease the likelihood that students will use alcohol, tobacco, or other psychoactive substances (Campello, Sloboda, Heikkil, & Brotherhood, 2014). The intentions of these approaches include:

- Support an orderly school climate and normal functioning
- Enhance teachers' ability to management their classrooms effectively
- Socialize children in their roles as students, and
- Support a positive school ethos and a commitment to school and student participation
- Reduce disruptive and aggressive behaviors.

The common elements of effective strategies to create a positive normative environment for children include the following (Fletcher, 2015).

- Ensuring the school environment is inclusive and emotionally and physically safe
- Promoting positive relationships between students, teachers, and other school staff in which there is mutual respect, caring and a shared sense of belonging and commitment to the school experience
- Setting and supporting health norms, behaviors and relationships including creating nonsubstance using settings.

In general the content of these approaches include strategies to respond to and correct inappropriate behavior and those that acknowledge and reward appropriate behavior. Training of school staff to implement these programs is required to assure fidelity, consistency, and sustainability.

One of the earliest programs designed to change school culture is the Child Development Project (CDP) (now termed Caring School Community Program) designed by Eric Schaps of the Developmental Studies Center. This program targets children when they are 5–12 years old. It is designed to promote school bonding, to enhance students' interpersonal skills and commitment to positive values, and to develop both a classroom and schoolwide atmosphere of caring (safety, respect, and helpfulness). The long-term outcomes are the reduction or elimination of the use of alcohol, tobacco, and marijuana and involvement in violent behaviors and other risky behaviors. The three program components consist of (1) intensive classroom activities that focus on cooperative learning, a literature-based reading and language arts curriculum, and developmental discipline; (2) schoolwide activities designed to involve teachers, parents, students, and extended family members in building a caring school community; and (3) family activities that are designed to bring classroom experiences into the home, promoting communication between students and their families. The program was evaluated in the 1990s using a quasi-experimental design with six demonstration and six comparison schools (Battistich, Schaps, Watson, Solomon, & Lewis, 2000).

Although programs to impact school culture also increase school bonding, there are a number of programs that focus primarily on school bonding per se. Common elements or principles of school bonding programs include the following:

- Focusing on early years; that is, preschool to middle school.
- Enhancing competency in reading and math.
- Providing interpersonal skills to enable students to relate positively with peers and adults.
- Involving parents in communication and parenting skills and in school activities.

There are several effective programs that emphasize school bonding. Among these are the Skills, Opportunities and Recognition (SOAR) program (Hawkins, Catalano, Kosterman, Abbott, & Hill, 1999), Incredible Years (Webster-Stratton, Reid, & Hammond, 2001), and Early Risers Skills for Success (August, Lee, Bloomquist, Realmuto, & Hektner, 2003).

The SOAR program developed at the University of Washington by the Social Development Research Group emphasizes positive personal development and academic success. This goal is achieved by providing opportunities for active involvement of elementary school aged-children in their family and in school with consistent positive recognition for their positive attitudes and behavior. The program has components for students, teachers, and parents. The student component is designed to develop acceptable social skills both in school and at home. The teacher component focuses on improving classroom management and instruction methods to increase academic skills and behavior. The parent component emphasizes developmentally appropriate parenting skills. Using a nonrandomized design with follow-up 6 years after the intervention, three treatment conditions were created: (1) full intervention group in which interventions occurred from grades 1 through 6; (2) late intervention group with interventions delivered in only grades 5 and 6; and (3) control group with no special intervention. Five hundred and ninety-eight students with parental consent were followed through age 18. It was found that students in the full implementation program had statistically significant improvements in their attachment to school and in their academic performance and had significantly lower rates of heavy drinking and violent behavior (Hawkins et al., 1999).

While these interventions address school climate and culture, there are interventions that address classroom climate. The most widely recognized intervention of this type is the Good Behavior Game. The purpose of this classroom management program, which targets children in elementary and early middle school, is to socialize them into their roles as students. In particular, the program seeks to reduce aggressive or otherwise disruptive classroom behavior by establishing a set of rules of appropriate conduct, teaching students how to behave and work together effectively as members of a team, and how to monitor their own as well as their team's behavior. The teacher also specifies incentives for positive behavior for both the individual student and the team as a whole. Evaluations have demonstrated that the program reduces substance use and violence, and enhances students' mental health (Kellam et al., 2014).

School Policy

Research examining school policies related to substance use within the school building have received relatively meager attention over the past two decades. School policies are especially appealing to address substance use as large numbers of the target population can be affected and the associated costs appear to be minimal. Evans-Whipp and colleagues (Evans-Whipp et al., 2004) conducted a review of school policies and found that most schools in developed countries have substance use policies that varied substantially in terms of how comprehensive they were and in how policies are enforced, whether punitive or remedial. They found that research studies that examined the outcomes from school policy focused on the use of tobacco that indicated the more comprehensive and enforced policies were related to lower rates of smoking.

Pentz (2003) suggests there are four types of formal regulations found in schools: (1) those that focus on the production or distribution of substances and those that regulate price and the conditions of use; (2) those that control the "flow of information" regarding substance use such as warning labels; (3) those that directly regulate consumption (e.g., use of prescriptions and monitoring use by physicians); and (4) those that declare use as illegal (e.g., minimum drinking age, sanctions against possession of illicit drugs.)

Common elements or principles of effective school policy approaches to impact substance use include the following:

- Reducing or eliminating access to and availability of tobacco, alcohol, or other drugs.
- Addressing infractions of policies with positive sanctions by providing counseling or treatment and special services to the students rather than punishing them through suspension or expulsion.
- Policies should not disrupt normal school functioning.
- Policies should address the full range of drug-using behaviors from initiation to progression to abuse and dependence and relapse.
- Policies should have a small number of focused goals.
- Policies should specify the substances that are targeted.
- Policies should reflect and be reflected in other community prevention efforts.
- The student body, faculty, and students should be involved in developing the policy.
- Policies should provide positive reinforcement for policy compliance.
- Policies should provide systematic training for policy administrators and educate the target population about participation in policy aims.

Direct interventions mentioned by Pentz (2003) with specific relevance for youth consist of drug testing in schools and athletic events. In 1995, the US Supreme Court upheld a school's right to conduct random drug tests of student athletes without any suspicion of use of drugs, and in 2002, the Supreme Court carried this decision further by upholding school districts' rights to extend testing to students participating in other extracurricular activities (Yamaguchi, Johnston, & O'Malley, 2003). However, to date there is no clear evidence that drug testing has an association with lower rates of substance use. The studies that were conducted have a number of methodological problems (Goldberg et al., 2003, 2007; James-Burdumy, Goesling, Deke, & Einspruch, 2010; Terry-McElrath, O'Malley, & Johnston, 2013; Yamaguchi et al., 2003). Goldberg and his group (Goldberg et al., 2003, 2007) have conducted two studies on the impact of drug testing on high school athletes, the Student Athlete Testing Using Random Notification. In the first study, although the researchers found that drug testing did result in decreased reported use of drugs, they caution against the use of this approach until a larger, randomized longitudinal study is conducted (Goldberg et al., 2003). The larger study was completed and the findings, based on self-report, indicate no differences between control and experimental students on past month drug use (Goldberg et al., 2007). The researchers conclude that drug testing is not an effective deterrent to drug use and actually may increase the risk factors that could be associated with future substance use.

Other environmental policies such as roadside testing for alcohol use; lower blood alcohol content (BAC) laws; higher minimum drinking laws; and drug and alcohol possession checks at school and public events can involve the school and other community organizations through direct involvement of school administrators in designing these policies or incorporating discussion of the legal consequences of alcohol use by minors in the school curriculum or special assemblies. Of these approaches, road-side checks and testing, lower BAC, higher minimum drinking age laws, and identification checks for the purchase of tobacco have been evaluated and found to be effective in decreasing alcohol-related accidents and tobacco purchases by youth (Callinan, Clarke, Doherty, & Kelleher, 2010; Forster, Wolfson, Murray, Wagenaar, & Claxton, 1997; Hingson et al., 1996; Hingson, Heeren, & Winter, 2000; Holder, 1993; Wagenaar, Salois, & Komro, 2009; Wolfson et al., 1996).

Other types of effective policies that extend beyond the school building but that can involve the school focus on the vendor controlling availability and access by youth. These include removal of cigarette vending machines, alerting parents about laws against serving alcohol to minors, local alcohol server and tobacco sales staff training to ensure understanding of sale restrictions to minors and the need to "card" customers, "sting" operations to determine that these deterrents are implemented, and follow through on penalties for sales of alcohol and tobacco to underage youth (Altman, Rasenick-Douss, Foster, & Tye, 1991; Forster et al., 1997; Forster & Wolfson, 1998).

Classroom Curriculum

Probably the most frequently occurring prevention approach is the use of a classroom curriculum that focuses on the prevention of substance use. A survey of Safe and Drug Free Schools Coordinators in a sample of 81 school districts in 11 states conducted in 1999 indicated that 80% delivered a prevention curriculum to their students. Of these 80%, 26% include elementary, middle, and high school programs, 42% reported that their districts focus primarily on the elementary school level (generally kindergarten through 5th or 6th grade), 26% on the middle school level (generally 6th or 7th grades to 8th grade), and 6% on the high school level (generally 9th through 12th grades) (Bruckner et al., 2014; Hallfors, Sporer, Pankratz, & Godette, 2000). As such, many types of classroom curricula have been developed and evaluated over the past 25 years. Several researchers have conducted meta-analyses of the data from studies of both universal and indicated programs (Durlak, Weissberg, Dymnicki, Taylor, & Schellinger, 2011; Faggiano, Minozzi, Versino, & Buscemi, 2014; Gottfredson & Wilson, 2003; Porath-Waller, Beasley, & Beimess, 2010; Tobler, 1986, 1992; Tobler, Lessard, Marshall, Ochshorn, & Roona, 1999) while others conducted program content analyses and surveys of prevention researchers (Dusenbury & Falco, 1995; Sloboda & David, 1997; United Nations Office on Drugs and Crime, 2013) to determine common elements of effective interventions. There have been consistent findings across all of these approaches.

Common elements of universal/indicated curriculum include the following:

- Dispelling misconceptions regarding the normative nature and expectancies of substance use (i.e., the prevalence and positive/negative effects of use).

- Impacting perceptions of risks associated with substance use for children and adolescents (i.e., emphasizing the effects students will experience now not when they are adults).
- Providing and practicing what are called life skills that include making decisions, especially about initiating or continuing substance use; communicating these decisions; and resistance skills to refuse the use of tobacco, alcohol, and illicit drugs using authentic scenarios.
- Providing interventions and boosters over multiple years into middle and high school when students are most at risk.

Most available evidence-based school curriculum programs are considered universal as they target general populations that include students at different levels of risk for initiating the use of alcohol, tobacco, or other psychoactive substances. There are a number of indicated programs that target students who are considered at higher risk to initiate the use of these substances because they are not doing well in school and are experiencing high numbers of absences, suspensions, or expulsions. There are few that could be considered selective programs, that is, that address students who may have initiated low levels of substance use or are expressing other problem behaviors.

There are several examples of effective universal curricula available. These include LST (Botvin, Baker, Dusenbury, Tortu, & Botvin, 1995), Project ALERT (Ellickson, Bell, & McGuigan, 1993), and Project STAR (Pentz et al., 1989). LST developed at Cornell University by Botvin and his group has been one of the most cited effective universal curricula in the USA. LST is a program that enhances competencies of the participants. It consists of a 24-session elementary school program delivered over 3 years (3rd or 4th to 6th grades) and/or a 30-session middle school also to be delivered over 3 years (6th or 7th to 8th grades). The three major aims of the program are to provide students with skills that enable them to challenge common misconceptions regarding the use of tobacco, alcohol, and other drugs and to learn the skills needed to resist pressures to engage in the use of these substances, personal self-management skills that help them set and keep personal goals and to make well-thought out decisions, and other social skills to communicate effectively and clearly with their peers and adults. LST has been evaluated with a number of diverse populations with consistently good results. For instance, in one evaluation study in which 56 public schools were randomized to an experimental or control condition, 3597 participating students were followed to the 12th grade. The study found that 44% fewer students exposed to a program of 15 lessons in the 7th grade, ten booster lessons in the 8th grade, and five booster lessons in the 9th grade used drugs and 66% fewer used a combination of tobacco, alcohol, and marijuana (Botvin et al., 1995). In other studies conducted by this same group of researchers, it was found that even without the boosters in the 8th and 9th grades there had been a reduction of between 56% and 67% in the number of students becoming smokers who were nonsmokers at baseline without the two additional years of booster lessons. When the 2 years of booster lessons are added, the percentage of nonuse of tobacco increased to 87% (Botvin & Griffin, 2003).

Another curriculum that we will describe is Project Toward No Drug Abuse (Project TND). The purpose of this curriculum is to teach a number of skills, including self-control, decision-making, and substance use resistance, and to strengthen motivations not to use substances, which is another way of saying to increase anti-substance use attitudes. Project TND, which uses interactive methods, is taught in 12 weekly sessions of about 40 min each, and is thus designed to fit comfortably within a traditional 45–50 min class period. While it has been tested on students from early adolescence through young adulthood, it is designed primarily for universal and selective populations of adolescents in school settings. We are paying particular attention to this curriculum because it is one of relatively few that are available adolescent populations. Project TND has conducted seven randomized field trials that evaluated the effectiveness of the program on teen substance use and violence. Overall in 1-year follow-up participants who received Project TND compared to comparison groups experienced reductions in cigarette, marijuana, and "hard drug" use.

Like all evidence-based substance use prevention curricula, these programs are manualized and require training by those implementing them.

Interventions That Do Not Work

Despite the clear evidence that there exists a range of effective substance use prevention interventions designed for the school and classroom-culture and climate, development of effective policies—when enforced appropriately, and prevention curricula, many policy makers and school administrators continue to implement interventions that have either been found not to be effective or even iatrogenic or if they do institute evidence-based interventions fail to implement with fidelity to the intent of the intervention.

As early as 2000, Tobler summarized what does and does not work in interventions. She found the following content and delivery features that do not work.

- Content
  - Failure to include short-term consequences
  - Failure to address perceptions of peer drug use
  - Failure to address media influences on prodrug attitudes
  - Addressing only ethical/moral decision-making
  - Teaching values only
  - Failure to provide interpersonal skills, particularly drug refusal skills
  - Having only an intrapersonal focus
  - Focusing only on self-esteem building
- Delivery
  - Passive participation primary delivery strategy
  - Didactic or lectures only

  - Having teacher-centered class discussions
  - Having unstructured dialogue sessions
  - Depending primarily on effective classroom management techniques without a drug program

  The International Standards adds to this list:

- Content
  - Providing information only on specific substances
  - Focus only on emotional education
  - Focus only on emotional education
  - Address only ethical/moral decision-making or values
- Structure
  - Fear arousal only
  - Unstructured dialogue sessions
- Delivery
  - Using untrained teachers
  - Using untrained teachers
  - Primarily using noninteractive methods
  - Use ex-drug users as testimonials

Recommendations for School-Based Prevention and Health Promotion

This chapter offers the following guidance to school administrators considering the implementation of substance use prevention programming in their schools.

1. Probably the most important recommendation is for the administrators to recognize that substance use is not the sole problem of the school. Findings from prevention research studies show that school-based programming is more effective when supported by community and/or family components such as PROSPER (Spoth et al., 2013) or Communities That Care (Hawkins, Oesterle, Brown, Abbott, & Catalano, 2014) that have demonstrated sustained effectiveness of prevention programming by building community prevention implementation systems.
2. In addition to what was presented above, there are a number of other issues that need to be thought about when selecting school-based substance abuse prevention interventions. Botvin and Griffin (2003) mention some key issues: timing of the interventions, delivery by peers and/or adults, use of interactive teaching approaches, targeting multiple substances, targeting minority groups, durability of interventions, and implementation fidelity.

Of particular importance is the last item, implementation fidelity. The issue of adaptation versus implementation fidelity is one of the great challenges to the prevention field. Implementation fidelity addresses the degree to which the curriculum content and delivery style consistently and completely match that of the original tested program. Often, a program taken from a research setting to the "real world" will undergo changes to meet the needs of the school or of the instructor. Understanding the curriculum design and key elements of the program is important. Sound training helps instructors comprehend why program design is essential and provides a basis for a commitment to prevention. The establishment of a monitoring system to assess program implementation and providing ongoing technical assistance would ensure fidelity of implementation. Tailoring or adapting an intervention by implementers or policy makers is a natural process. Such tailoring increases the likelihood that the participants will view the program as relevant and that our desired outcomes will be achieved. Tailoring includes addressing cultural beliefs, values, language, and visual images but does not mean altering the theoretical foundation of the intervention. It is important to remember, particularly for evidence-based interventions, to maintain the intent of the program by maintaining the full program. This represents a balance between fidelity, the delivery of a prevention intervention program as prescribed or designed by those who developed the program and adaptation, the modification of program content to accommodate the needs of a specific consumer or target group (Castro, Barrera, & Martinez, 2004). The Substance Abuse and Mental Health Services Administration (2017) has some pointers about adapting a program for a new community:

- Change capacity before changing the program. It may be easier to change the program, but changing local capacity to deliver it as it was designed is a safer choice.
- Consult with the program developer. Consult with the program developer to determine what experience and/or advice he or she has about adapting the program to a particular setting or circumstance.
- Retain core components. There is a greater likelihood of effectiveness when a program retains the core component(s) of the original intervention.
- Be consistent with evidence-based principles. There is a greater likelihood of success if an adaptation does not violate an established evidence-based prevention principle.
- Add, rather than subtract. It is safer to add to a program than to modify or subtract from it.

3. There is agreement in the prevention field that prevention is a process that takes place across the lifespan. The factors related to increasing the risks for initiating substance use occur across developmental stages suggesting that interventions should take place at key developmental points including infancy, early childhood, childhood, preadolescence, and adolescence. Early interventions with identified vulnerable children may be most effective in the long term. Yet the expected outcomes from interventions for each developmental stage are not clear.

4. Several studies and meta-analyses (Tobler, 1986, 1992; Tobler et al., 1999) suggest that interventions delivered by same age or slightly older peer leaders are more effective than when delivered by adults. On the other hand, as Botvin and Griffin (2003) point out peer leaders alone may not have the maturity to manage a classroom or to engage students in small group or open discussion, particularly when the program heavily emphasizes skills building. Their suggestion is to use peer leaders in supportive roles such as assisting with program activities with adults taking the lead in delivery. The information of peer-led substance use interventions is weak at this time. Experience with such programs as Sources of Strength, a peer-led suicide prevention program, supports this intervention structural suggestion (Wyman et al., 2010).
5. The sequencing of substance use suggests that the risk for using marijuana is increased if a young adolescent has used alcohol or tobacco, particularly if this use was initiated in childhood or early adolescence. Therefore, prevention programs should address multiple substances. The social tolerance is unequal for each of these substances and some programs may be less effective for one or more of these substances (Werch & Owen, 2002).
6. Finally, school administrators should be mindful of the fact that the field of psychoactive substance use prevention is relatively new. The knowledge that is accumulating from prevention researchers changes as intervention strategies and statistical methodologies become more sophisticated. In addition, the research that serves to guide prevention intervention development, that is, epidemiology and behavioral science, is also evolving, and, finally, our children's cultural worlds and influences are ever changing. What programs may be effective for adolescents today may not be as effective for their younger siblings when they enter their teen years. Such changes suggest constant attention to updating prevention messages and strategies.

References

Altman, D. G., Rasenick-Douss, L., Foster, V., & Tye, J. B. (1991). Sustained effects of an educational program to reduce sales of cigarettes to minors. *American Journal of Public Health, 81*(5), 891–893.

Ashe, M., Jernigan, D., Kline, R., & Galaz, R. (2003). Land use planning and the control of alcohol, tobacco, firearms, and fast food restaurants. *American Journal of Public Health, 93*(9), 1404–1408.

August, G. J., Lee, S. S., Bloomquist, M. L., Realmuto, G. M., & Hektner, J. M. (2003). Dissemination of an evidence-based prevention innovation for aggressive children living in culturally diverse, urban neighborhoods: The Early Risers effectiveness study. *Prevention Science, 4*(4), 271–286.

Battistich, V., Schaps, E., Watson, M., Solomon, D., & Lewis, C. (2000). Effects of the Child Development Project on students' drug use and other problem behaviors. *The Journal of Primary Prevention, 21*(1), 75–99.

Bloom, B. S., Engelhart, M. D., Furst, E. J., Hill, W. H., & Krathwohl, D. R. (1956). *Taxonomy of educational objectives: The classification of educational goals. Handbook 1: Cognitive domain*. New York, NY: David McKay.

Bosworth, K., & Sloboda, Z. (2015). Prevention science 1970-Present. In K. Bosworth (Ed.), *Prevention science in school settings: Complex relationships and processes* (pp. 125–149). New York, NY: Springer.
Botvin, G. J., Baker, E., Dusenbury, L., Tortu, S., & Botvin, E. M. (1995). Long-term follow-up results of a randomized drug abuse prevention trial in a White middle-class population. *Journal of the American Medical Association, 273*(14), 1106–1112.
Botvin, G. J., & Griffin, K. W. (2003). Drug abuse prevention curricula in schools. In Z. Sloboda & W. J. Bukoski (Eds.), *Handbook of drug abuse prevention: Theory, science, and practice* (pp. 45–74). New York, NY: Kluwer Academic/Plenum Publishers.
Bruckner, T. A., Domina, T., Hwang, J. K., Gerlinger, J., Carpenter, C., & Wakefield, S. (2014). State-level education standards for substance use prevention programs in schools: A systematic content analysis. *Journal of Adolescent Health, 54*(4), 467–473.
Bruner, J. S. (1960). *The process of education*. Cambridge, MA: Harvard University Press.
Bukoski, W. J. (2003). The emerging science of drug abuse prevention. In Z. Sloboda & W. J. Bukoski (Eds.), *Handbook of drug abuse prevention: Theory, science, and practice* (pp. 3–26). New York, NY: Kluwer Academic/Plenum Publishers.
Callinan, J. E., Clarke, A., Doherty, K., & Kelleher, C. (2010). Legislative smoking bans for reducing secondhand smoke exposure, smoking prevalence and tobacco consumption. *Cochrane Database of Systematic Reviews*, (4), CD005992. https://doi.org/10.1002/14651858.CD005992.pub2
Campello, G., Sloboda, Z., Heikkil, H., & Brotherhood, A. (2014). International standards on drug use prevention: The future of drug use prevention world-wide. *International Journal of Prevention and Treatment of Substance Use Disorders, 1*(2), 6–27.
Castro, F. G., Barrera, M., Jr., & Martinez, C. R., Jr. (2004). The cultural adaptation of prevention interventions: Resolving tensions between fidelity and fit. *Prevention Science, 5*(1), 41–45.
Coie, J. D., Watt, N. F., West, S. G., Hawkins, J. D., Asarnow, J. R., Markman, H. J., … Long, B. (1993). The science of prevention: A conceptual framework and some directions for a national research program. *American Psychologist, 48*(10), 1013–1022.
Colombo Plan International Centre for Credentialing and Education of Addiction Professionals (ICCE). (2015). *Introduction to the universal prevention curriculum series for implementers* (p. 229). Colombo, Sri Lanka: Colombo Plan.
Crowley, D. M., Greenberg, M. T., Feinberg, M. E., Spoth, R. L., & Redmond, C. R. (2012). The effect of the PROSPER Partnership model on cultivating local stakeholders' knowledge of evidence-based programs: A five-year longitudinal study of 28 communities. *Prevention Science., 13*(1), 96–105.
Durlak, J. A., & Dupre, E. P. (2008). Implementation matters: A review of research on the influence of implementation on program outcomes and the factors affecting implementation. *American Journal of Community Psychology, 41*, 327–350.
Durlak, J. A., Weissberg, R. P., Dymnicki, A. B., Taylor, R. D., & Schellinger, K. B. (2011). The impact of enhancing students' social and emotional learning: A meta-analysis of school-based universal interventions. *Child Development, 82*(1), 405–432.
Dusenbury, L., & Falco, M. (1995). Eleven components of effective drug abuse prevention curricula. *Journal of School Health, 65*(10), 420–425.
Ellickson, P. L., Bell, R. M., & McGuigan, K. (1993). Preventing adolescent drug use: Long term results of a junior high program. *American Journal of Public Health, 83*(6), 856–861.
European Monitoring Centre for Drugs and Drug Addiction. (2011). *European drug prevention quality standards*. Lisbon, Portugal: European Drug Prevention Monitoring Centre for Drugs and Drug Addiction (EMCDDA).
Evans-Whipp, T., Beyers, J. M., Lloyd, S., Lafazia, A. N., Toumbourou, J. W., Arthur, M. W., & Catalano, R. F. (2004). A review of school drug policies and their impact on youth substance use. *Health Promotion International, 19*(2), 227–234.
Faggiano, F., Minozzi, S., Versino, E., & Buscemi, D. (2014). Universal school-based prevention for illicit drug use. *Cochrane Database of Systematic Reviews*, (12), CD003020. https://doi.org/10.1002/14651858.CD003020.pub3

Fishbein, D. H., Rose, E. J., Darcey, V., Belcher, A., & VanMeter, J. (2016, June). Neurodevelopmental precursors and consequences of substance use during adolescence: Promises and pitfalls of longitudinal neuroimaging strategies. *Frontiers in Human Neuroscience, 10*, 296. https://doi.org/10.3389/fnhum.2016.00296

Fletcher, A. (2015). School culture and classroom climate. In K. Bosworth (Ed.), *Prevention science in school settings: Complex relationships and processes* (pp. 273–286). New York, NY: Springer.

Forster, J. L., & Wolfson, M. (1998). Youth access to tobacco: Policies and politics. *Annual Review of Public Health, 19*, 203–2335.

Forster, J. L., Wolfson, M., Murray, D. M., Wagenaar, A. C., & Claxton, A. J. (1997). Perceived and measured availability of tobacco to youths in 14 Minnesota communities: The TPOP Study. Tobacco Policy Options for Prevention. *American Journal of Preventive Medicine, 13*(3), 167–174.

Goldberg, L., Elliot, D. L., MacKinnon, D. P., Moe, E., Kuehl, K. S., Nohre, L., & Lockwood, C. M. (2003). Drug testing athletes to prevent substance abuse: Background and pilot study results of the SATURN (Student Athlete Testing Using Random Notification) study. *Journal of Adolescent Health, 32*(1), 16–25.

Goldberg, L., Elliot, D. L., MacKinnon, D. P., Moe, E. L., Kuehl, K. S., Yoon, M., … Williams, J. (2007). Outcomes of a prospective trial of student-athlete drug testing: The Student Athlete Testing Using Random Notification (SATURN) study. *Journal of Adolescent Health, 41*(5), 421–429.

Gordon, R. (1983). An operational classification of disease prevention. *Public Health Reports, 98*(2), 107–109.

Gottfredson, D. C., & Wilson, D. B. (2003). Characteristics of effective school-based substance abuse prevention. *Prevention Science, 4*(1), 27–38.

Gottfredson, G. D., & Gottfredson, D. C. (2001). What schools do to prevent problem behavior and promote safe environments. *Journal of Educational and Psychological Consultation, 12*(4), 313–344.

Green, L. W., & Kreuter, M. W. (2005). *Health program planning: An educational and ecological approach* (4th ed.). Columbus, OH: McGraw Hill.

Hallfors, D., Sporer, A., Pankratz, M., & Godette, D. (2000). *Drug free schools survey: Report of results*. Unpublished manuscript, School of Public Health, Department of Maternal and Child Health, University of North Carolina, Chapel Hill, North Carolina.

Hawkins, J. D., Catalano, R. F., Kosterman, R., Abbott, R., & Hill, K. G. (1999). Preventing adolescent health-risk behaviors by strengthening protection during childhood. *Archives of Pediatric and Adolescent Medicine, 153*, 226–234.

Hawkins, J. D., Catalano, R. F., & Miller, J. Y. (1992). Risk and protective factors for alcohol and other drug problems in adolescence and early adulthood: Implications for substance abuse prevention. *Psychological Bulletin, 112*(1), 64–105.

Hawkins, J. D., Oesterle, S., Brown, E., Abbott, R., & Catalano, R. F. (2014). Youth problem behaviors 8 years after implementing the Communities That Care prevention system. A community randomized trial. *Journal of the American Medical Association Pediatrics, 168*(2), 122–129.

Hingson, R., Heeren, T., & Winter, M. (2000). Effects of recent 0.08% legal blood alcohol limits on fatal crash involvement. *Injury Prevention, 6*(2), 109–114.

Hingson, R., McGovern, T., Howland, J., Heeren, T., Winter, M., & Zakocs, R. (1996). Reducing alcohol-impaired driving in Massachusetts: The Saving Lives Program. *American Journal of Public Health, 86*(6), 791–797.

Holder, H. D. (1993). Prevention of alcohol-related accidents in the community. *Addiction, 88*(7), 1003–1012.

Holder, H. D. (2000). Community prevention of alcohol problems. *Addictive Behaviors, 25*(6), 843–859.

Holder, H. D. (2001). Prevention of alcohol problems in the 21st century: Challenges and opportunities. *American Journal on Addictions, 10*(1), 1–15.

James-Burdumy, S., Goesling, B., Deke, J. & Einspruch, E. (2010). *The effectiveness of mandatory-random student drug testing* (NCEE 2010-4025). Washington, DC: National Center for Education Evaluation and Regional Assistance, Institute of Education Sciences, U.S. Department of Education.

Kellam, S. G., Wang, W., Mackenzie, A. C. L., Brown, C. H., Ompad, D. C., Or, F., … Windham, A. (2014). The impact of the Good Behavior Game, a universal classroom based preventive intervention in first and second grades, on high risk sexual behaviors and drug abuse and dependence disorders in young adulthood. *Prevention Science, 15*(Suppl 1), S6–S18.

Liang, L., Chaloupka, F., Nichter, M., & Clayton, R. (2003). Prices, policies and youth smoking. *Addiction, 98*(Suppl. 1), 105–122.

Luke, D. A., Stamatakis, K. A., & Brownson, R. C. (2000). State youth-access tobacco control policies and youth smoking behavior in the United States. *American Journal of Preventive Medicine, 19*(3), 180–187.

Mrazek, P. J., & Haggerty, R. J. (1994). *Reducing risks for mental disorders*. Washington, DC: National Academy Press.

Payne, A. A., Gottfredson, D. C., & Gottfredson, G. D. (2006). School predictors of the intensity of implementation of school-based prevention programs: Results from a national study. *Prevention Science, 7*(2), 225–237.

Pentz, M. A. (2003). Anti-drug-abuse policies as prevention strategies. In Z. Sloboda & W. J. Bukoski (Eds.), *Handbook of drug abuse prevention: Theory, science, and practice* (pp. 217–244). New York, NY: Kluwer Academic/Plenum Publishers.

Pentz, M. A., Dwyer, J. H., MacKinnon, D. P., Flay, B. R., Hansen, W. B., Wang, E. Y., & Johnson, C. A. (1989). A multi-community trial for primary prevention of adolescent drug abuse: Effects on drug use prevalence. *Journal of the American Medical Association, 261*(2), 3259–3266.

Porath-Waller, A., Beasley, E., & Beimess, D. J. (2010). A meta-analytic review of school-based prevention for cannabis use. *Health Education Behavior, 37*(5), 709–723.

Powers, J. D., Bowen, N. K., & Bowen, G. L. (2010). Evidence-based programs in school settings: Barriers and recent advances. *Journal of Evidence-Based Social Work, 7*, 313–331.

Renner, J., Stafford, D., Lawson, A., McKinnon, J., Friot, E., & Kellogg, D. (1976). *Research, teaching, and learning with the Piaget model*. Norman, OK: University of Oklahoma Press.

Ringwalt, C., Hanley, S. M., Vincus, A. A., Ennett, S. T., Rohrbach, L. A., & Bowling, J. M. (2008). The prevalence of effective substance use prevention curricula in the Nation's high schools. *Journal of Primary Prevention, 29*(6), 479–488.

Ringwalt, C., Vincus, A. A., Hanley, S. M., Ennett, S. T., Bowling, J. M., & Haws, S. W. (2010). The prevalence of evidence-based prevention curricula in U.S. middle schools in 2008. *Prevention Science, 12*, 63–69.

Ringwalt, C. L., Ennett, S. T., Vincus, A. A., Rohrbach, L. A., & Simons-Rudolph, A. (2004). Who's calling the shots? Decision-makers and the adoption of effective school-based substance use prevention curricula. *Journal of Drug Education, 34*(1), 19–31.

Ringwalt, C. L., Ennett, S. T., Vincus, A. A., Thorne, J., Rohrbach, L. A., & Simons-Rudolph, A. (2002). The prevalence of effective substance use prevention curricula in U.S. middle schools. *Prevention Science, 3*(4), 257–265.

Ringwalt, C. L., Vincus, A. A., Ennett, S. T., Hanley, S., Bowling, J. M., & Rohrbach, L. A. (2009). The prevalence of evidence-based substance use prevention curricula in U.S. middle schools in 2005. *Prevention Science, 10*(1), 33–40.

Rohrbach, L. A. (2014). Design of prevention interventions. In Z. Sloboda & H. Petras (Eds.), *Defining prevention science* (pp. 275–292). New York, NY: Springer.

Rohrbach, L. A., & Dyal, S. R. (2015). Scaling up evidence-based prevention interventions. In K. Bosworth (Ed.), *Prevention science in school settings: Complex relationships and processes* (pp. 175–197). New York, NY: Springer.

Rohrbach, L. A., Ringwalt, C. L., Ennett, S. T., & Vincus, A. A. (2005). Factors associated with adoption of evidence-based substance use prevention curricula in U.S. school districts. *Health Education Research, 20*(5), 514–526.

Ross, H., & Chaloupka, F. J. (2003). The effect of cigarette prices on youth smoking. *Health Economics, 12*(3), 217–230.
Sackett, D. L., Rosenberg, W., McGray, J. A., Haynes, R. B., & Richardson, W. S. (1996). Evidence-based medicine: What it is and what it isn't. *British Medical Journal, 312*, 71–72.
Schaps, E., & Solomon, D. (2003). The role of the school's social environment in preventing student drug use. *The Journal of Primary Prevention, 23*(3), 299–328.
Sherman, L. W. (2000). The safe and drug-free schools program. In D. Ravitch (Ed.), *Brookings papers on education policy* (pp. 125–156). Washington, DC: Brookings Institution Press.
Shonkoff, J. (2010). Building a new biodevelopmental framework to guide the future of early childhood policy. *Child Development, 81*(1), 357–367.
Sloboda, Z. (2015). Vulnerability and risks: Implications for understanding etiology and drug use prevention. In L. M. Scheier (Ed.), *Handbook of adolescent drug use prevention: Research, intervention strategies, and practice* (pp. 85–100). Washington, DC: American Psychological Association.
Sloboda, Z., & David, S. L. (1997). *Preventing drug abuse among children and adolescents: A research-based guide* (NIH Publication No. 97–4212). Washington, DC: National Institute of Health.
Sloboda, Z., Dusenbury, L., & Petras, H. (2014). Implementation science and the effective delivery of evidence-based prevention. In Z. Sloboda & H. Petras (Eds.), *Defining prevention science* (pp. 293–314). New York, NY: Springer.
Sloboda, Z., Glantz, M. D., & Tarter, R. E. (2012). Revisiting the concepts of risk and protective factors for understanding the etiology and development of substance use and substance use disorders: Implications for prevention. *Substance Use and Misuse, 47*(8-9), 1–19.
Sloboda, Z., Pyakuryal, A., Stephens, P., Teasdale, B., Forrest, D., Stephens, R. C., & Grey, S. F. (2008). Reports of substance abuse programming available in schools. *Prevention Science., 9*(4), 276–287.
Society for Prevention Research. (2011). *Standards of knowledge for the science of prevention*. Retrieved from http://www.preventionresearch.org/advocacy/#SofK.
Spoth, R., Redmond, C., Shin, C., Greenberg, M., Feinberg, M., & Schainker, L. (2013). PROSPER community-university partnerships delivery system effects on substance misuse through 6½ years past baseline from a cluster randomized controlled intervention trial. *Preventive Medicine, 56*(4), 190–196.
Substance Abuse and Mental Health Services Administration. (2017). *Applying the Strategic Prevention Framework (SPF)*. Retrieved from https://www.samhsa.gov/capt/applying-strategic-prevention-framework.
Tarter, R., Vanyukov, M., Giancola, P., Dawes, M., Blackson, T., Mezzich, A., & Clark, D. B. (1999). Etiology of early age onset substance use disorder: A maturational perspective. *Development and Psychopathology, 11*(4), 657–683.
Terry-McElrath, Y. M., O'Malley, P. M., & Johnston, L. D. (2013). Middle and high school drug testing and student illicit drug use: A national study 1998-2011. *The Journal of Adolescent Health, 52*(6), 707–715.
Tobler, N. S. (1986). Meta-analysis of 143 adolescent drug prevention programs: Quantitative outcome results of program participants compared to a control or comparison group. *Journal of Drug Issues, 16*(4), 537–567.
Tobler, N. S. (1992). Drug prevention programs can work: Research findings. *Journal of Addictive Diseases, 11*(3), 1–28.
Tobler, N. S. (2000). Lessons learned. *The Journal of Primary Prevention, 20*(4), 261–274.
Tobler, N. S., Lessard, T., Marshall, D., Ochshorn, P., & Roona, M. (1999). Effectiveness of school-based drug prevention programs for marijuana use. *School Psychology International, 20*(1), 105–137.
U.S. Department of Education. (1998). Notice of final principles of effectiveness. *Federal Register, 63*(104), 29902–29906.

United Nations Office on Drugs and Crime. (2013/2015). *International standards for drug use prevention*. Retrieved from https://www.unodc.org/unodc/en/prevention/prevention-standards.html

Wagenaar, A. C., Salois, M. J., & Komro, K. A. (2009). Effects of beverage alcohol price and tax levels on drinking: A meta-analysis of 1003 estimates from 112 studies. *Addiction, 104*(2), 179–190.

Webster-Stratton, C., Reid, J., & Hammond, M. (2001). Preventing conduct problems, promoting social competence: A parent and teacher training partnership in Head Start. *Journal of Clinical Child Psychology, 30*(3), 282–302.

Wenter, D. L., Ennett, S. T., Ribisl, K. M., Vincus, A. A., Rohrbach, L., Ringwalt, C. L., & Jones, S. M. (2002). Comprehensiveness of substance use prevention programs in U.S. middle schools. *Journal of Adolescent Health, 30*(6), 455–462.

Werch, C. E., & Owen, D. M. (2002). Iatrogenic effects of alcohol and drug programs. *Journal of Studies of Alcohol, 63*(5), 581–590.

Wolfson, M., Toomey, T. L., Forster, J. L., Wagenaar, A. C., McGovern, P. G., & Perry, C. L. (1996). Characteristics, policies and practices of alcohol outlets and sale to underage persons. *Journal of Studies on Alcohol, 57*(6), 670–674.

Wyman, P. A., Brown, C. H., LoMurray, M., Schmeelk-Cone, K., Petrova, M., Yu, Q., … Wang, W. (2010). An outcome evaluation of the sources of strength suicide prevention program delivered by adolescent peer leaders in high schools. *American Journal of Public Health, 100*(9), 1653–1661.

Yamaguchi, R., Johnston, L. D., & O'Malley, P. M. (2003). Relationship between student illicit drug use and school drug-testing policies. *Journal of School Health, 3*(4), 159–164.

Evidence-Based Practices: Community-Based Interventions to Reduce Alcohol Use and Misuse

Pamela S. Imm, Matthew Chinman, Magdalena Kulesza, Sarah Hunter, and Joie Acosta

Introduction

This chapter focuses on community-based prevention initiatives for reducing and preventing adolescent substance use. It is an update of the research literature from the initial chapter published in 2009 (e.g., D'Amico, Chinman, Stern, & Wandersman, 2009). The reader is encouraged to review this initial chapter for foundational reading in important areas such as pathways into alcohol and drug use and theories that ground community interventions. Updated findings are presented from the research literature on multicomponent prevention initiatives and environmental strategies/policies implemented by communities that have a consistent evidence base of positive results—in other words, programs or initiatives that are run by communities that target whole communities. For these sections, the authors integrate findings from two recent publications, (1) Planning Alcohol Interventions Using NIAAA's

P. S. Imm (✉)
LRADAC, Columbia, SC, USA

M. Chinman
RAND Corporation, Pittsburgh, PA, USA
e-mail: chinman@rand.org

M. Kulesza
RAND Corporation, Santa Monica, CA, USA
e-mail: mkulesza@rand.org

S. Hunter
RAND, Santa Monica, CA, USA
e-mail: shunter@rand.org

J. Acosta
RAND Arlington, VA, USA
e-mail: jacosta@rand.org

C. G. Leukefeld, T. P. Gullotta (eds.), *Adolescent Substance Abuse*, Issues in Children's and Families' Lives, https://doi.org/10.1007/978-3-319-90611-9_14

College AIM Alcohol Interventions Matrix (2015), and (2) Facing Addiction in America: The Surgeon General's Report on Alcohol, Drugs, and Health (US Department of Health and Human Services, 2016).

This update also includes a brief review of research literature on positive youth development (PYD), a holistic approach that focuses on developmental characteristics that can lead to positive outcomes including a reduction in negative behaviors among youth such as substance use (Durlak et al., 2007). We conclude by providing some recommendations to promote high-quality implementation to increase the likelihood of positive results. As funding for comprehensive evaluation efforts of community-based efforts becomes scarce, a communities' capacity to ensure high-quality implementation should be prioritized.

What Is Community Prevention for Adolescent Substance Abuse?

In the field of prevention, drug and alcohol programs are typically classified as *universal*, designed for the general population; *selective*, designed for subgroups at risk for substance use, such as youth who have parents who abuse substances or who are already experimenting with substances themselves; or *indicated*, designed for youth who have been treated but are at high risk for relapse (Institute of Medicine, 1994; National Institute on Drug Abuse, 1997; National Research Council and Institute of Medicine, 2009). Universal or primary prevention oriented activities remain the most frequently used approach with young people.

Adolescence is a time when many biological, social, and cognitive changes take place which may be associated with initiation and maintenance of alcohol and drug use (Lanza & Collins, 2002; Tarter, 2002; Tschann et al., 1994). Prevention programming content for youth must address these developmental changes in order to be effective (D'Amico & Stern, 2008; US Department of Health and Human Services, 2016). Community-based interventions are one effective way to address these many changes as they typically target multiple factors (e.g., individual, community, peer) at once. When discussing community-based interventions, the word "community" can have different meanings. Ultimately, all types of interventions aimed at preventing youth substance abuse typically take place in a community. For example, programs delivered in schools could still be considered to take place in the community. However, for this chapter, a clearer operationalization of community-based is needed. Here, we focus primarily on interventions that are *delivered by whole communities* that *target whole communities*. Interventions that fall into this category include (a) substance abuse prevention programs that use multiple components to target multiple sectors of the community, and (b) those that are designed to prevent underage drinking through environmental prevention strategies and policies.

Given the increasing recognition that successful transitioning from adolescence to adulthood requires more than avoiding problematic behavior (Catalano, Berglund,

Ryan, Lonczak, & Hawkins, 2004; US Department of Health and Human Services, 2016), we also highlight promising practices for how communities organize to promote positive attributes and prevent problematic behaviors through initiatives designed to build positive youth development (Hilliard et al., 2014). Curriculum and training materials to build capacities for youth workers in the areas of positive youth development are available from the ACT for Youth Center for Excellence at Cornell University and from, www.actforyouth.net/youth_development/professionals/manual.cfm.

What Is the Estimated Number of Adolescents Using/Misusing Substances Yearly?

It is well known that alcohol and other drug use increases during adolescence (D'Amico et al., 2005; Johnston, O'Malley, Bachman, & Schulenberg, 2007; US Department of Health and Human Services, 2016) and is often associated with a host of problems, including school dropout (Muthén & Muthén, 2000), delinquency (Bui, Ellickson, & Bell, 2000), psychological distress (Hansell & White, 1991), and accidents or injury (Hingson, Heeren, Jamanka, & Howland, 2000). While there are recent data showing decreases in adolescent use of tobacco and alcohol, existing and newer threats have emerged such as e-cigarettes/vaping, marijuana (including synthetic marijuana), opioids, and heroin.

According to the Monitoring the Future Survey (MTF), rates of tobacco and alcohol use among adolescents are the lowest since the survey began tracking adolescent perceptions and behaviors over 40 years ago (Johnston, O'Malley, Miech, Bachman, & Schulenberg, 2016). Nevertheless, the use of these and other substances is still unacceptably high with six out of every ten students (61%) having consumed alcohol (more than just a few sips) by the end of high school, and about a quarter (23%) has done so by eighth grade. Almost half of 12th grade students and 10% of 8th grade students reported having been drunk at least once in their life (Johnston et al., 2016). Approximately 13% of 12th grade students report 30-day use of e-cigarettes/vaping, which outpaces the use of cigarettes (e.g., 11%). Marijuana is the most frequently used illicit drug with 14% of 12th grade students reporting past month use and 6% reporting daily marijuana use (Johnston et al., 2016). Because of the downward trend of the perceived levels of risk of harm of marijuana, there is some anticipation that the prevalence of marijuana use will rise. The legalization of medical and recreational marijuana is likely to be contributing to these trends of acceptability of use and decreased perceptions that the drug is harmful.

Furthermore, alcohol and drug use during adolescence can adversely impact functioning across several different areas. Because the adolescent brain is not fully developed (Sowell, Thompson, Holmes, Jernigan, & Toga, 1999), alcohol and drug use may disrupt this maturation process and impair brain function over the long term (Chambers, Taylor, & Potenza, 2003; Tapert, Caldwell, & Burke, 2004–2005). Heavy drinking during this time period can affect memory function and may also impair the growth and integrity of certain brain structures (De Bellis et al., 2000; Tapert et al., 2004–2005). Early initiation of marijuana and frequent use during this time period is associated with lower grades, dropping out of school, lower life satisfaction, and earning less money in young adulthood (Brook, Balka, & Whiteman, 1999; Ellickson, Martino, & Collins, 2004). Research shows that for those who meet criteria for a substance use disorder, the majority began using substances during adolescence (Hasin, Stinson, Ogburn, & Grant, 2007) highlighting the need to ensure that effective prevention programs and strategies are available and widely disseminated in communities.

Table 1 highlights risk and protective factors associated with alcohol and drug use during adolescence.

Community Coalitions as a Mechanism for Preventing Substance Use

Given the environment's impact on youth drinking, it is believed that it takes an entire community to enact effective and meaningful change in underage drinking (Holder, 2000). Community coalitions are one vehicle that can be used to implement community-based initiatives (USDHHS, 2016; Imm et al., 2007; Zakocs & Edwards, 2006). Coalitions can be used to assess problems facing their community, develop a plan to address the needs identified, implement strategies to address the problems, and evaluate these strategies (Butterfoss & Kegler, 2002). Although coalitions are often viewed as an intervention themselves, they are actually a delivery vehicle or catalyst for many types of interventions. We therefore describe coalitions in the current chapter, but we do not evaluate the many different community coalitions that focus on the prevention of alcohol use and misuse.

Coalitions are defined as "inter-organizational, cooperative, and synergistic working alliances" of individuals and/or organizations (Butterfoss, Goodman, & Wandersman, 1993, p. 316). Community coalitions tend to concentrate on community planning, increasing public participation, and changing public policy. These coalitions can play an important coordinating role, "bringing together community institutions and residents to develop comprehensive, integrated approaches" (Join Together, 1999, p. 12). Mobilizing at the community level requires a variety of activities, including the development of a diverse membership, ongoing mobilization to promote true collaboration, and systematic processes to strengthen community resources and infrastructures. Media advocacy, in which coalitions work directly with local news and social media platforms to increase local attention to a specific public health problem is a common way coalitions work to build momentum and support alcohol policy change (Holder & Treno, 1997). In short, environmental strategies require collaboration across diverse members of a community.

Butterfoss et al. (1993) suggest that coalitions are ideal for large-scale community change because they can provide an avenue for recruiting participants from

Table 1 Risk and protective factors for alcohol and drug use

Domain	Risk factors	Protective factors
Individual	• Biological and psychological dispositions • Positive beliefs about alcohol and other drug (AOD) use • Early initiation of AOD use • Negative relationships with adults • Risk-taking propensity/ impulsivity	• Opportunities for prosocial involvement • Rewards/recognition for prosocial involvement • Healthy beliefs and clear standards for behavior • Positive sense of self • Negative beliefs about AOD • Positive relationships with adults
Peer	• Association with peers who use or value AOD use • Association with peers who reject mainstream activities and pursuits • Susceptibility to negative peer pressure • Easily influenced by peers	• Association with peers who are involved in school, recreation service, religion, or other organized activities • Resistance to negative peer pressure • Not easily influenced by peers
Family	• Family history of AOD use • Family management problems • Family conflict • Parental beliefs about AOD	• Bonding (positive attachments) • Healthy beliefs and clear standards for behavior • High parental expectations • A sense of basic trust • Positive family dynamics
School	• Academic failure beginning in elementary school • Low commitment to school	• Opportunities for prosocial involvement • Rewards/recognition for prosocial involvement • Healthy beliefs and clear standards for behavior • Caring and support from teachers and staff • Positive instructional climate
Community	• Availability of AOD • Community laws, norms favorable toward AOD • Extreme economic and social deprivation • Transition and mobility • Low neighborhood attachment and community disorganization	• Opportunities for participation as active members of the community • Decreasing AOD accessibility • Cultural norms that set high expectations for youth • Social networks and support systems within the community
Society	• Impoverishment • Unemployment and underemployment • Discrimination • Pro-AOD-use messages in the media	• Media literacy (resistance to pro-use messages) • Decreased accessibility • Increased pricing through taxation • Raised purchasing age and enforcement • Stricter driving-under-the-influence laws

This table is adapted from:

1. Substance Abuse and Mental Health Services Administration (SAMHSA). (2001). *Science-based substance abuse prevention: A guide* (DHHS Publication No. SMA d-3505). Rockville, MD: Substance Abuse and Mental Health Services Administration

2. Chinman, M., Imm, P., & Wandersman, A. (2004). *Getting to Outcomes 2004: Promoting accountability through methods and tools for planning, implementation, and evaluation*, No. TR-TR101. Santa Monica, CA: RAND Corporation. Retrieved from http://www.rand.org/publications/TR/TR101/

diverse constituencies, help mobilize more resources than any single organization can achieve alone, minimize duplication of efforts, maximize the power of individuals and groups by increasing the "critical mass" and develop widespread public support. Literature reviews and research conducted on community coalitions have consistently found similar factors associated with community effectiveness, including formalization of rules and procedures, leadership style, member participation, membership diversity, agency collaboration, and group cohesion (Butterfoss, 2007; Zakocs & Edwards, 2006). Certainly, coalitions are in a unique position to bring about community change in that their formation requires the inclusions of various stakeholder groups that can help garner support and funding for community awareness, community concern, and community action. The Community Anti-Drug Coalitions of America (CADCA) and their partners have provided training and technical assistance to over 900 previous and current drug free communities coalitions who work nationwide to address communities' underlying needs and conditions that promote underage drinking and alcohol misuse among adults.

What Types of Preventive/Promotive Interventions Are Presently Used in Communities?

Multicomponent initiatives: While there are many types of prevention programs targeted toward adolescents, we update research on substance abuse prevention programs that use multiple components and changes in environmental policies. Multicomponent programs target the behavior of interest using multiple interventions across multiple settings Wandersman & Florin, 2003; Nation et al., 2003). As such, these programs tend to address multiple protective and risk factors at once: individual, peer, family, school, community, and society. The components used are usually designed to complement one another over time. For example, policy change efforts are designed to have impacts on all other sectors. Media advocacy efforts can support policy change and serve to cue peers and families to make use of school and family based services and make healthier choices (Pentz, 2003). Multicomponent initiatives tend to yield larger and longer lasting effects than other programs because they are best able to simultaneously address the various influences of youth drug use (peer, family, school, societal norms). Research has shown that multicomponent initiatives also provide longer-lasting exposure to the components than single component programs (Hawkins et al., 2012; Pentz et al., 1989; Sagrestano & Paikoff, 1997).

NIDA published its "Red Book" that presents a series of "prevention principles" (National Institute on Drug Abuse, 2003). These principles are essentially propositions about effective prevention that are based on years of research. NIDA published this book to serve as a guide to communities implementing prevention programs. While the Red Book's 16 principles address many issues regarding prevention, three principles specifically talk about the benefit of using programs with multiple components whenever possible:

- "Community prevention programs that combine two or more effective programs, such as family-based and school-based programs, can be more effective than a single program alone" (Battistich, Solomon, Watson, & Schaps, 1997, p. 11).
- "Community prevention programs reaching populations in multiple settings—for example, schools, clubs, faith-based organizations, and the media—are most effective when they present consistent, community-wide messages in each setting" (Chou et al., 1998, p. 11).
- "Prevention programs should be long-term with repeated interventions (i.e., booster programs) to reinforce the original prevention goals. Research shows that the benefits from middle school prevention programs diminish without follow up programs in high school" (Scheier, Botvin, Diaz, & Griffin, 1999, p. 11).

While clearly advantageous, Kumpfer and colleagues (Kumpfer, Whiteside, & Wandersman, 1997) point out that community interventions can also be more costly to implement in terms of both funds and personnel time.

Environmental Alcohol Policies: There are also a variety of environmental strategies and policies to reduce or prevent alcohol use that, by definition, are implemented to modify the underlying needs and conditions of the community that contribute to alcohol and drug use. In this chapter, we also update the research on evidence-based environmental strategies designed to prevent underage drinking in Table 2. This includes well-documented strategies/policies, a summary of the evidence, and an effectiveness rating. The table is organized by the strength of the evidence (e.g., high, moderate, etc.) and updated references are provided. These strategies have been evaluated by at least one of the following sources: (a) the National Institute on Alcohol Abuse and Alcoholism (NIAAA; 2015): *Planning Alcohol Interventions Using NIAAA's College AIM Alcohol Interventions Matrix, 2015*; and (b) the Surgeon General: *Facing Addiction in America: The Surgeon General's Report on Alcohol, Drugs, and Health* (US Department of Health and Human Services, 2016).

Youth Development Approaches to Prevent Underage Alcohol Use: The use of positive youth development (PYD) approaches has been suggested as a promising strategy for preventing adolescent substance use (Masten, 2014; Schwartz et al., 2010). PYD programs have grown in popularity because they offer a holistic alternative to programs that target only a single risk or protective factor or a handful of factors. Instead of developing separate interventions for each risk factor, PYD approaches focus on promoting healthy development and thus the prevention of multiple risk behaviors. PYD focuses on building assets rather than reducing deficits, and builds youth competencies by using a holistic developmental perspective focused on achieving healthy personal growth (Amodeo & Collins, 2007).

While there are varying models and definitions of PYD, one common focus is building young people's positive personal competencies and assets through increased positive relationships, social supports, and opportunities that strengthen assets (Taylor, Oberle, Durlak, & Weissberg, 2017). There is not a lot of empirical

Table 2 Evidence based strategies and policies for preventing underage drinking and alcohol misuse

Strategy	Definition	Evidence	Effectiveness
Alcohol compliance checks[a]	Law enforcement officials supervise undercover youth who attempt to purchase alcohol, penalizing establishments for successful attempts	• Checks reduced number of outlets selling to minors: – in Concord, NH: from 28% to 10% (Centers for Disease Control and Prevention, 2004) – in Denver, CO: from 60% to 26% (Drug Strategies, 1999)	• High[b]
Increase alcohol taxes[a]	Raise taxes on alcohol, for example by pegging it to inflation	• Higher alcohol taxes lead to: – reductions in the levels and frequency of drinking and heavy drinking among youth (Coate & Grossman, 1988) (see following literature reviews: Elder et al., 2010; Wagenaar, Salois, & Komro, 2009; Xu & Chaloupka, 2011) – lower traffic crash fatality rates (Ruhm, 1996) (see following literature reviews: Elder et al., 2010; Wagenaar, Tobler, & Komro, 2010; Xu & Chaloupka, 2011) – reduced incidence of some types of crime (Cook & Moore, 1993) (see following literature reviews: Elder et al., 2010; Wagenaar et al., 2010; Xu & Chaloupka, 2011) • Five states with the lowest beer tax have double the percent of 18–20-year-olds binge drinkers compared to the five with the highest tax (Imm et al., 2007)	• High[b]
Restrictions on "happy hour" drink discounts	Restrict the use of happy hour or other discounted pricing schemes	• Alcohol consumption strongly related to consumption (Chaloupka, Grossman, & Saffer, 2002), especially among minors (Chaloupka et al., 2002; Grossman & Chaloupka, 1998) • Lower drink prices found to be related to binge drinking alcohol (Wechsler et al., 2003)	• High[b]
Dram Shop Liability Laws[a]	Holds commercial servers of alcohol liable when they provide alcohol to a minor or adult drunk customer, who later causes harm to another	• States with Dram Shop Liability Laws have significantly lower rates of alcohol-related crash fatalities across all drinkers (Rammohan et al., 2011) and among adolescents (Fell, Scherer, Thomas, & Voas, 2016).	• Moderate[b]

(continued)

Table 2 (continued)

Strategy	Definition	Evidence	Effectiveness
Limit the density of alcohol outlets[a]	Density is the number of alcohol merchants available to a particular population or in a particular area	• Higher alcohol outlet density is associated with drinking and driving and riding with drinking drivers, especially for youth (Treno & Lee, 2002) • US cities with higher densities had more alcohol-related traffic fatalities (Cohen, Mason, & Scribner, 2002) • Density is strongly related to binge drinking (Weitzman, Folkman, Folkman, & Wechsler, 2003) • Reductions in alcohol density are significantly associated with lower rates of violent crime in the area (Xu et al., 2012; Zhang et al., 2015) • Higher alcohol outlet density is significantly related to higher rates of underage drinking (Paschall, Grube, Thomas, Cannon, & Treffers, 2012; Reboussin, Song, & Wolfson, 2011) and more alcohol-related negative consequences (Reboussin et al., 2011).	• Moderate[b]
Responsible beverage service (RBS) programs	Require training for servers and merchants on responsible serving practices (i.e., not serving obviously intoxicated patrons)	• RBS implementation lead to: – an 11.5% reduction in sales to underage youth, and a decrease in sales to intoxicated patrons, compared to establishments that did not receive the training (Alcohol Epidemiology Program, 2000) – 23% fewer single-vehicle nighttime crashes in Oregon (Holder & Wagenaar, 1994) – States with RBS laws had significantly lower rates of fatal car crashes among underage youth; however, significantly higher beer consumption among youth was also observed in these states (Fell et al., 2016).	• Moderate[b]

(continued)

Table 2 (continued)

Strategy	Definition	Evidence	Effectiveness
Restrict hours of alcohol sales[a]	Laws limiting the hours that alcohol is permitted for commercial sale.	• Significant alcohol-related harm associated with 2 or more hour increases in alcohol sales (see Hahn et al., 2010 for review) • Policies allowing for 2 or more hours of alcohol sale were significantly associated with: alcohol-related injuries (Newton, Sacker, Pahal, van der Bergh, & Young, 2007; Smith, 1988, 1990), alcohol-related assault (Newton et al., 2007).	• Moderate[b]
Social host laws[a]	Holds noncommercial servers of alcohol (e.g., parents), liable when they provide alcohol to a minor or drunk individual who later causes injury or death to another	• Social host liability laws have found to: – lower the probability of binge drinking and drinking and driving among all drinkers (Dills, 2010; Stout, Sloan, Liang, & Davies, 2000) – decrease adult alcohol-related traffic deaths across all states for the years 1984–1995 (Whetten-Goldstein, Sloan, Stout, & Liang, 2000) as well as underage drunk-driving fatality rates (Dills, 2010; Fell et al., 2016). – While social host laws were significantly related to lower drinking rates, these laws were not significantly related to underage drunk-driving fatality rates (Fell, Scherer, Thomas, & Voas, 2014)	• Moderate[b]

(continued)

Table 2 (continued)

Strategy	Definition	Evidence	Effectiveness
Keg registration laws	Require kegs of beer to be tagged with an ID number and information to be recorded about the purchaser	• US cities with a keg registration law had fewer alcohol-related traffic fatalities (Cohen et al., 2002). However, other studies reported that states with keg registration laws had significantly higher fatal crash ratios among underage drinkers (Fell et al., 2016; Fell, Fisher, Voas, Blackman, & Tippetts, 2009). At the same time, these laws were associated with significant decreases of beer consumption among underage drinkers (Fell et al., 2009, 2016). • The passage of states' keg registration laws were not significantly related to underage binge drinking rates or driving after drinking (Ringwalt & Paschall, 2011)	• Low[b]
Limit alcohol at sports and community events	Limit or ban alcohol consumption at sporting or other public events	• Banning alcohol at football games led to a reduction of arrests, assaults, ejections, and student referrals to the judicial affairs (Bormann & Stone, 2001) • US cities with more restrictions on alcohol consumption in public places had less alcohol-related traffic fatalities (Cohen et al., 2002)	• Too few robust studies to rate effectiveness or mixed results[b]
Sobriety and traffic safety checkpoints[a]	Law enforcement stops drivers to determine if they are driving under the influence of alcohol or drugs	• Three literature reviews on checkpoint studies found: – Reductions in alcohol-related fatalities ranged from 8% to 71% (Peek-Asa, 1999; and 9% (Bergen et al., 2014) – Reductions in alcohol-related fatal crashes of 22% (Shults et al., 2001) and 20% (Fell, Ferguson, Williams, & Fields, 2001) States with sobriety checkpoints had significantly lower rates of underage alcohol consumption and fatal car crashes (Fell et al., 2016). While sobriety checkpoint laws were associated with 18% reduction in drinking and driving, states that conducted sobriety checks reported 41% lower rates of drinking and driving (Lenk, Nelson, Toomey, Jones-Webb, & Erickson, 2016)	• Well Supported[a]

(continued)

Table 2 (continued)

Strategy	Definition	Evidence	Effectiveness
Use/Lose Laws[a]	Allows authorities to suspend individual's driver's license for underage alcohol violations	States with Use and Lose Laws had significantly lower rates of: underage alcohol consumption (Cavazos-Rehg et al., 2012; Fell et al., 2016), driving after drinking (Cavazos-Rehg et al., 2012), and fatal car crashes (Fell et al., 2009, 2016).	• Well Supported[a]
Zero Tolerance Laws[a]	Illegal for an underage driver to drive under the influence of any amount of alcohol	States with Zero Tolerance Laws had significantly lower rates of underage alcohol consumption (Fell et al., 2016) and fatal car crashes (Fell et al., 2009, 2016).	• Well Supported[a]
Graduated drivers' license (GDLs) laws	Requiring youth to progress through stages of driving privileges starting with a highly supervised permit to a supervised license with restrictions and then to a full-privileged drivers' license	• Passing GDLs have led to reductions in crashes among young drivers in: – California: 17–28% (Cooper, Gillen, & Atkins, 2004; Rice, Peek-Asa, & Kraus, 2004); – Michigan: 19% (Shope & Molnar, 2004); and – Utah: 16% (Hyde, Cook, Knight, & Olson, 2005) Significant (13%) reduction of fatal car crashes, among underage drinkers, across states with GDL laws (Fell, Todd, & Voas, 2011). However, two other studies found no effect of GDL laws on fatal car crash rates among underage drinkers (Fell et al., 2009, 2016).	• Rating not included

This table is an updated version of the original chapter from the first edition of this book with the "effectiveness" column added and content taken from the Matrix Report (NIAAA, 2015) and the US Surgeon General's Report (2016) (cited in USDHHS, 2016)

[a]Indicates interventions included in the US Surgeon General's Report (2016) (cited in USDHHS, 2016) where "well supported" was defined as evidence derived from multiple controlled trials or large-scale population studies

[b]Ratings included in Matrix Report (NIAAA, 2015) which were based on the percentage of studies reporting positive outcomes, possible ratings were high, moderate and low. Strategies with three or fewer studies were not rated for effectiveness

evidence for the causal relationship between implementation of community-based PYD initiatives and reduced alcohol and drug use among youth despite resources to help promote evaluation (e.g., Fisher, Imm, Chinman, & Wandersman, 2006). We include a brief summary on PYD research findings as a promising approach for building youth assets and supports, and therefore, potentially reducing rates of alcohol and drug use in communities.

Research on Community-Based Preventive Interventions

In this section, we describe research on community-based interventions that use various combinations of multicomponent interventions to improve various alcohol-related outcomes (see Table 3). Many of the community-based interventions occur in different cities/settings and also assess many different outcomes, such as underage drinking, alcohol sales, or traffic fatalities due to alcohol. Thus, one large trial may have been implemented only once, but in 20 cities. It may have shown success on some variables (e.g., traffic fatalities due to alcohol) but not others (e.g., heavy drinking among high school youth).

Many of these interventions were included in the *Facing Addiction in America: The Surgeon General's Report on Alcohol, Drugs, and Health* (US Department of Health and Human Services, 2016) and are noted as such for the empirical support for their effectiveness. For each, we provide a brief description and then the most updated evaluation findings.

Saving Lives Program

Brief Description: The Saving Lives Program (Hingson et al., 1996) (SLP) organized community task forces in six mid-size towns in Massachusetts to reduce driving after drinking and improve traffic safety. Intervention communities received a full-time municipal-based coordinator charged with convening the task forces, which consisted of private citizens and representatives from different city departments (e.g., school, police, health, recreation). The communities, not state or federal agencies developed most of the program initiatives. The task forces oversaw various interventions including media advocacy campaigns, business information programs, speeding and drunk driving awareness days, speed watch telephone hotlines, high school peer-led education, alcohol-free prom nights, college prevention programs, enhanced police enforcement, responsible server training, alcohol outlet surveillance, and keg registration. For funding, each community received ~$1 per town inhabitant per year.

Research Findings: The SLP evaluation utilized a quasi-experimental design (Hingson et al., 1996). The six program communities selected for funding were compared with the rest of the state of Massachusetts and also with five other cities that also prepared high quality proposals but were not funded. Comparisons were made using data from 5 preprogram years compared to the 5 program years. SLP examined fatal and injury crash monitoring, direct observation of safety belt use and speeding, conducted telephone surveys, and monitored traffic citations. In SLP cities, fatal crashes that involved alcohol declined from 69 crashes to 36 crashes during the program years, which is equivalent to a 42% decline. In addition, the number of fatally injured drivers with positive blood alcohol levels declined in the SLP cities by 47% compared to the rest of the state. Safety belt use increased and the proportion of vehicles observed traveling at 10 or more miles over the speed limit declined in the SLP cities compared to the state. Finally, SLP communities experienced statistically significant declines in self-reported driving after drinking among 16–19 year-olds compared to the rest of the state. When compared to the five other cities that were not funded, SLP cities had fewer fatal crashes and fewer alcohol-related fatal crashes.

Project Northland

Brief Description: Project Northland is a multilevel, multiyear program that targeted 6th to 12th graders from 1991 to 1998 in 24 school districts in northeastern Minnesota (Komro, Perry, Veblen-Mortenson, & Williams, 1994; Perry et al., 2000, 2002, 1996). Phase I occurred from 1991 to 1994 when the cohort was in 6th to 8th grade and consisted of 3 years of social-behavioral curricula in the classroom, parent involvement programs, peer leadership opportunities, and community task forces. During 1994–1996, the cohort was in 9th and 10th grade and there was an interim phase in which 9th graders received a brief five-session classroom program. This program focused on pressures to drink and drive or ride with a drunk driver as well as the influential pressures of alcohol advertising. No programming was conducted in 10th grade. During Phase II from 1996 to 1998 when the cohort was in 11th and 12th grade, a six-session classroom curriculum was implemented in 11th grade, which focused on the social and legal responsibilities concerning alcohol use. In addition, parents received behavioral tips through postcards, print media campaigns occurred, peer action teams were created at each high school to develop and promote alcohol-free activities, and community action teams were formed to help reduce commercial and social access to alcohol among minors (Komro et al., 1994; Perry et al., 2000, 2002).

Research Findings: For Project Northland, students in the intervention and control school districts were surveyed at baseline in 1991 and followed up each spring from 1992 to 1998. Results from Phase I indicated that youth in the intervention schools were less likely to increase their tendency to drink in the past month and to binge drink than the control schools. Past week alcohol use was not significantly different between the Project Northland and control schools. Intervention youth also were less likely to increase their perceptions of peer influence to use alcohol and

Table 3 Community-based program trials and outcomes

Study name	Study type	Population	No. of communities	Major outcomes				Effectiveness[a]
Communities Mobilizing for Change on Alcohol (CMCA) (Wagenaar et al., 2000)	Community mobilizing via local public officials, enforcement agencies, alcohol merchants, the media, schools, and other community institutions to change community policies and practices	Socially and geographically diverse communities in Minnesota and Wisconsin (avg. pop. = 20,000)	$N = 15$	Several trends emerged at 3-year follow-up. Alcohol merchants in the intervention community increased ID checks and reduced alcohol sales to minors. 18–20-year-olds reduced their likelihood of trying to buy alcohol and fewer 18–20-year-olds in the intervention community reported 30 day drinking.				Well Supported
				% alcohol merchants ID checks at on-sale establishments				
					Intervention	**Control**	***p*-value**	
				1992	60.2	49.1	$p = 0.06$	
				1995	78.1	56.5		
				% 18–20 year olds trying to buy alcohol				
					Intervention	**Control**	***p*-value**	
				1992	10.4	10.9	$p = 0.06$	
				1995	7.5	10.7		
				% 18–20 year olds 30-day drinking prevalence				
					Intervention	**Control**	***p*-value**	
				1992	56.3	55.7	$p = 0.07$	
				1995	59.5	62.5		

(continued)

Table 3 (continued)

<table>
<tr><th>Study name</th><th>Study type</th><th>Population</th><th>No. of communities</th><th>Major outcomes</th><th>Effectiveness[a]</th></tr>
<tr><td>Communities Mobilizing for Change on Alcohol (CMCA) (Komro et al., 2017)</td><td>Community mobilizing via local public officials, enforcement agencies, alcohol merchants, the media, schools, and other community institutions to change community policies and practices</td><td>Cherokee Nation citizens, who reside in NE Oklahoma.</td><td>$N = 6$</td><td>Over the 3-year study period, youth enrolled in all three active intervention conditions (CMCA-only, CONNECT-only, and combined), showed significantly greater reduction in past month alcohol use and heavy episodic drinking, compared to the control group. While, no direct statistical tests were performed, youth in the CMCA-only group (compared to CONNECT-only or Combined) reported higher treatment gains on both alcohol outcomes.
Reductions in drinking rates (from baseline to 3-year follow-up) for CMCA-only, CONNECT-only and Combined groups.<table><tr><th></th><th>CMCA</th><th>CONNECT</th><th>Combined</th></tr><tr><td>30-day drinking</td><td>25%***</td><td>22%**</td><td>12%*</td></tr><tr><td>Heavy episodic drinking</td><td>24%***</td><td>19%*</td><td>13%*</td></tr></table>*Note, all significance levels reflect comparisons between each intervention group and control.* $^{*}p < 0.05$, $^{**}p < 0.01$, $^{***}p < 0.001$.</td><td>Well Supported</td></tr>
</table>

<table>
<tr><th>Study name</th><th>Study type</th><th>Population</th><th>No. of communities</th><th colspan="4">Major outcomes</th><th>Effectiveness[a]</th></tr>
<tr><td rowspan="10">Communities that Care (CTC; Hawkins et al., 2009)</td><td rowspan="10">Community mobilizing via local public officials, enforcement agencies, alcohol merchants, the media, schools, and other community institutions to implement evidence-based policies and practices.</td><td rowspan="10">Communities in seven states: Colorado, Illinois, Kansas, Maine, Oregon, Utah, and Washington</td><td rowspan="10">N = 24</td><td colspan="4">In 8th grade, students in the CTC communities, compared to control condition, reported significantly lower past month prevalence of alcohol and smokeless tobacco use. However, intervention groups did not differ significantly in the prevalence of cigarette, marijuana, inhalant, or prescription drug use in the past month.</td><td rowspan="10">Well Supported</td></tr>
<tr><td colspan="4">Observed prevalence rates (%) of past month substance use in Grade 8th and AORs comparing CTC and Control groups.</td></tr>
<tr><td></td><td>CTC</td><td>Control</td><td>AOR</td></tr>
<tr><td>Alcohol</td><td>16%</td><td>21%</td><td>1.25*</td></tr>
<tr><td>Cigarettes</td><td>6%</td><td>8%</td><td>1.21</td></tr>
<tr><td>Smokeless tobacco</td><td>2%</td><td>4%</td><td>1.79**</td></tr>
<tr><td>Inhalants</td><td>5%</td><td>5%</td><td>1.11</td></tr>
<tr><td>Marijuana</td><td>5%</td><td>6%</td><td>1.15</td></tr>
<tr><td>Prescription drugs</td><td>3%</td><td>3%</td><td>1.30</td></tr>
<tr><td colspan="4">AOR = Adjusted odds ratio. Adjustments were made for: baseline prevalence, age, sex, race/ethnicity, parental educational achievement, religious attendance, rebelliousness, and student population in the community. *p < 0.05, **p < 0.01.</td></tr>
</table>

(continued)

Table 3 (continued)

<table>
<tr><th>Study name</th><th>Study type</th><th>Population</th><th>No. of communities</th><th>Major outcomes</th><th>Effectiveness[a]</th></tr>
<tr><td>Communities that Care (CTC; Hawkins et al., 2012)</td><td>Community mobilizing via local public officials, enforcement agencies, alcohol merchants, the media, schools, and other community institutions to implement evidence-based policies and practices.</td><td>Communities in seven states: Colorado, Illinois, Kansas, Maine, Oregon, Utah, and Washington</td><td>$N = 24$</td><td>In 10th grade, students in the CTC communities, compared to control condition, reported significantly lower past month prevalence of cigarettes use. However, intervention groups did not differ significantly in the prevalence of any other drug use in the past month.
Observed prevalence rates (%) of past month substance use in Grade 10th and AORs comparing CTC and Control groups.
<table>
<tr><th></th><th>CTC</th><th>Control</th><th>AOR</th></tr>
<tr><td>Alcohol</td><td>29%</td><td>30%</td><td>1.10*</td></tr>
<tr><td>Cigarettes</td><td>13%</td><td>16%</td><td>0.79</td></tr>
<tr><td>Smokeless tobacco</td><td>6%</td><td>7%</td><td>0.85</td></tr>
<tr><td>Inhalants</td><td>3%</td><td>2%</td><td>1.50</td></tr>
<tr><td>Marijuana</td><td>14%</td><td>15%</td><td>0.99</td></tr>
<tr><td>Prescription drugs</td><td>6%</td><td>5%</td><td>1.15</td></tr>
</table>
AOR = Adjusted odds ratio. Adjustments were made for: baseline prevalence, age, sex, race/ethnicity, parental educational achievement, religious attendance, rebelliousness, and student population in the community. *$p < 0.05$.</td><td>Well Supported</td></tr>
</table>

<table>
<tr><th>Study name</th><th>Study type</th><th>Population</th><th>No. of communities</th><th>Major outcomes</th><th>Effectiveness[a]</th></tr>
<tr><td>Communities that Care (CTC; Hawkins, Oesterle, Brown, Abbott, & Catalano, 2014)</td><td>Community mobilizing via local public officials, enforcement agencies, alcohol merchants, the media, schools, and other community institutions to implement evidence-based policies and practices.</td><td>Communities in seven states: Colorado, Illinois, Kansas, Maine, Oregon, Utah, and Washington</td><td>$N = 24$</td><td>By 12th grade, significantly fewer CTC students started drinking or smoking cigarettes for the first time, and fewer initiated any delinquent or violent behavior. Except for ecstasy use, there were no significant differences between study groups in either past month or past year substance use prevalence. Students in the CTC communities, compared to control, reported significantly higher past month prevalence of ecstasy use.
Observed prevalence rates (%) of past month substance use in Grade 12th and AORs comparing CTC and Control groups.<table>
<tr><th></th><th>CTC</th><th>Control</th><th>AOR</th></tr>
<tr><td>Alcohol</td><td>36%</td><td>36%</td><td>1.04</td></tr>
<tr><td>Cigarettes</td><td>23%</td><td>24%</td><td>0.94</td></tr>
<tr><td>Ecstasy</td><td>2.6%</td><td>1.4%</td><td>1.89*</td></tr>
<tr><td>Inhalants</td><td>2%</td><td>1%</td><td>1.37</td></tr>
<tr><td>Marijuana</td><td>22%</td><td>20%</td><td>1.09</td></tr>
<tr><td>Prescription drugs</td><td>7%</td><td>5%</td><td>1.44</td></tr>
</table>AOR = Adjusted odds ratio. Adjustments were made for student and community characteristics. *$p < 0.05$.</td><td>Well Supported</td></tr>
</table>

(continued)

Table 3 (continued)

Study name	Study type	Population	No. of communities	Major outcomes	Effectiveness[a]
Midwestern Prevention Project (locally called Project STAR or I-STAR) (Pentz et al., 1989)	Classroom curricula (grades 6–7); mass media programming; parent program; community organization; and health policy change	Middle school students in Kansas City, MO and KS	$N = 15$ (42 schools)	At 1-year follow-up, results showed decreases in cigarette, alcohol, and marijuana use for the intervention group relative to the delayed intervention condition. Prevalence rates for each substance increased over the 1 year period across all groups; however the net increase in drug use among intervention schools was half that of delayed intervention schools. Prevalence rates, 1-year follow-up (columns: Intervention / Intervention-delayed) Cigarettes: 17% / 24% Alcohol: 11% / 16% Marijuana: 7% / 10%	Well Supported
Midwestern Prevention Project (locally called Project STAR or I-STAR) (Chou et al., 1998)	Classroom curricula (grades 6–7); mass media programming; parent program; community organization; and health policy change	Middle school students in Indianapolis, IN	$N = 12$ school districts (57 schools)	Across all follow-up points (up to 3.5 years) baseline users decreased their use of cigarettes, alcohol, and marijuana in the program relative to the control group. Odds ratios for decreasing use among baseline users in the program relative to the control group, at all 4 follow-ups with repeated measures (columns: Odds ratio / *p*-value) Baseline cigarette users: 1.53 / $p < 0.05$ Baseline alcohol users: 1.54 / $p < 0.005$ Baseline marijuana users: 3.96 / $p < 0.05$ *Note: Odds ratios were repeated were adjusted for ethnicity, socioeconomic status, gender, school type (public or private), grade, and time trend.*	Well Supported

<table>
<tr><th>Study name</th><th>Study type</th><th>Population</th><th>No. of communities</th><th colspan="3">Major outcomes</th><th>Effectiveness[a]</th></tr>
<tr><td rowspan="7">Midwestern Prevention Project (locally called Project STAR or I-STAR) (Riggs, Chou, & Pentz, 2009)</td><td rowspan="7">Classroom curricula (grades 6–7); mass media programming; parent program; community organization; and health policy change</td><td rowspan="7">Middle school students in Kansas City, MO</td><td rowspan="7">N = 8 schools; # of school districts not reported</td><td colspan="3">Intervention group participants, relative to the control group, had reduced growth (slope) in amphetamine use during high school and these group differences were maintained (intercept) continuously through both emerging adulthood and early adulthood periods.</td><td rowspan="7">Well Supported</td></tr>
<tr><td colspan="3">Program effects on amphetamine use prevalence from high school to early adulthood.</td></tr>
<tr><td></td><td>Intercept</td><td>Slope</td></tr>
<tr><td>High school</td><td>−0.05</td><td>−0.07*</td></tr>
<tr><td>Emerging adulthood</td><td>−0.07*</td><td>0.00</td></tr>
<tr><td>Early adulthood</td><td>−0.09*</td><td>0.06</td></tr>
<tr><td colspan="3">Note: Analyses were adjusted for baseline substance use, ethnicity, gender, and grade. *p < 0.05</td></tr>
</table>

(continued)

Table 3 (continued)

<table>
<tr><th>Study name</th><th>Study type</th><th>Population</th><th>No. of communities</th><th colspan="4">Major outcomes</th><th>Effectiveness[a]</th></tr>
<tr><td rowspan="15">Project Northland (Perry et al., 1996)</td><td rowspan="15">Classroom behavioral curricula (grades 6–8); parent involvement programs; community task forces (e.g., government officials, law enforcement, health professionals, school personnel, youth workers, clergy, parents, and adolescents).</td><td rowspan="15">School districts and adjacent rural Minnesota communities</td><td rowspan="15">$N = 24$</td><td colspan="4">At 3-year follow-up, students in intervention districts had statistically significant lower scores on likelihood of drinking, onset of alcohol use, and prevalence of alcohol use (shown) than students who did not participate in Project Northland. Students in the intervention showed lower scores on prevalence of cigarette and marijuana use.</td><td rowspan="15">Well Supported</td></tr>
<tr><td colspan="4">% past month alcohol use for all students</td></tr>
<tr><td></td><td>Intervention</td><td>Control</td><td>p-value</td></tr>
<tr><td>1991</td><td>$M = 6.9$</td><td>$M = 3.9$</td><td></td></tr>
<tr><td>1994</td><td>$M = 23.6$</td><td>$M = 29.2$</td><td>$p < 0.05$</td></tr>
<tr><td colspan="4">% cigarette use for all students</td></tr>
<tr><td></td><td>Intervention</td><td>Control</td><td>p-value</td></tr>
<tr><td>1991</td><td>$M = 6.9$</td><td>$M = 4.7$</td><td></td></tr>
<tr><td>1994</td><td>$M = 24.8$</td><td>$M = 30.7$</td><td>ns</td></tr>
<tr><td colspan="4">% marijuana use for all students</td></tr>
<tr><td></td><td>Intervention</td><td>Control</td><td>p-value</td></tr>
<tr><td>1991</td><td>$M = 0.7$</td><td>$M = 0.4$</td><td></td></tr>
<tr><td>1994</td><td>$M = 7.4$</td><td>$M = 8.6$</td><td>ns</td></tr>
<tr><td colspan="4">The project was more successful with those students who were nonusers at baseline compared with those who had already initiated use.</td></tr>
</table>

<table>
<tr><th>Study name</th><th>Study type</th><th>Population</th><th>No. of communities</th><th>Major outcomes</th><th>Effectiveness[a]</th></tr>
<tr><td>Project Northland (Perry et al., 2002)</td><td>Follow-up of 1996 study cohort: Classroom curricula (grades 11–12); parent education; print media campaigns; youth development and community organizing via peer action and community action teams.</td><td>School districts and adjacent rural Minnesota communities</td><td>$N = 24$</td><td>During the interim phase (grades 9 and 10) alcohol use rates increased among students in the intervention schools. During grades 11 and 12, there was a reduced tendency to use alcohol, binge drinking, and ability to obtain alcohol.
<table>
<tr><td colspan="4">Changes in past month alcohol use</td></tr>
<tr><td></td><td>Intervention</td><td>Control</td><td>p-value</td></tr>
<tr><td>1996</td><td>$M = 1.96$ (0.07)</td><td>$M = 1.83$ (0.07)</td><td>$p = 0.08$</td></tr>
<tr><td>Growth rate</td><td>0.13</td><td>0.20</td><td>$p = 0.07$</td></tr>
<tr><td colspan="4">Changes in binge drinking (5+ drinks)</td></tr>
<tr><td></td><td>Intervention</td><td>Control</td><td>p-value</td></tr>
<tr><td>1996</td><td>$M = 1.60$ (0.06)</td><td>$M = 1.45$ (0.05)</td><td>$p = 0.02$</td></tr>
<tr><td>Growth rate</td><td>0.09</td><td>0.18</td><td>$p = 0.02$</td></tr>
<tr><td colspan="4">Mean success rates for ability to obtain alcohol, all outlets (analyzed at community level)</td></tr>
<tr><td></td><td>Intervention</td><td>Control</td><td>p-value</td></tr>
<tr><td>1991</td><td>$M = 42.3$</td><td>$M = 47.9$</td><td>$p = 0.57$</td></tr>
<tr><td>1998</td><td>$M = 13.6$</td><td>$M = 25.4$</td><td>$p = 0.05$</td></tr>
</table></td><td>Well Supported</td></tr>
</table>

(continued)

Table 3 (continued)

<table>
<tr><th>Study name</th><th>Study type</th><th>Population</th><th>No. of communities</th><th colspan="4">Major outcomes</th><th>Effectiveness[a]</th></tr>
<tr><td rowspan="11">Saving Lives Program (Hingson et al., 1996)</td><td rowspan="11">Media campaigns, business information programs, speeding and drunk driving awareness days, telephone hotlines, police training, high school peer-led education, Students Against Drunk Driving chapters, college prevention programs, alcohol-free prom nights, beer keg registration, and increased surveillance for liquor stores.</td><td rowspan="11">Massachusetts communities varying in population size and geographic location within the state</td><td rowspan="11">$N = 6$</td><td colspan="4">At 9-year follow-up, compared with the rest of Massachusetts (the control group), program cities had a decline in fatal crashes (25%), fatal crashes involving alcohol (42%), visible injuries per 100 crashes (5%), proportion of vehicles observed speeding (50%), proportion of teenagers who drove after drinking (50%), and number of fatal crashes involving drivers 15–25 years of age (39%). Among teenagers, the proportion who believed the license of a person caught drinking and driving could be suspended before a trial increased (from 61% to 76%) while it did not change statewide.</td><td rowspan="11">Well Supported</td></tr>
<tr><td colspan="4"># of fatal crashes</td></tr>
<tr><td></td><td>Intervention</td><td>Control</td><td>p-value</td></tr>
<tr><td>1984</td><td>$M = 178$</td><td>$M = 3030$</td><td>$p = 0.02$</td></tr>
<tr><td>1993</td><td>$M = 120$</td><td>$M = 2707$</td><td></td></tr>
<tr><td colspan="4"># of alcohol-involved fatal crashes</td></tr>
<tr><td></td><td>Intervention</td><td>Control</td><td>p-value</td></tr>
<tr><td>1984</td><td>$M = 69$</td><td>$M = 1162$</td><td>$p = 0.01$</td></tr>
<tr><td>1993</td><td>$M = 36$</td><td>$M = 1039$</td><td></td></tr>
<tr><td colspan="4">Note: A log scale was used to compare percentage changes between the intervention area and control area.</td></tr>
</table>

<table>
<tr><th>Study name</th><th>Study type</th><th>Population</th><th>No. of communities</th><th colspan="4">Major outcomes</th><th>Effectiveness[a]</th></tr>
<tr><td rowspan="5">Community Trials Intervention to Reduce High-Risk Drinking (RHRD) (Grube, 1997)</td><td rowspan="5">Enforcement of underage alcohol sales laws; responsible beverage service (RBS) training for off-sale clerks, managers, and owners; and media advocacy designed for awareness of enforcement and increased public support for intervention activities.</td><td rowspan="5">Intervention and comparison communities in northern California, southern California, and South Carolina (pop. = ~100,000 ea.)</td><td rowspan="5">$N = 6$</td><td colspan="4">At 10 month follow-up, more citations were given to beverage outlets in the intervention communities. Of 148 outlets, 22 citations were given during the 10 months of the intervention versus 4 during the previous nonintervention year.
Sales of alcohol to minors were significantly reduced after the intervention. Intervention communities had fewer sales of alcohol to minors compared to the control communities at posttest.</td><td rowspan="5">Rating not included</td></tr>
<tr><td colspan="4">% outlets selling alcohol to underage buyers, all communities combined</td></tr>
<tr><td></td><td>All three interventions</td><td>Control</td><td>p-value</td></tr>
<tr><td>1995</td><td>45</td><td>47</td><td>$p < 0.0001$</td></tr>
<tr><td>1996</td><td>16</td><td>35</td><td></td></tr>
</table>

(continued)

Table 3 (continued)

Study name	Study type	Population	No. of communities	Major outcomes		Effectiveness[a]
Community Trials Intervention to Reduce High-Risk Drinking (RHRD) (Holder et al., 2000)	Enforcement of underage alcohol sales laws; responsible beverage service (RBS) training for off-sale clerks, managers, and owners; and media advocacy designed for awareness of enforcement and increased public support for intervention activities.	Intervention and comparison communities in northern California, southern California, and South Carolina (pop. = ~100,000 ea.)	$N = 6$	At 5 year follow-up, traffic data for the intervention communities showed a decline in nighttime injury crashes (10%), crashes in which the driver had been drinking (6%), and assault injuries observed in emergency departments (43%). Population surveys showed a decline in alcohol consumption per drinking occasion and driving after drinking versus the comparison communities (*p*-values and control group means not reported in study).		
				Self-reported # of drinks of alcohol consumed per drinking occasion		
					Intervention	
				1992	$M = 1.37$	
				1996	$M = 1.29$	
				Self-reported rate of driving after too much to drink, # times per 6-month period		
					Intervention	
				1992	$M = 0.43$	
				1996	$M = 0.22$	
				Self-reported driving when over the legal limit, # times per 6-month period		
					Intervention	
				1992	$M = 0.77$	
				1996	$M = 0.38$	

Study name	Study type	Population	No. of communities	Major outcomes	Effectiveness[a]
Project SixTeen (Biglan, Ary, Smolkowski, Duncan, & Black, 2000)	Classroom curricula addressing tobacco use (grades 6–9); mass media programming; youth community activities; family communications training; and merchant education to restrict sales to minors	7th and 9th grade students in small Oregon communities	$N = 8$	The figures only provided covariate adjusted prevalence rates, thus it was not possible to estimate the numeric value and provide data for this study. Results indicated that smoking did not increase as significantly among youth in the communities that received the community intervention compared to the school-based intervention. Use of smokeless tobacco among boys decreased for the community intervention but not the school-based intervention. Weekly alcohol use increased significantly over 5 years for those who participated in the school-based intervention compared to the community intervention which did not see an increase.	Rating not included

This table is an updated version of the original chapter from the first edition of this book with the "effectiveness" column added and content taken from the Matrix Report (NIAAA, 2015) and the US Surgeon General's Report (2016) (cited in the USDHHS, 2016).

[a]Ratings included in the Surgeon General's Report (2016) (cited in the USDHHS, 2016) where "well supported" was defined as evidence derived from multiple controlled trials or large-scale population studies

their perceived access to alcohol. There were no significant differences in rates of alcohol purchases at the end of Phase I.

During the interim phase, when little programming occurred, many of these positive effects were reversed. Adolescents in the intervention schools increased their tendency to use alcohol, past month alcohol use, past week alcohol use, and binge drinking. They also increased their perceptions of peer use during this time and decreased their self-efficacy to refuse alcohol.

Phase II results indicated that the intervention was again successful in reducing adolescents' tendency to use alcohol and to binge drink. No differences were found on perceptions of peer use, perceived access to alcohol, or self-efficacy to refuse alcohol. Phase II results also indicated a large reduction in underage alcohol purchases in the intervention communities.

The lack of intervention when youth were in 9th and 10th grade was associated with increases in alcohol use. Despite this negative impact, when the additional intervention activities were implemented 2 years after this hiatus, alcohol use among this cohort decreased again. Overall, these results highlight the importance of continuing prevention programming throughout the period of adolescence (Perry et al., 2002).

Communities Mobilizing for Change on Alcohol (CMCA)

Brief Description: Communities Mobilizing for Change on Alcohol (CMCA) is a community-based initiative designed to reduce youth access to alcohol by changing community policies and practices. The first CMCA study involved 15 communities, with seven communities randomly assigned to receive the intervention and eight communities serving as control communities (Wagenaar et al., 1999; Wagenaar, Murray, Wolfson, Forster, & Finnegan, 1994). During the first phase of the intervention period, meetings were conducted with leaders and citizens to help build personal and political relationships, gain an understanding of individuals' commitments, and identify individuals for recruitment into the core leadership group. During Phase II, a local core leadership group and a larger base of active citizens were developed. Baseline surveys were conducted in 1992 and each survey was repeated 3 years later in 1995 (Wagenaar et al., 1999). Data were collected through self-administered surveys of 9th graders and 12th graders at baseline and a follow-up of the 9th graders 3 years later, telephone surveys of youth aged 18–20 years, telephone surveys of alcohol retailers, alcohol purchase attempts, content analysis of media coverage of alcohol issues, archival data, such as arrest and crash indicators, and process records (Wagenaar et al., 1994, 1999). The program collaborated with local public officials, enforcement agencies, alcohol merchants, the media, schools, and other community institutions that influence the environment.

In the second study, six communities in the NE Oklahoma Cherokee Nation, were randomly assigned to: (a) community intervention (CMCA-only); (b) individual intervention (CONNECT-only); (c) Combined CMCA and CONNECT;

and (d) control group (Komro et al., 2017). Data were collected through quarterly surveys (between 2012 and 2015) from students in 9th–10th grades through 11th–12th grades. The program collaborated with local public officials, enforcement agencies, alcohol merchants, the media, schools, and other community institutions that influence the environment. CMCA implementation was documented by each CMCA team member electronically by recording daily work tasks such as team meetings, actions taken as a result of team meetings and their outcomes (Komro et al., 2017).

Research Findings: Overall, many of the results from the first CMCA trial were not statistically significant at the $p < 0.05$ level; however, reductions were seen in the accessibility to alcohol, which is clinically important. For example, in the intervention communities, for alcohol purchase attempts, both on-sale (e.g., bars, restaurants) and off-sale (e.g., liquor and convenience stores) establishments which sold alcohol were more likely to check ID and less likely to sell to underage buyers. However, the intervention did not affect reports from alcohol retailers about checking ID for customers; that is; there was no increase in reports of checking IDs among merchants in the intervention communities. Telephone surveys of 18–20 year olds indicated a 25% decrease in the number of youth attempting to buy alcoholic beverages ($p = 0.06$). In contrast to this favorable result, high school seniors reported an increase of 30% in the proportion who tried to buy alcoholic beverages. In terms of drinking behavior, the proportion of 18- to 20-year olds who reported drinking alcohol in the past 30 days decreased by 7%, although this change was not statistically significant ($p = 0.07$). There was also no statistically significant effect of the intervention on the high school seniors who were 9th graders when the project began (Wagenaar et al., 2000). Overall, the CMCA did report some positive changes in the community, although the majority of the effects did not reach statistical significance. Thus, replication of this intervention is needed to determine whether this type of programming can significantly reduce access to alcohol and subsequent drinking among youth. In study 2, CMCA was implemented among underserved population of the Cherokee Nation, and implementation results were encouraging. Specifically, CMCA action teams reported organizing between 38 and 85 actions per community (i.e., increasing police patrols and police alcohol compliance checks), which led to significant number (between 23 and 43 per community) of sustained community changes such as enactment of new police procedures. Regarding intervention outcomes, the proportion of youth, who reported drinking alcohol in the past 30 days, decreased significantly in all intervention groups (ps < 0.05), compared to control. Likewise, the proportion of youth, who reported heavy episodic drinking, decreased significantly in all intervention groups (ps < 0.05), compared to control. Finally, the proportion of youth, who reported negative alcohol-related consequences, decreased significantly in all intervention groups (ps < 0.05), compared to control (Komro et al., 2017).

Community Trials Intervention to Reduce High-Risk Drinking

Brief Description: The Community Trials Intervention to Reduce High-Risk Drinking (RHRD) is a community-based program that targeted all ages and implemented five broad prevention activities. These activities were: (1) community mobilization (e.g., increase community awareness; increase community support for prevention approaches); (2) responsible beverage service (e.g., reduce the likelihood of customer intoxication at licensed establishments); (3) focus on drinking and driving (e.g., increase community support for enforcement of driving while intoxicated laws; increase enforcement efficiency); (4) focus on underage drinking (e.g., enforcement of underage alcohol sales, media advocacy to bring attention to issue of underage drinking); and (5) reduced alcohol access (e.g., increasing restrictions on access to alcohol (Holder et al., 1997). The project took place over 5 years from 1992 to 1996 in three intervention communities. The intervention and comparison communities were not randomized, but they were matched on the basis of similar local geographic area characteristics, industrial/agricultural bases and minority compositions (Holder et al., 1997). Outcomes were assessed by conducting 120 general population telephone surveys of randomly selected individuals per month for 66 months, examining traffic data on motor vehicle crashes, and conducting emergency department surveys in one intervention and one control site (Holder et al., 2000).

Research Findings: Findings from the RHRD indicated that people in the intervention communities reported less heavy drinking. In addition, there were declines in night time crashes (from 8 pm to 4 am), driving after drinking crashes, and assault injuries observed in the emergency departments in the intervention communities when compared to the control sites (Holder et al., 2000). The RHRD intervention did not report any measurement or outcomes for youth substance use; thus the program is promising, but its effectiveness in changing youth behavior has not been established.

Project SixTeen

Project SixTeen involved a randomized controlled trial to assess whether a comprehensive community wide prevention effort was more effective than a school-based program in reducing tobacco use among youth (Biglan et al., 2000). Eight pairs of Oregon communities were randomly assigned to receive each program and effects were assessed by analyzing five annual surveys of 7th and 9th grade students. The school-based program, Project Programs to Advance Teen Health (PATH) consisted of nine levels of instruction, with four levels developed for use with 6th–9th grade, which included materials and videos that complemented the health program. Five levels were developed for use with 10th through 12th grade and were designed to address issues related to tobacco in health, social studies, biology, and English classes. The PATH curriculum was presented in five sessions over a 1-week period.

The community intervention was conducted by a paid community coordinator and youth and adult volunteers from the community. It included a media advocacy component, which was designed to publicize the tobacco problem and included newspaper articles and presentations to local civic groups. There was also a youth antitobacco component, which was designed to help coordinators and youth develop antitobacco activities to engage young people. A family communication component incorporated activities to help parents communicate with their children that they did not want them to use tobacco. The ACCESS component focused on decreasing the proportion of stores selling tobacco to minors.

Research Findings: Project SixTeen outcomes focused on cigarette and alcohol use. For smoking prevalence, both groups increased prevalence over time; however smoking prevalence did not increase as significantly among youth in the communities that received the community intervention compared to the school-based intervention (Biglan et al., 2000). Results also indicated that prevalence of smokeless tobacco use in the past month among boys decreased for the community intervention but not the school-based intervention. For alcohol use, 9th graders who participated in the school-based intervention increased their weekly alcohol use significantly over the 5 years whereas youth who participated in cities that received the community intervention did not increase their weekly alcohol use during this time (Biglan et al., 2000). Overall, the intervention mainly influenced smoking prevalence—it did not decrease prevalence, but did slow the increase of smoking prevalence during this time period. Findings from this study were not strong and results were not consistent for reducing tobacco and alcohol use. Further evaluation of both the school-based and community-based interventions is necessary before substantive conclusions can be made about their potential efficacy in reducing smoking and drinking behaviors.

Midwestern Prevention Project

The Midwestern Prevention Project (MPP) targeted avoidance and reduction of cigarette, alcohol, and marijuana use among youth in middle/junior high school (Chou et al., 1998; Pentz et al., 1989). MPP implemented five components: (1) mass media coverage, promotional videotapes, and commercials about each program component; (2) a school-based program that included homework sessions that involved parents; (3) a parent organization program; (4) a community organization program; and (5) drug use policy change. The purpose of MPP was to reduce the prevalence of cigarettes, alcohol, and marijuana among adolescents, using the school-based program to help build skills to support resistance of drug use via interactive role play and other engaging sessions. Additional program components, such as mass media programming and parent involvement in homework, were planned to aid in these efforts. Intervention components were introduced into 15 communities in the Kansas City metropolitan area over a 6-year period (1984–1990) with randomized intervention and delayed intervention groups. A second study was implemented in Indianapolis, Indiana in 12 school districts in Marion County, IN (1987–1991) and also used a randomized experimental design. Annual assessments were conducted of youth in the schools assigned to both the immediate and delayed intervention groups (Pentz et al., 1990). A third study examined long-term effects of the MPP program on amphetamine use trajectories from early adolescence to early adulthood (Riggs et al., 2009). This longitudinal study presents data from eight randomly selected schools in Kansas City over a 17-year period (ages 11–28 years).

Research Findings: The MPP involved two cohorts of youth. For the Kansas City cohort, at the 1-year follow-up, the intervention schools had reduced rates of increase for cigarettes, alcohol, and marijuana compared to the control schools (Pentz et al., 1989). For the Indiana cohort, results indicated that across all four follow-up time points (up to 3.5 years) baseline substance users consistently demonstrated lower levels of cigarettes and alcohol use (Chou et al., 1998). Both studies showed slower growth or decreased use of all substances among baseline users, suggesting that this type of program can affect both initiation and escalation of use. Results have also indicated that after 3 years, compared to school-based or other single channel programs, the MPP found greater and more sustained effects on daily cigarette use, monthly drunkenness, and heavy marijuana use (Pentz, 1998). Analyses of the eight randomly selected schools from the Kansas City cohort demonstrated program effects on amphetamine use in high school, specifically reduced growth in lifetime amphetamine use prevalence rates. Further, program gains in lower amphetamine use prevalence rates among the intervention group were maintained into early and emerging adulthood (Riggs et al., 2009).

Communities That Care Communities That Care (CTC)

Brief Description: The CTC is a system for guiding communities in development and implementation of evidence-based prevention program whose goal is to (a) promote positive development and healthy behaviors; and (b) prevent substance use and other harmful behaviors such as delinquency and violence. The CTC process typically provides funding for a full-time local coordinator and $75,000 annually to engage entire communities (youth, parents, policy makers, police, schools, businesses, etc.) to assess and prioritize substance use as well as risk and protective factors among students in grades 6–12. Based on these priorities, appropriate interventions are implemented by the community and tested over time (Hawkins et al., 2008).

The CTC was tested in a 24-community trial (Colorado, Illinois, Kansas, Maine, Oregon, Utah, and Washington), where 12 communities were randomly assigned to receive the CTC intervention while the remaining 12 were assigned to the control condition (Hawkins et al., 2009, 2012; 2014). Data were collected through annual self-administered surveys of youth assigned to both the intervention and control conditions. Study 1 (2004–2007) presents CTC intervention outcomes (i.e., substance use and delinquent behavior) from youth in grades 5 through 8 (Hawkins et al., 2009). In study 2, (2004–2009) intervention outcomes through grade 10th are presented (Hawkins et al., 2012) while study 3 (2004–2011) presents CTC intervention outcomes up to grade 12th (Hawkins et al., 2014).

Research Findings: Four years after the initial implementation of the CTC system, 8th graders enrolled in the intervention were less likely to report past month substance use (i.e., alcohol, cigarettes and smokeless tobacco) and engagement in delinquent behavior such as property damage, stealing, and being arrested (Hawkins et al., 2009). Study 2 results indicated that 10th graders enrolled in the CTC system were significantly less likely, compared to a control condition, to initiate cigarette smoking (CTC group = 45% lower odds, $p < 0.01$) and alcohol use (CTC group = 38% lower odds, $p < 0.05$), but no significant differences in initiation rates were observed for other drugs (marijuana, smokeless tobacco, inhalants, and prescription drugs). Further, students in the CTC system had significantly lower prevalence rates of past month cigarette use while prevalence rates of other drugs (i.e., alcohol, marijuana, smokeless tobacco, inhalants, prescription drugs) were not significantly different between the CTC and control group. Still, students in the CTC system had 17% lower odds of engaging in any delinquent behavior in the past year, $p < 0.05$ (Hawkins et al., 2012). Study 3 results indicated that by 12th grade, CTC students were more likely, compared to control communities, to report lifetime abstinence from any drug use (24% and 18% for CTC and control groups respectively, $p < 0.05$), alcohol (32% and 23% respectively, $p < 0.05$), cigarettes (50% and 43% respectively, $p < 0.05$), and marijuana (53% and 48% respectively, $p < 0.05$). Likewise, youth in the CTC communities were significantly more likely to avoid ever engaging in any delinquent behavior (43% and 33% for CTC and control communities respectively, $p < 0.05$). However, past month and past year prevalence rates of substance use were not significantly different (except for ecstasy which was higher in the CTC group) between youth enrolled in the CTC system compared to a control condition (Hawkins et al., 2014).

Environmental Strategies/Policies That Address Alcohol Use and Misuse

There are a variety of environmental strategies/policies that are aimed to prevent underage drinking; however, not all of these strategies are evidence based. For this chapter, we update the literature on the 13 evidence-based strategies/policies shown to be effective at reducing underage drinking and alcohol misuse among adults. Table 2 integrates findings from NIAAA's College AIM Alcohol Intervention Matrix and the 2016 Surgeon General's Report. Ratings included in the Matrix Report (NIAAA, 2015) were based on the percentage of studies reporting positive outcomes, with possible ratings being high, moderate, and low. The category of "well-supported" is language used in the 2016 Surgeon General's report and is defined as evidence derived from multiple controlled trials or large-scale population studies.

Summary Research on Positive Youth Development

Positive youth development promotes a developmental trajectory of adaptive functioning including social connections and self-confidence that can serve to buffer youth against substance abuse risks (Toumbourou et al., 2007). Bonell et al. (2016) reviewed and then synthesized the literature on PYD to develop a theory of change showing how PYD can result in reduced substance abuse (Fig. 1). Based on the positive expectations, relationships, and opportunities offered as part of a PYD approach, a youth develops intentional self-regulation and positive assets that compensates for individual risk and that acts as a buffer against risks in the environment, ultimately reducing substance use.

A 2007 meta-analysis of PYD approaches found that many PYD interventions incorporate social system change as a mechanism to promote positive development (64% of the 526 reviewed approaches; Durlak et al., 2007). This is much greater than other prevention approaches. For example, a 1997 review of primary prevention programs for children and adolescents found that only 15% of the 177 programs incorporated a focus on systems-levels change. In addition, the PYD approaches that measures these system-level changes have achieve positive effects on classrooms, whole schools, families, communities, and across families, schools, and communities. Durlak et al. (2007) found effect sizes ranging from 0.34 to 0.78 at post. However, the evidence base on PYD approaches is still fairly scant. Fewer than a quarter of the studies Durlak et al. (2007) examined had any quantitative data on systems change and only 3% of studies had data on how linkages across systems were affected.

Promising Approaches for Prevention

The Building Assets Reducing Risk (BARR) program is one example of a systems-level focused PYD approach that is building evidence of its effectiveness to reduce the likelihood of decreased high-risk behaviors among youth. Specifically, the model incorporates eight individual and school-wide strategies to support students and enhance student development by improving the school setting. The program focuses on building relationships with students to promote outcomes such as student achievement and school-related outcomes (e.g., attendance). The eight core components of BARR are as follows:

1. Provide professional development for teachers, counselors and administrators to use student–teacher relationships to enhance achievement;
2. Cultivate connections through creating a student cohort where students schedules are aligned so students take three core subjects with only other students in their cohort;
3. Engage families in student learning through a parent advisory council and regular calls and meetings;

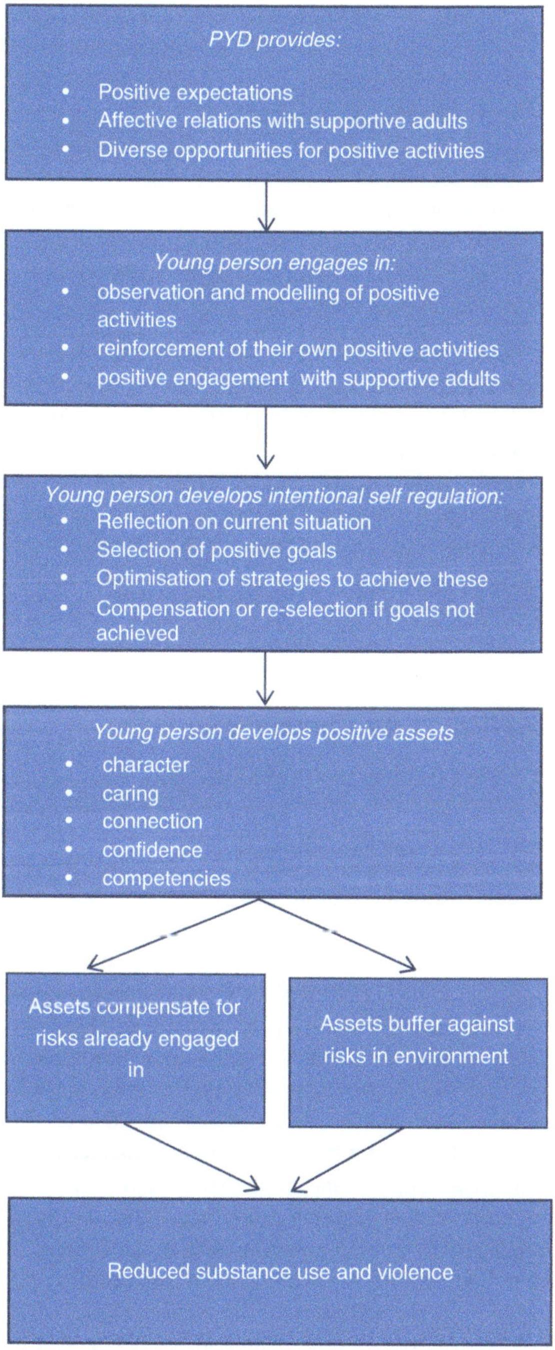

Fig. 1 Theory of Change Showing How Positive Youth Development May Effect Substance Use. This figure operationalizes the links between positive youth development, changes in youth behaviors that affect risk and protective factors, and youth substance use and violence. From "What is positive youth development and how might it reduce substance use and violence? A systematic review and synthesis of theoretical literature," by C. Bonell, K. Hinds, K. Dickson, J. Thomas, A. Fletcher, S. Murphy, … R. Campbell, 2016, *BMC Public Health, 16*, p. 143. Copyright 2016 by Chris Bonell. Reprinted with permission

4. Use I-Time, a 30-min weekly lesson with a social-emotional focus, to address important issues (e.g., substance abuse, bullying) and set personal goals;
5. Hold regular meetings of the cohort teacher teams to determine how to best intervene and support students;
6. Conduct risk-review meetings with persistently low-performing students to help them get essential external supports;
7. Focus on the whole student (academic, emotional, social, physical, etc.) and work to better understand student strengths during each interaction
8. Engage administrators to support, become involved, and communicate with the BARR team in their school.

BARR was first implemented at Saint Louis Park High School in Minnesota and after 1 year of implementation, course failure rates fell from 44% to 47% down to 28% and then held steadily at 20% or lower for the next 15 years (Evans, Sharma, & Jerabek, 2013). A 2015 within-school randomized controlled trial of BARR with 555 9th grade students in California found that after 1-year BARR students had earned significantly more course credits, had higher grade point averages, and had a lower course failure rate than non-BARR students. BARR students also scored significantly higher on standardized math and reading tests than non-BARR students (Corsello & Sharma, 2015).

Challenges for Communities

Communities have benefitted from decades of research on how to best organize individual and groups to address issues of alcohol and drug use in various settings such as schools and communities. However, communities often face difficulty in implementing these strategies with quality and achieving outcomes demonstrated by prevention researchers. This gap between research and practice (e.g., Green, 2001; Wandersman & Florin, 2003) is often the result of limited resources in real world settings. For example, the typical settings in which these strategies are delivered often lack resources (i.e., tools or funding) or capacity (i.e., knowledge, attitudes, skills) to adapt and implement strategies that have been developed in resource-intense research settings. Common ways to bridge this gap, such as information dissemination, fail to change practice or outcomes at the local level in part because they do not sufficiently build capacity or use community stakeholder input to address adoption and implementation barriers.

In one review (Durlak & DuPre, 2008), identified 23 different factors that were important to implementation. These factors cut across five different categories including community level factors (e.g., politics and funding), provider characteristics (e.g., perceived need for innovation, self-efficacy) characteristics of the innovation (e.g., compatibility, adaptability), organizational capacity (e.g., positive work climate, norms regarding change), and factors related to the prevention support system (e.g., training, technical assistance).

What can help communities implement these programs and strategies effectively is to receive support in their prevention work from a "Prevention Support System." Wandersman and colleagues (Wandersman et al., 2008) describe an Interactive Systems Framework for disseminating and implementing preventive innovations. In this framework, researchers develop interventions which are readied for use in a "Prevention Synthesis and Translation System" and then communities put them into practice in a "Prevention Delivery System." A "Prevention Support System" plays the key role of linking these two systems, facilitating the process of translation within the Synthesis and Translation System and implementation within the Prevention Delivery System in order to improve outcomes.

One example of a Prevention Support System that has been specifically applied to the types of strategies described above is Getting To Outcomes™ (GTO). GTO was developed to address the gap between prevention research and practice by building capacity (self-efficacy, attitudes, and behaviors) at the individual and program levels for effective prevention practices (e.g., choosing evidence-based practices; and planning, implementing, evaluating, and sustaining those practices). The GTO model provides communities a manual that offers guidance and tools, training, and on-site technical assistance. Relevant to this chapter are two specific applications of GTO. The first was the development of a GTO manual for communities working to promote positive youth development in their communities (Fisher et al., 2006). In a randomized control trial of 12 community coalitions, the coalitions that utilized the GTO system and customized tools improved their capacities and performance to carry out high quality prevention in the area of positive youth development (Acosta et al., 2013). The second application was to environmental prevention strategies to reduce and prevent underage drinking (Imm et al., 2007). In a small randomized control trial, coalitions who utilized the GTO system and customized tools show improvement in some key prevention activities (e.g., compliance checks) and increased rates of merchants refusing to sell alcohol to minors (e.g., Chinman et al., 2014). As shown, GTO can help organizations build capacities to put prevention interventions into place. It is in this vein that we offer the following recommendations.

- Communities could benefit from continued support to implement community-based prevention initiatives designed to address large-scale, community change (e.g., reduced alcohol and drug use rates). This involves providing the knowledge and skills necessary to complete core components such as needs/resource assessments, setting priorities and high-quality program delivery. This also involves helping communities obtain buy-in from stakeholders, such as law enforcement, on and off premises alcohol establishments, schools, media, and parents.
- Communities need more support to ensure that community-based initiatives are implemented with fidelity. The concept of fidelity is relatively clear in school-based programs where most program developers have made fidelity monitoring tools available. However, with many multicomponent underage drinking initiatives, some components may be quite complicated and do not easily lend themselves to tracking fidelity. For example, what does it mean to

have fidelity with the component of "community mobilization," which is one of the key components of the Community Trials Intervention program? How are environmental strategies such as limiting "happy hour" discounts and other promotions to be monitored to ensure that establishments are uniform in their approach? For these types of challenges, it may be helpful to contact program developers for guidance or establish a network of communities that all use similar approaches so that the lessons learned can be easily shared (e.g., "practice collaboratives," Wilson, Berwick, & Cleary, 2003). In addition, manuals such as GTO can offer tools to assist communities with planning, implementation, and self-evaluation to improve quality of implementation (Fisher et al., 2006; Imm et al., 2007).

- Strategies to promote a systematic approach to continuous quality improvement (CQI) should be helpful to ensure ongoing improvement. This model may include regular performance monitoring, testing small changes or potential improvements, and then assessing the impact of those improvements similar to a Plan Do Study Act (PDSA) cycle. While CQI strategies are common in medical and business settings, they are not typically utilized in community-based prevention to ensure high-quality implementation to reach desired outcomes. Tools do exist that offers practical steps for conducting CQI in community-based organizations (Hunter, Ebener, Chinman, Ober, & Huang, 2015).
- To complement the CQI process, all programs need assistance with conducting their own program evaluations. Evidence shows that when programs implement self-monitoring processes, they are more likely to achieve better outcomes regardless of their program (Durlak & DuPre, 2008).

Summary

This chapter highlights research literature and updated findings about community-based environmental initiatives that have shown to be effective at reducing alcohol use and misuse. Many of the initiatives are well-established programs in which data have been collected over time with sustained positive results. Summary research and references on environmental strategies/policies to reduce underage drinking are also highlighted we well as promising programs in the area of positive youth development. Communities continue to work toward implementing evidence-based community prevention but are frequently challenged to ensure high-quality implementation that lead to positive outcomes. Comprehensive prevention systems (e.g., GTO) that help to build capacities of practitioners and community members to implement high-quality programming have showed promising results.

References

Acosta, J., Chinman, M., Ebener, P., Malone, P., Paddock, S., Phillips, A., ... Slaughter, M. (2013, August). An intervention to improve program implementation. Findings from a two-year cluster randomized trial of Assets-Getting to Outcomes. *Implementation Science*, 887. https://doi.org/10.1186/1748-5908-8-87. PMCID: PMC3751245.

Alcohol Epidemiology Program. (2000). *Alcohol compliance checks: A procedures manual for enforcing alcohol age-of-sale laws*. Minneapolis, MN: University of Minnesota.

Amodeo, M., & Collins, M. E. (2007). Using a positive youth development approach in addressing problem-oriented youth behavior. *Families in Society: The Journal of Contemporary Social Services, 88*(1), 75–85.

Battistich, V., Solomon, D., Watson, M., & Schaps, E. (1997). Caring school communities. *Educational Psychologist, 32*(3), 137–151.

Bergen, G., Pitan, A., Qu, S., Shults, R. A., Chattopadhyay, S. K., Elder, R. W., ... Nichols, J. L. (2014). Publicized sobriety checkpoint programs: A community guide systematic review. *American Journal of Preventive Medicine, 46*(5), 529–539.

Biglan, A., Ary, D. V., Smolkowski, K., Duncan, T., & Black, C. (2000). A randomised controlled trial of a community intervention to prevent adolescent tobacco use. *Tobacco Control, 9*(1), 24–32.

Bonell, C., Hinds, K., Dickson, K., Thomas, J., Fletcher, A., Murphy, S., ... Campbell, R. (2016, February). What is positive youth development and how might it reduce substance use and violence? A systematic review and synthesis of theoretical literature. *BMC Public Health, 16*, 135–147. https://doi.org/10.1186/s12889-016-2817-3

Bormann, C. A., & Stone, M. H. (2001). The effects of eliminating alcohol in a college stadium: The Folsom Field beer ban. *Journal of American College Health, 50*(2), 81–88.

Brook, J. S., Balka, E. B., & Whiteman, M. (1999). The risks for late adolescence of early adolescent marijuana use. *American Journal of Public Health, 89*(10), 1549–1554.

Bui, K. V. T., Ellickson, P. L., & Bell, R. M. (2000). Cross-lagged relationships among adolescent problem drug use, delinquent behavior, and emotional distress. *Journal of Drug Issues, 30*(2), 283–303.

Butterfoss, F. D. (2007). *Coalitions and partnerships in community health*. San Francisco, CA: Jossey-Bass.

Butterfoss, F. D., Goodman, R. M., & Wandersman, A. (1993). Community coalitions for prevention and health promotion. *Health Education Research, 8*(3), 315–330.

Butterfoss, F. D., & Kegler, M. C. (2002). Toward a comprehensive understanding of community coalitions. In R. DiClemente, R. A. Crosby, & M. C. Kegler (Eds.), *Emerging theories in health promotion practice and research* (pp. 157–193). San Francisco, CA: Jossey-Bass.

Catalano, R. F., Berglund, M. L., Ryan, J. A., Lonczak, H. S., & Hawkins, J. D. (2004). Positive youth development in the United States: Research findings on evaluation of positive youth development programs. *Annals of the American Academy of Political and Social Science, 591*, 98–204. https://doi.org/10.1177/0002716203260102

Cavazos-Rehg, P. A., Krauss, M. J., Spitznagel, E. L., Chaloupka, F. J., Schootman, M., Grucza, R. A., & Bierut, L. J. (2012). Associations between selected state laws and teenagers' drinking and driving behaviors. *Alcoholism: Clinical and Experimental Research, 36*(9), 1647–1652.

Centers for Disease Control and Prevention. (2004). *WebBased injury statistics query and reporting system (WISQARS)*. Retrieved from http://www.cdc.gov/ncipc/wisqars/default.htm.

Chaloupka, F. J., Grossman, M., & Saffer, H. (2002). The effects of price on alcohol consumption and alcohol-related problems. *Alcohol Research & Health, 26*(1), 22–34.

Chambers, R. A., Taylor, J. R., & Potenza, M. N. (2003). Developmental neurocircuitry of motivation in adolescence: A critical period of addiction vulnerability. *American Journal of Psychiatry, 160*(6), 1041–1052.

Chinman, M., Ebener, P., Burkhart, Q., Osilla, K., Imm, P., Paddock, S., & Wright, P. (2014). Evaluating the impact of Getting to Outcomes—Underage drinking on prevention capacity and alcohol merchant attitudes and selling behaviors. *Prevention Science, 15*(4), 485–496.

Chinman, M., Imm, P., & Wandersman, A. (2004). *Getting to Outcomes 2004: Promoting accountability through methods and tools for planning, implementation, and evaluation* (No. TR-TR101). Santa Monica, CA: RAND Corporation.

Chou, C. P., Montgomery, S., Pentz, M. A., Rohrbach, L. A., Johnson, C. A., Flay, B. R., … MacKinnon, D. (1998). Effects of a community-based prevention program on decreasing drug use in high-risk adolescents. *American Journal of Public Health, 88*(6), 944–948.

Coate, D., & Grossman, M. (1988). Effects of alcoholic beverage prices and legal drinking ages on youth alcohol use. *The Journal of Law and Economics, 31*(1), 145–171.

Cohen, D. A., Mason, K., & Scribner, R. (2002). The population consumption model, alcohol control practices, and alcohol-related traffic fatalities. *Preventive Medicine, 34*(2), 187–197.

Cook, P. J., & Moore, M. J. (1993). Drinking and schooling. *Journal of Health Economics, 12*(4), 411–429.

Cooper, D., Gillen, D., & Atkins, F. (2004). *Impacts of California's graduated licensing law of 1998*. Berkeley, CA: University of California Institute of Transportation Studies.

Corsello, M., & Sharma, A. (2015). The building assets-reducing risks program: Replication and expansion of an effective strategy to turn around low-achieving schools. i3 Development Grant Final Report to the U.S. Department of Education, Washington, DC. Retrieved from https://static1.squarespace.com/static/5613cb59e4b009e45cc5c677/t/56fee985b6aa6038541b7c36/1459546503250/Final+report+for+BARR+i3+Development+grant+-+ERIC+upload.pdf.

D'Amico, E., Chinman, M., Stern, S., & Wandersman, A. (2009). Community prevention handbook on adolescent substance abuse prevention and treatment. Evidence-based practices. In C. G. Leukefeld, T. P. Gullotta, & M. Staton-Tindall (Eds.), *Adolescent substance abuse: Evidence-based approaches to prevention and treatment* (pp. 213–249). New York, NY: Springer.

D'Amico, E. J., Ellickson, P. L., Wagner, E. F., Turrisi, R., Fromme, K., Ghosh-Dastidar, B., … Wright, D. (2005). Developmental considerations for substance use interventions from middle school through college. *Alcoholism: Clinical and Experimental Research, 29*(3), 474–483.

D'Amico, E. J., & Stern, S. A. (2008). Preventing alcohol and drug use. In J. A. Trafton & W. T. Gordon (Eds.), *Best practices in the behavioral management of health from preconception to adolescence* (Vol. 3, pp. 341–401). Los Altos, CA: Institute for Disease Management.

De Bellis, M. D., Clark, D. B., Beers, S. R., Soloff, P. H., Boring, A. M., Hall, J. H., … Keshauvan, M. S. (2000). Hippocampal volume in adolescent-onset alcohol use disorders. *American Journal of Psychiatry, 157*, 737–744.

Dills, A. K. (2010). Social host liability for minors and underage drunk-driving accidents. *Journal of Health Economics, 29*(2), 241–249.

Drug Strategies. (1999). *Keeping score on alcohol. Drug strategies*. Retrieved from http://drugstrategies.org/keepingscore1999/Score99.pdf.

Durlak, J. A., & DuPre, E. P. (2008). Implementation matters: A review of research on the influence of implementation on program outcomes and the factors that affect implementation. *American Journal of Community Psychology, 41*(3-4), 327–350.

Durlak, J. A., Taylor, R. D., Kawashima, K., Pachan, M. K., DuPre, E. P., Celio, C. I., … Weissberg, R. P. (2007). Effects of positive youth development programs on school, family, and community systems. *American Journal of Community Psychology, 39*(3-4), 269–286.

Elder, R. W., Lawrence, B., Ferguson, A., Naimi, T. S., Brewer, R. D., Chattopadhyay, S. K., … Task Force on Community Preventive Services. (2010). The effectiveness of tax policy interventions for reducing excessive alcohol consumption and related harms. *American Journal of Preventive Medicine, 38*(2), 217–229.

Ellickson, P. L., Martino, S. C., & Collins, R. L. (2004). Marijuana use from adolescence to young adulthood: Multiple developmental trajectories and their associated outcomes. *Health Psychology, 23*(3), 299–307.

Evans, J., Sharma, A., & Jerabek, A. (2013, April). Building assets reducing risks: Whole 9th grade strategy reduces coursework failure for students of color. Paper presented at the American Educational Research Association 2013 Annual Meeting. San Francisco, CA.

Fell, J. C., Ferguson, S. A., Williams, A. F., & Fields, M. (2001). Why aren't sobriety checkpoints widely adopted as an enforcement strategy in the United States? *Proceedings for the Association for the Advancement of Automotive Medicine, 45*, 425–428.

Fell, J. C., Fisher, D. A., Voas, R. B., Blackman, K., & Tippetts, A. S. (2009). The impact of underage drinking laws on alcohol-related fatal crashes of young drivers. *Alcohol, Clinical and Experimental Research, 33*(7), 1208–1219.

Fell, J. C., Scherer, M., Thomas, S., & Voas, R. B. (2014). Effects of social host and fake identification laws on reducing underage drinking driver fatal crashes. *Traffic Injury Prevention, 15*(Suppl. 1), S64–S73.

Fell, J. C., Scherer, M., Thomas, S., & Voas, R. B. (2016). Assessing the impact of twenty underage drinking laws. *Journal of Studies on Alcohol and Drugs, 77*(2), 249–260.

Fell, J. C., Todd, M., & Voas, R. B. (2011). A national evaluation of the nighttime and passenger restriction components of graduated driver licensing. *Journal of Safety Research, 42*(4), 283–290.

Fisher, D., Imm, P., Chinman, M., & Wandersman, A. (2006). *Getting to outcomes with developmental assets*. Minneapolis, MN: Search Institute.

Green, L. W. (2001). From research to "best practices" in other settings and populations. *American Journal of Health Behavior, 25*(3), 165–178.

Grossman, M., & Chaloupka, F. J. (1998). The demand for cocaine by young adults: A rational addiction approach. *Journal of Health Economics, 17*(4), 427–474.

Grube, J. W. (1997). Preventing sales of alcohol to minors: Results from a community trial. *Addiction, 92*(Suppl. 2), S251–S260.

Hahn, R. A., Kuzara, J. L., Elder, R., Brewer, R., Chattopadhyay, S., Fielding, J., ... Lawrence, B. (2010). Effectiveness of policies restricting hours of alcohol sales in preventing excessive alcohol consumption and related harms. *American Journal of Preventive Medicine, 39*(6), 590–604.

Hansell, S., & White, H. R. (1991). Adolescent drug use, psychological distress, and physical symptoms. *Journal of Health and Social Behavior, 32*, 288–301.

Hasin, D. S., Stinson, F. S., Ogburn, E., & Grant, B. F. (2007). Prevalence, correlates, and disability, and comorbidity of DSM-IV alcohol abuse and dependence in the United States: Results from the National Epidemiologic Survey on alcohol and related conditions. *Archives of General Psychiatry, 64*(7), 830–842.

Hawkins, J. D., Catalano, R. F., Arthur, M. W., Egan, E., Brown, E. C., Abbott, R. D., & Murray, D. M. (2008). Testing communities that care: The rationale, design and behavioral baseline equivalence of the community youth development study. *Prevention Science, 9*(3), 178–190.

Hawkins, J. D., Oesterle, S., Brown, E. C., Abbott, R. D., & Catalano, R. F. (2014). Youth problem behaviors 8 years after implementing the Communities That Care prevention system: A community-randomized trial. *JAMA Pediatrics, 168*(2), 122–129.

Hawkins, J. D., Oesterle, S., Brown, E. C., Arthur, M. W., Abbott, R. D., Fagan, A. A., & Catalano, R. F. (2009). Results of type 2 translational research trial to prevent adolescent drug use and delinquency: A test of Communities That Care. *Archives of Pediatrics & Adolescent Medicine, 163*, 789–798.

Hawkins, J. D., Oesterle, S., Brown, E. C., Monahan, K. C., Abbott, R. D., Arthur, M. W., & Catalano, R. F. (2012). Sustained decreases in risk exposure and youth problem behaviors after installation of the Communities That Care prevention system in a randomized trial. *Archives of Pediatrics & Adolescent Medicine, 166*(2), 141–148.

Hilliard, L. J., Bowers, E. P., Greenman, K. N., Hershberg, R. M., Geldhof, G. J., Glickman, S. A., ... Lerner, R. M. (2014). Beyond the deficit model: Bullying and trajectories of character virtues in adolescence. *Journal of Youth and Adolescence, 43*(6), 991–1006.

Hingson, R., McGovern, T., Howland, J., Heeren, T., Winter, M., & Zakocs, R. (1996). Reducing alcohol-impaired driving in Massachusetts: The Saving Lives Program. *American Journal of Public Health, 86*(6), 791–797.

Hingson, R. W., Heeren, T., Jamanka, A., & Howland, J. (2000). Age of drinking onset and unintentional injury involvement after drinking. *Journal of the American Medical Association, 284*(12), 1527–1533.

Holder, H. (2000). Community prevention of alcohol problems. *Addictive Behaviors, 25*(6), 843–859.

Holder, H., & Treno, J. (1997). Media advocacy in community prevention: News as a means to advance policy change. *Addiction, 92*(suppl. 2), S189–S199.

Holder, H. D., Gruenewald, P. J., Ponicki, W. R., Treno, A. J., Grube, J. W., Saltz, R. F., … Roeper, P. (2000). Effect of community-based interventions on high-risk drinking and alcohol related injuries. *Journal of the American Medical Association, 284*(18), 2341–2347.

Holder, H. D., Saltz, R. F., Grube, J. W., Voas, R. B., Gruenewald, P. J., & Treno, A. J. (1997). A community prevention trial to reduce alcohol-involved accidental injury and death: Overview. *Addiction, 92*, S155–S171.

Holder, H. D., & Wagenaar, A. C. (1994). Mandated server training and reduced alcohol-involved traffic crashes: A time series analysis of the Oregon experience. *Accident Analysis and Prevention, 26*(1), 89–97.

Hunter, S., Ebener, P., Chinman, M., Ober, J., & Huang, C. (2015). *Promoting success: A getting to outcomes guide to implementing continuous quality improvement for community service organizations* (RAND, TL-179-NIDA). Santa Monica, CA: RAND Corporation.

Hyde, L. K., Cook, L. J., Knight, S., & Olson, L. M. (2005). Graduated driver licensing in Utah: Is it effective? *Annals of Emergency Medicine, 45*(2), 147–154.

Imm, P., Chinman, M., Wandersman, A., Rosenbloom, D., Guckenburg, S., & Leis, R. (2007). *Preventing underage drinking: Using getting to outcomes with the SAMHSA strategic prevention framework to achieve results* (No. TR-403-SAMHSA). Santa Monica, CA: RAND Corporation.

Institute of Medicine. (1994). *Reducing risks for mental disorders: Frontiers for preventive intervention research*. Washington, DC: Academy Press.

Johnston, L. D., O'Malley, P. M., Bachman, J. G., & Schulenberg, J. E. (2007). *Monitoring the Future national survey results on drug use, 1975-2006. Volume I: Secondary school students*. Bethesda, MD: National Institute on Drug Abuse.

Johnston, L. D., O'Malley, P. M., Miech, R. A., Bachman, J. G., & Schulenberg, J. E. (2016). *Monitoring the Future national survey results on drug use, 1975-2016. Key Findings on adolescent drug use*. Ann Arbor, MI: Institute for Social Research, The University of Michigan.

Join Together. (1999). *Promising strategies: Results of the fourth national survey on community efforts to reduce substance abuse and gun violence*. Boston, MA: Boston University School of Public Health.

Komro, K. A., Livingston, M. D., Wagenaar, A. C., Kominksy, T. K., Pettigrew, D. W., Garrett, B. A., & The Cherokee Nation Prevention Trial Team. (2017). American. *Journal of Public Health, 107*(3), 453–459.

Komro, K. A., Perry, C. L., Veblen-Mortenson, S., & Williams, C. L. (1994). Peer participation in Project Northland: A community-wide alcohol use prevention project. *The Journal of School Health, 64*(8), 318–322.

Kumpfer, K., Whiteside, H., & Wandersman, A. (1997). *Community readiness for drug abuse prevention: Issues, tips and tools*. Rockville, MD: National Institute of Drug Abuse.

Lanza, S. T., & Collins, L. M. (2002). Pubertal timing and the onset of substance use in females during early adolescence. *Prevention Science, 3*(1), 69–82.

Lenk, K. M., Nelson, T. F., Toomey, T. L., Jones-Webb, R., & Erickson, D. J. (2016, November). Sobriety checkpoint and open container laws in US: Associations with reported drinking-driving. *Traffic Injury Prevention, 17*(18), 782–787. https://doi.org/10.1080/15389588.2016.1161759

Masten, A. S. (2014). *Ordinary magic: Resilience in development*. New York, NY: Guilford Press.
Muthén, B. O., & Muthén, L. K. (2000). The development of heavy drinking and alcohol-related problems from ages 18 to 37 in a U. S. national sample. *Journal of Studies on Alcohol, 61*(2), 290–300.
Nation, M., Crusto, C., Wandersman, A., Kumpfer, K. L., Seybolt, D., Morrissey-Kane, E., & Davino, K. (2003). What works in prevention: Principles of effective prevention programs. *American Psychologist, 58*(6-7), 449–456.
National Institute on Alcohol Abuse and Alcoholism (NIAAA). (2015). *Planning alcohol interventions using NIAAA's College AIM Alcohol Interventions Matrix* (NIH Publication No. 15-AA-8017). Bethesda, MD: National Institutes of Health. Retrieved from http://www.collegedrinkingprevention.gov/CollegeAIM/Resources/NIAAA_College_Matrix_Booklet.pdf.
National Institute on Drug Abuse. (1997). *Drug abuse prevention for at risk groups*. Rockville, MD: U.S. Department of Health and Services, National Institutes of Health, National Institute on Drug Abuse, Office of Science Policy and Communications.
National Institute on Drug Abuse. (2003). Preventing drug use among children and adolescents (Vol. 04-4212 (B). Bethesda, MD: National Institutes of Health.
National Research Council and Institute of Medicine. (2009). Committee on the prevention of mental disorders and substance abuse among children, youth, and young adults: Research advances and promising interventions. Preventing mental, emotional, and behavioral disorders among young people: Progress and possibilities. Washington DC: The National Academies Press.
Newton, A., Sacker, S. J., Pahal, G. S., van der Bergh, E., & Young, C. (2007). Impact of the new UK licensing law on emergency hospital attendance: A cohort study. *Journal of Emergency Medicine, 24*(8), 531–536.
Paschall, M. J., Grube, J. W., Thomas, S., Cannon, C., & Treffers, R. (2012). Relationships between local enforcement, alcohol availability, drinking norms, and adolescent alcohol use in 50 California cities. *Journal of Studies on Alcohol and Drugs, 73*(4), 657–665.
Peek-Asa, C. (1999). The effect of random alcohol screening in reducing motor vehicle crash injuries. *American Journal of Preventive Medicine, 16*(1), 57–67.
Pentz, M. A. (1998). *Preventing drug abuse through the community: Multicomponent programs that make a difference* (NIDA Publication No. 98-4293). Rockville, MD: National Institute on Drug Abuse.
Pentz, M. A. (2003). Evidence-based prevention: Characteristics, impact, and future direction. *Journal of Psychoactive Drugs, 35*(Suppl. 1), 143–152.
Pentz, M. A., Dwyer, J. H., MacKinnon, D. P., Flay, B. R., Hansen, W. B., Wang, E. Y., & Johnson, C. A. (1989). A multicommunity trial for primary prevention of adolescent drug abuse: Effects on drug use prevalence. *Journal of the American Medical Association, 261*(22), 3259–3266.
Pentz, M. A., Trebow, E. A., Hansen, W. B., MacKinnon, D. P., Dwyer, J. H., Flay, B. R., … Johnson, C. A. (1990). Effects of program implementation on adolescent drug use behavior: The Midwestern Prevention Project (MPP). *Evaluation Review, 14*(3), 264–289.
Perry, C. L., Williams, C. L., Komro, K. A., Veblen-Mortenson, S., Forster, J. L., Bernstein-Lachter, R., … McGovern, P. (2000). Project Northland high school interventions: Community action to reduce adolescent alcohol use. *Health Education and Behavior, 27*(1), 29–49.
Perry, C. L., Williams, C. L., Komro, K. A., Veblen-Mortenson, S., Stigler, M. H., Munson, K. A., … Forster, J. (2002). Project Northland: Long-term outcomes of community action to reduce adolescent alcohol use. *Health Education Research, 17*(1), 117–132.
Perry, C. L., Williams, C. L., Veblen-Mortenson, S., Toomey, T. L., Komro, K. A., Anstine, P. S., … Wolfson, M. (1996). Project Northland: Outcomes of community-wide alcohol use prevention program during early adolescence. *American Journal of Public Health, 7*(86), 956–965.
Rammohan, V., Hahn, R. A., Elder, R., Brewer, R., Fielding, J., Naimi, T. S., … Task Force on Community Preventive Services. (2011). Effects of dram shop liability and enhanced over-service law enforcement initiatives on excessive alcohol consumption and related harms:

Two community guide systematic reviews. *American Journal of Preventive Medicine, 41*(3), 334–343.

Reboussin, B. A., Song, E. Y., & Wolfson, M. (2011). The impact of alcohol outlet density of the demographic clustering of underage drinking behaviors within census tracts. *Alcoholism: Clinical & Experimental Research, 35*(8), 1541–1549.

Rice, T. M., Peek-Asa, C., & Kraus, J. F. (2004). Effects of the California graduated driver licensing program. *Journal of Safety Research, 35*(4), 375–381.

Riggs, N. R., Chou, C. P., & Pentz, M. A. (2009). Preventing growth in amphetamine use: Longterm effects of the Midwestern Prevention Project (MPP) from early adolescence to early adulthood. *Addiction, 104*(10), 1691–1699.

Ringwalt, C. L., & Paschall, M. J. (2011). The utility of Keg Registration Laws: A cross-sectional study. *The Journal of Adolescent Health, 48*(1), 106–108. https://doi.org/10.1016/j.jadohealth.2010.05.012

Ruhm, C. J. (1996). Alcohol policies and highway vehicle fatalities. *Journal of Health Economics, 15*(4), 435–454.

Sagrestano, L., & Paikoff, R. L. (1997). Preventing high risk sexual behavior, sexually transmitted diseases, and pregnancy among adolescents. In R. Weissberg, T. P. Gullotta, R. L. Hampton, B. A. Ryan, & G. R. Adams (Eds.), *Enhancing children's wellness* (pp. 76–104). Newbury Park, CA: Sage.

Scheier, L. M., Botvin, G. J., Diaz, T., & Griffin, K. W. (1999). Social skills, competence, and drug refusal efficacy as predictors of adolescent alcohol use. *Journal of Drug Education, 29*(3), 251–278.

Schwartz, S. J., Phelps, E., Lerner, J. V., Huang, S., Brown, C. H., Lewin-Bizan, S., … Lerner, R. M. (2010). Promotion as prevention: Positive youth development as protective against tobacco, alcohol, illicit drug, and sex initiation. *Applied Developmental Science, 14*, 197–211. https://doi.org/10.1080/10888691.2010.516186

Shope, J. T., & Molnar, L. J. (2004). Michigan's graduated driver licensing program: Evaluation of the first four years. *Journal of Safety Research, 35*(3), 337–344.

Shults, R. A., Elder, R. W., Sleet, D. A., Nichols, J. L., Alao, M. O., Carande-Kulis, V., … Thompson, R. S. (2001). Reviews of evidence regarding interventions to reduce alcohol-impaired driving. *American Journal of Preventive Medicine, 21*(4 Suppl), 66–88.

Smith, D. I. (1988). Effectiveness on restrictions of availability as a means of preventing alcohol-related problems. *Contemporary Drug Problems, 15*(4), 627–684.

Smith, D. I. (1990). Effect on casualty traffic accidents of changing Sunday alcohol sales legislation in Victoria, Australia. *Journal of Drug Issues, 20*(3), 417–426.

Sowell, E. R., Thompson, P. M., Holmes, C. J., Jernigan, T. L., & Toga, A. W. (1999). In vivo evidence for post-adolescent brain maturation in frontal and striatal regions. *Nature Neuroscience, 2*(10), 859–861.

Stout, E. M., Sloan, F. A., Liang, L., & Davies, H. H. (2000). Reducing harmful alcohol-related behaviors: Effective regulatory methods. *Journal of Studies on Alcohol, 61*(3), 402–412.

Substance Abuse and Mental Health Administration (SAMHSA). (2001). *Science-based substance abuse prevention: A guide* (HHS Publication No. SMA d-3505). Rockville, MD: Substance Abuse and Mental Health Administration.

Tapert, S. F., Caldwell, L., & Burke, M. A. (2004–2005). Alcohol and the adolescent brain--Human studies. *Alcohol Research & Health, 28*(4), 205–212.

Tarter, R. E. (2002). Etiology of adolescent substance abuse: A developmental perspective. *American Journal on Addictions, 11*(3), 171–191.

Taylor, R. D., Oberle, E., Durlak, J., & Weissberg, R. (2017). Promoting positive youth development through school-based social and emotional learning interventions. A meta-analysis of follow-up effects. *Child Development, 88*(4), 1156–1171.

Toumbourou, J. W., Stockwell, T., Neighbors, C., Marlatt, G. A., Sturge, J., & Rehm, J. (2007). Interventions to reduce harm associated with adolescent substance use. *The Lancet, 369*(9570), 1391–1401.

Treno, A. J., & Lee, J. P. (2002). Approaching alcohol problems through local environmental interventions. *Alcohol Research & Health, 26*(1), 35–40.

Tschann, J. M., Adler, N. E., Irwin, C. E., Jr., Millstein, S. G., Turner, R. A., & Kegeles, S. M. (1994). Initiation of substance use in early adolescence: The roles of pubertal timing and emotional distress. *Health Psychology, 13*(4), 326–333.

U.S. Department of Health and Human Services, Office of the Surgeon General. (2016, November). *Facing addiction in America: The Surgeon General's report on alcohol, drugs, and health.* Washington, DC: U.S. Department of Health and Human Services.

Wagenaar, A. C., Gehan, J. P., Jones-Webb, R., Toomey, T. L., Forster, J. L., Wolfson, M., … Murray, D. (1999). Communities mobilizing for change on alcohol: Lessons and results from a 15-community randomized trial. *Journal of Community Psychology, 27*(3), 315–326.

Wagenaar, A. C., Murray, D. M., Gehan, J. P., Wolfson, M., Forster, J. L., Toomey, T. L., … Jones-Webb, R. (2000). Communities mobilizing for change on alcohol: Outcomes from a randomized community trial. *Journal of Studies on Alcohol, 61*(1), 85–94.

Wagenaar, A. C., Murray, D. M., Wolfson, M., Forster, J. L., & Finnegan, J. R. (1994). Communities mobilizing for change on alcohol: Design of a randomized community trial. *Journal of Consulting Psychology, 22*(CSAP Special Issue), 79–101.

Wagenaar, A. C., Salois, M. J., & Komro, K. A. (2009). Effects of beverage alcohol price and tax levels on drinking: A meta-analysis of 1003 estimates from 112 studies. *Addiction, 104*(2), 179–190.

Wagenaar, A. C., Tobler, A. L., & Komro, K. A. (2010). Effects of alcohol tax and price policies on morbidity and mortality. A systematic review. *American Journal of Public Health, 100*(11), 2270–2278.

Wandersman, A., Duffy, J., Flaspohler, P., Noonan, R., Lubell, K., Stillman, L., … Saul, J. (2008). Bridging the gap between prevention research and practice: The interactive systems framework for dissemination and implementation. *American Journal of Community Psychology, 41*(3-4), 171–181.

Wandersman, A., & Florin, P. (2003). Community interventions and effective prevention. *American Psychologist, 58*(6-7), 441–448.

Wechsler, H., Nelson, T. F., Lee, J. E., Seibring, M., Lewis, C., & Keeling, R. P. (2003). Perception and reality: A national evaluation of social norms marketing interventions to reduce college students' heavy alcohol use. *Quarterly Journal of Studies on Alcohol, 64*(4), 484–494.

Weitzman, E. R., Folkman, A., Folkman, M. P., & Wechsler, H. (2003). The relationship of alcohol outlet density to heavy and frequent drinking and drinking-related problems among college students at eight universities. *Health Place, 9*(1), 1–6.

Whetten-Goldstein, K., Sloan, F. A., Stout, E., & Liang, L. (2000). Civil liability, criminal law, and other policies and alcohol-related motor vehicle fatalities in the United States: 1984-1995. *Accident Analysis and Prevention, 32*(6), 723–733.

Wilson, T., Berwick, D. M., & Cleary, P. D. (2003). Performance improvement - What do collaborative improvement projects do? Experience from seven countries. *Joint Commission Journal on Quality and Safety, 29*(2), 85–93.

Xu, X., & Chaloupka, F. J. (2011). The effects of prices on alcohol use and its consequences. *Alcohol Research and Health, 34*(2), 236–245.

Xu, Y., Yu, Q., Scribner, R., Theall, K., Scribner, S., & Simonsen, N. (2012). Multilevel spatio-temporal change-point models for evaluating the effect of an alcohol outlet control policy on changes in neighborhood assaultive violence rates. *Spatiotemporal Epidemiology, 3*(2), 121–128.

Zakocs, R. C., & Edwards, E. M. (2006). What explains community coalition effectiveness? *American Journal of Preventive Medicine, 30*(4), 351–361.

Zhang, X., Hatcher, B., Clarkson, L., Holt, J., Bagchi, S., Kanny, D., & Brewer, R. (2015, May). Changes in density of on-premises alcohol outlets and impact on violent crime, Atlanta, Georgia, 1997–2007. *Preventing Chronic Disease, 12*(140317), E84. https://doi.org/10.5888/pcd12.140317

Epilogue: The Present State of Adolescent Substance Abuse Treatment and Prevention Practice

Thomas P. Gullotta and Carl G. Leukefeld

The inscription on my mirror says: "Your looking at the only problem you'll have today."

(Anonymous)

Unfortunately some adolescents do not take time to think about problems, particularly how to solve their own, but forge ahead into high-risk and risky behaviors including substance abuse. Our hope is that readers come to share our remarkable learning process from the conceptualization of this second edition through the writing process to this final chapter. In our journey we uncovered the recipe for brewing Chicha, discovered the reasons why tobacco is so addictive that half of the smokers continue their destructive habit despite losing a lung to cancer, why there is our current widespread opioid abuse despite the increased number of recent opioid overdoses and deaths, came to better understand the value of some therapeutic techniques, and the harm that other interventions can have. In this epilogue, we revisit some of our discoveries and share our understanding of adolescence treatment and prevention interventions in a field progressing from an art in which the personal magnetism of the healer is being replaced by science in which such enemas are no longer seen as powerful medicine and scare approaches are limited.

T. P. Gullotta
Child and Family Agency of Southeastern Connecticut
New London, CT, USA
e-mail: tpgullotta@aol.com

C. G. Leukefeld
University of Kentucky
Department of Behavioral Science
Center on Drug and Alcohol Research
Lexington, KY, USA
e-mail: cleukef@uky.edu

C. G. Leukefeld, T. P. Gullotta (eds.), *Adolescent Substance Abuse*, Issues in Children's and Families' Lives, https://doi.org/10.1007/978-3-319-90611-9

Evidence-Based Practice

Recent interest in evidence-based practice can be traced to the publication of *Effectiveness and Efficiency: Random Reflections on Health Services* by the Scottish epidemiologist Archie Cochrane (1972/1999). His pioneering efforts led to the establishment of a medical research database that has grown into an international collaboration directed at identifying medical practices that actually work. Cochrane's interest began with the recognition that much of medical practice was rooted in oral tradition. That is, clinical reports based on personal experience were the means by which knowledge was transferred from one healer to the other. Thus, Joseph Lister's positive experience in treating the deadly illness "Milk Fever,"[1] which afflicted new mothers, with washing one's hands before examining the new mom, was shared with his colleagues. Now, depending on the persuasiveness of the healer and the reported experiences of other doctors, a new treatment, *if it did not disturb the existing social reality*, gradually became a part of medical practice. In Joseph Lister's case, this was initially not to be. He was ridiculed for his ludicrous beliefs that cleanliness mattered and the practice of examining new mothers with soiled hands continued much to the dismay of orphans who lost their mothers to infectious "Milk Fever." Therein rested the problem of oral tradition. If the new information challenged an existing cherished belief, say, for example, Hippocrates four humors (black bile, yellow bile, phlegm, and blood which Galen repopularized and whose medical theories dominated medical treatment for centuries), then the information was rejected and existing treatments derived from humoral theory, namely, bloodletting, purging (vomiting), blistering, and enemas, to balance the humors and return the patient to health continued. From this example, realize that the conceptualization of an issue, which is imaging how something behaves, is more important then how it actually operates!

This paradigm shift in physical medicine from thinking something works to evidence that it actually works extends today into the treatment and prevention of behavioral disorders to include science-based interventions, technology transfer, and the novel idea that practitioners should be helpful.

The Institute of Medicine (IOM, 2001) defined evidence-based practice as "the integration of best research evidence with clinical practice and patient values" (IOM, 2001, p. 47). This definition not only recognizes that clinical observations give rise to suspicions (hypothesizes) that can then be tested but also goes further to embrace the critical role the client has in this process because (and this is not attended to enough) it is the client's life!

[1] In Lister's time (1860s) the high fever some women experienced shortly after the birth of their child was attributed to the start of lactation. No one thought that the filthy hands of the attending physician examining the new mother's bruised and damaged birth area was in any way related to the infection "Milk Fever."

Impressions

Treatment

Adolescence is a time of change, experimentation and perhaps pushing boundaries. The talented group of authors brought together for this project explored these areas, accomplished their assignment of providing readers with the current state of knowledge on the bio-psycho-social-environmental dimensions of adolescent substance abuse and evidence-based practices for its treatment and prevention. From their work, we saw that substance misuse led to several negative health and social consequences for adolescents. Further, these researchers and practitioners identified a number of social factors contributing to adolescent misuse including family environment and family relationships, peer associations, religious involvement, and school and community settings.

In these chapters, we discovered the current state of knowledge about evidence-based practices that "work" for adolescents across different treatment modalities. One intriguing observation from our reading was that while some therapeutic approaches are considered "evidence-based" for outpatient or family therapy, they have not been "proven" in another setting (residential for example). Clearly, much work remains to be done. Table 1 summarizes our understanding of suitable evidence-based practices in different therapeutic settings for adolescent substance users:

Evidence-based practices for residential treatment among adolescent substance users are less defined and supported by the clinical and empirical literature. Although there is tremendous variation in the approach taken to the residential treatment of adolescent substance abuse, researchers have begun to identify common key elements and features related to positive outcomes. From the Lichvar and colleagues chapter (in press; in this volume), we offer these observations:

1. Treatment retention—Adolescents who remain longer in residential substance abuse treatment have demonstrated more positive treatment outcomes.
2. Family involvement—Working with the family as a unit and including the family members in residential treatment interventions has been associated with positive outcomes.
3. Therapeutic milieu—Developing a therapeutic environment that is a good fit for adolescents that includes a motivational approach focused on harm reduction has been associated with positive outcomes.
4. Medications assisted therapy—Physician-prescribed medications off label to reduce opioid relapse including methadone, naltrexone, and other drugs to reduce craving and relapse.

Building on these key components of success in residential treatment, a number of interventions that have demonstrated effectiveness in home and community settings are being modified and integrated into residential modalities. In particular, Cognitive behavioral approaches (CBT), Motivational Enhancement Therapy (MET), and family-based and/or multisystemic approaches including multiple systemic therapy (MST), functional family therapy (FFT), brief strategic family ther-

Table 1 Summary of adolescent substance interventions

Intervention	Goal	Use
Cognitive Behavioral Therapy (CBT)	Improves the patient's cognitive (i.e., attitudes, values) and behavioral skills for changing his/her problematic drug use.	Individual, Outpatient
Behavioral Therapy	Emphasizes overcoming skill deficits and strengthening the patient's ability to cope with high-risk situations.	Individual, Outpatient
Brief Intervention	Involves a small number of sessions, which capitalize on the readiness of individuals to change their behavior (i.e., Motivational Enhancement Therapy, MET).	Individual, Outpatient
Node-Link Mapping	Incorporates visual representations of the range of difficulties, issues, and their potential solutions.	Individual, Outpatient
Relapse Prevention Therapy (RPT)	Identifies and changes problematic behavior through examining positive and negative consequences of continued drug use.	Individual, Outpatient
Trauma-Focused Cognitive Behavioral Therapy (TF-CBT)	Adapts CBT for use among children who have been exposed to such traumatic experiences as physical abuse.	Individual, Outpatient
Multidimensional Treatment Foster Care (MTFC)	Involves a behavioral intervention for delinquent youths and youths in need of out-of-home placement.	Individual, Outpatient
Multisystemic Therapy (MST)	Reduces drug use problems through interventions with the adolescent, family, and extrafamilial systems.	Family-based
Multidimensional Family Therapy (MDFT)	Focuses on reducing drug use by tailoring treatment to the characteristics of the adolescent, family, and their involvement with extrafamilial systems.	Family-based
Functional Family Therapy (FFT)	Emphasizes that the family's interactions are central to problem development and change occurs through family-based interventions.	Family-based
Medications Assisted Therapy	Reduces drug use relapse with off label physician prescribed medications for adolescents.	Individual, Outpatient

Suitable Evidence-Based Practices Presented by Author
Created by Authors Leukefeld & Gullotta, 2017

apy (BSFT), and multidimensional family therapy (MDFT) are being incorporated into residential care. The current state of research and knowledge is developing in this area to understand whether these approaches should be considered promising for adolescents in residential substance abuse treatment.

In addition to spotlighting practices that worked, we asked authors to identify practices that were not effective in treating adolescent substance misusers. Authors identified individual or group (supportive) therapy, and interactional therapy because there is a lack of skill-building to enable adolescents to handle high-risk situations. In addition, group therapy has been associated with negative outcomes for adolescents. The primary reason group therapy is ineffectual is that participants associate with deviant peers in the context of the group environment encouraging their dysfunctional behavior. With regard to residential programs, intervention with negative outcomes included boot camps, Scared Straight Programs, and treatment approaches that incorporated punishment as a consequence for noncompliance.

Prevention

In addition to a focus on evidence-based interventions for adolescent substance use, this volume examined approaches to prevent substance misuse. With roots in the Quaker tradition of helping individuals with social problems that were largely believed to be tied to poverty, a number of successful prevention efforts have been launched over the last 200 years to address substance abuse. The reality is that alcohol and drug abuse remain significant social problems which have largely been unchanged by large-scale (Prohibition) or small-scale (state laws) policy changes. Nonetheless, the call for continued evidence-based prevention interventions remains and this volume offers several promising avenues to achieve that end.

Bloom and Gullotta (2018; in this volume) states that primary prevention involves planned actions focusing on (1) predictable problems in relatively healthy individuals and groups, (2) protecting existing states of health and healthy functioning, and (3) promoting desired future states not yet attained. One of the most important venues for substance abuse prevention interventions is the school. The need for school-based prevention and evidence-based practices is important because of the harmful effects of substance use for adolescents, the fact that possession of tobacco and alcohol products by persons under the age of 18 is illegal, and research which suggests that use of tobacco and alcohol may increase risk for later, more extensive drug use. School-based prevention interventions have been shown to be effective, due in large part because adolescents spend a significant amount of time in school, schools provide an environment conducive to enforcing social norms, and schools are a safe place for adolescents and children. In addition to school-based prevention interventions that are delivered by whole communities that target whole community have also demonstrated effectiveness for adolescent substance abuse.

Whether evidence-based prevention interventions are delivered in schools or in the community, the use of technology is critical to the development, implementation, and dissemination of prevention practices for adolescent substance users. Bloom described five technologies to consider as fundamental elements of any adolescent substance abuse prevention effort: education, promotion of self-competency, connections with natural caregivers, impacting change at the community organization and systems level, and redesigning the social environment.

Final Thoughts

We end this book on two hopeful notes and a challenge for graduate programs and academicians. Encouragingly, the psychological bloodletting, purging, blistering, and enemas of yesteryear have been replaced with more successful interventions. Still, too many youth do not respond to current treatments and too many return to dysfunctional behaviors too quickly. We do not seek a utopia in which self-destructive behavior does not exist. We are too old for that dream. Rather, we seek a society that acknowledges the pathway it has paved for bio-psycho-social-environmentally vulnerable youth to walk and to better attend to environmental controls to limit the number of those who fall prey to the misuse of legal and illegal substances. We are encouraged by the progress that those who seek to promote resiliency and prevent substance misuse in schools and other settings have made, but these remain baby steps and more remains to be done particularly with harm risk reduction and distribution of consumption models. Further, the first generation of evidence-based models in treatment and prevention is just that–first generation. Improvements to these approaches and the development of still more robust actions that can withstand the inevitable tinkering that occurs in the field must be encouraged. We urge those who would fund these new developments to invest their dollars in a variety of approaches that are both interdisciplinary and multifactorial. If we have learned anything from the field of prevention, it is that single technology approaches are of limited, if any, value.

Toward that end, we have challenged graduate programs to reengineer the process by which doctoral degrees are conferred (Gullotta & Blau, 2008). Presently, the system is built around a course of study and the undertaking of a dissertation of marginal value that will reside forlorn in some neglected corner of cyberspace. Imagine instead a school, ideally many schools in an international collaboration, embarking on a behavioral research database developing, testing, refining, and disseminating practices that work. We have no shortage of theories (psychoanalytic, behavioral, humanistic, transpersonal) offering a multitude of approaches for helping those in need. Are the adherents of logotherapy, gestalt, analysis, behaviorism, theosophy, and a thousand other interventions blowing worthless smoke over and into those seeking their help? Are new "DARE," carding, and traffic stop points effective prevention efforts? Granted, there are beginning databases collecting information. But these are potentially flawed efforts packed with programs that have been well funded by the maintainers of the database. Recall our earlier observation about social reality. Change in practice occurred if it did not disturb the existing pattern of social beliefs. The creation, maintenance, and entry into a database maintained by Gallen would value the humors, by Freud it would favor the Oedipal complex, or by behavioral analysts it would omit feelings. Transpersonal approaches would find no place in their databases, and yet in the new North America where both Canada and the USA are in the midst of ethnic and cultural transformation theosophical approaches matter. This could be a time of psychological renaissance across schools of higher learning and the field identifying *effective* approaches to maintain existing health, foster new health abilities, prevent distress, and successfully treat illness when it develops. We know there is no magic silver bullet to achieve this. We suspect this behavioral formulary will be as large as it is for pharmacology. Still, it needs to be undertaken and now is the time.

References

Bloom, M., & Gullotta, T. P. (2018). Primary prevention in adolescent substance abuse. In C. G. Leukefeld & T. P. Gullotta (Eds.), *Adolescent substance abuse: Evidence-based approaches to prevention and treatment* (2nd ed., pp. 277–292). New York, NY: Springer.

Cochrane, A. (1972/1999). *Effectiveness and efficiency: Random reflections on health services*. London, UK: Royal Society of Medicine.

Gullotta, T. P., & Blau, G. M. (2008). Epilogue. In T. P. Gullotta & G. M. Blau (Eds.), *Handbook of childhood behavioral issues: Evidence-based approaches to prevention and treatment* (pp. 399–401). New York, NY: Routledge.

Institute of Medicine (IOM). (2001). *Crossing the quality chasm: A new health system for the 21st century*. Washington, DC: National Academy Press.

Leukefeld, C. G., & Gullotta, T. P. & (Eds.). (2018). *Adolescent substance abuse: Evidence-based approaches to prevention and treatment* (2nd Ed.). New York, NY: Springer.

Lichvar, E. K., Stilwell, S., Ajmera T., Alexander, A. L., Plant, R. W., Panzarella, P., & Blau, G. M. (2018). Residential treatment of adolescents with substance use disorders: Evidence-based approaches and best practice recommendations. In C. G. Leukefeld & T. P. Gullotta (Eds.), *Adolescent substance abuse: Evidence-based approaches to prevention and treatment* (2nd ed., pp. 191–213). New York, NY: Springer.

Index

C. G. Leukefeld, T. P. Gullotta (eds.), *Adolescent Substance Abuse*, Issues in Children's and Families' Lives, https://doi.org/10.1007/978-3-319-90611-9

D

E

U

V

Y

GPSR Compliance
The European Union's (EU) General Product Safety Regulation (GPSR) is a set of rules that requires consumer products to be safe and our obligations to ensure this.

If you have any concerns about our products, you can contact us on

ProductSafety@springernature.com

In case Publisher is established outside the EU, the EU authorized representative is:

Springer Nature Customer Service Center GmbH
Europaplatz 3
69115 Heidelberg, Germany

www.ingramcontent.com/pod-product-compliance
Ingram Content Group UK Ltd.
Pitfield, Milton Keynes, MK11 3LW, UK
UKHW020712071026
15590UKWH00010B/476
* 9 7 8 3 0 3 0 0 8 0 5 4 9 *